THE DUKE DIET

BALLANTINE BOOKS

NEW YORK

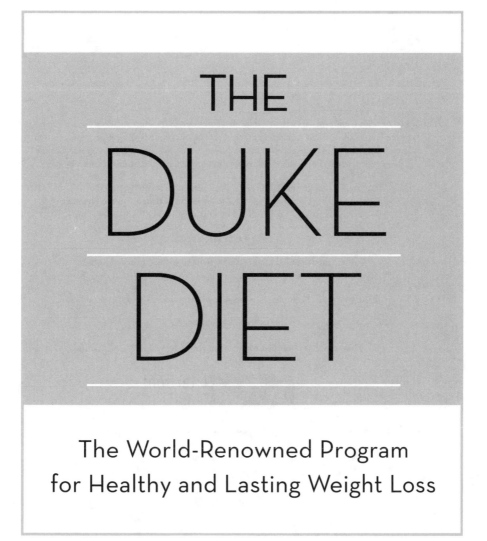

THE
DUKE
DIET

The World-Renowned Program
for Healthy and Lasting Weight Loss

HOWARD J. EISENSON, M.D.,
and
MARTIN BINKS, PH.D.
OF THE DUKE DIET & FITNESS CENTER

Author's Note: This book proposes a program of diet and exercise recommendations for the reader to follow. However, you should consult a qualified medical professional (and, if you are pregnant, your ob/gyn) before starting this or any other diet or fitness program. As with any health program, if at any time you experience any discomfort or unease, stop immediately and consult your physician.

Published in the United States by Ballantine Books, an imprint of
The Random House Publishing Group, a division of Random House, Inc., New York.

BALLANTINE and colophon are registered trademarks of Random House, Inc.

ISBN 978-0-345-49903-5

This edition is published by arrangement with Waterfront Media, Inc.

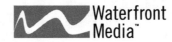

Printed in the United States of America on acid-free paper

www.ballantinebooks.com

2 4 6 8 9 7 5 3 1

First Edition

Book Design by Stephanie Huntwork

To my parents, Vel and Sam, for gifts beyond measure,
to Heather and Vince, who make me very proud,
and to Beth—with gratitude, and with love, always.

—Howard J. Eisenson, M.D.

In loving memory of "Grammy," Eleanor M Wilson;
and to my parents, John and Kathleen Binks.
Your belief in me throughout my life has been my inspiration.

—Martin Binks, Ph.D.

SPECIAL ACKNOWLEDGMENT

We wish to provide special acknowledgment to Duke Diet & Fitness Center (DFC) fitness manager Gerald Endress, M.S., R.C.E.P., and nutrition manager Elisabetta Politi, M.P.H., R.D., C.D.E. They provided invaluable assistance to ensure that the materials in this book and the companion website accurately represent the curriculum used with our clients at the DFC.

Contents

THE DUKE DIET

PART ONE

A University Medical Diet Goes Mainstream

CHAPTER ONE

The Duke Difference

What's different about the Duke Plan? That's easy—it's not a diet! Our "diet" is really a self-care plan—a plan that can help you not only lose weight but also improve your overall quality of life. The plan has been developed and refined, over nearly four decades, by a team of professionals dedicated to educating and empowering the clients we serve, with the latest and most authoritative scientific information and time-tested, practical tools. You won't get a "one size fits all" approach from us or a false promise that weight control is easy—it isn't, for the vast majority of us. But we know, from the thousands of clients who've tried the Duke Plan, that weight loss *is* achievable and, what's more, can be sustained—for a lifetime.

It's very gratifying that so many patients, after just a few weeks at the Duke Diet & Fitness Center, or even long after their first visit, tell us that their new, healthier lifestyle choices have made them feel so much better— some say, better than they've felt in years—and more energized and optimistic about the future.

Surely you've tried other diets. The truth is that nearly all diets can work. They all have one thing in common: calorie reduction. In fact, even the most ridiculous and unhealthy gimmicks, such as wearing a weight loss suit or eating nothing but cabbage soup for a week, will knock off pounds—for a while. But the weight loss achieved with fad diets almost never sticks because most diets have a fundamental flaw: an on-off switch. You go on the diet and follow it for a limited time—often, for as long as you can stand it—and then you go *off* the diet. Chances are, once you resume your old habits, you gain back all the weight and, for good measure, perhaps an extra ten or fifteen or more pounds. Honestly, very few diets are designed to help you maintain your weight loss over the long haul.

Almost every dieter we've worked with knows this yo-yo pattern all too well. Many of our patients see the weight-loss-and-rebound cycle as a nightmare that makes them feel desperate and out of control. Like them, you may define your life in terms of your struggle with weight loss and consider yourself a failure. But that harsh self-assessment is way off base and definitely not helpful. First of all, there's a heck of a lot more to success in life than weight control! But even if weight control were the most important thing in life, you still didn't fail. You dieted and may even have succeeded at losing weight for a while. But ultimately, the diets, with their time-limited approach, failed you!

In our years of working with patients and *specializing* in weight loss, we've learned firsthand the range of challenging problems associated with weight control. We work every day with people like you—people who are tired of dieting and frustrated with their lack of success, but, just as important, people who have not given up and are ready to learn a reasonable approach to shedding the pounds and inches and to claim (or reclaim) good health.

Our plan helps you lose weight by teaching you good habits that last—not by insisting that you starve yourself, give up carbs or fats or any other food group, forgo all your favorite dishes forever, or become a slave to rigid discipline. As Dr. Eisenson is fond of saying, "We are more likely to be successful with achieving long-term weight control if we outsmart the problem, rather than try to defeat it with brute force, or sheer willpower, alone."

We'll help you outsmart this problem by providing you with the knowledge and the tools to make healthier choices, for life. This is the Duke difference! We'll share recipes from the renowned Duke Diet & Fitness Center chefs and registered dietitians to help you prepare meals that will surprise you because they're so filling and delicious, despite being considerably lower in calories than your usual fare. And here's another Duke difference: Unlike most weight loss programs, we appreciate that there is no dietary plan that's right for everyone—so we offer you more options.

Some patients select our Traditional Meal Plan—lower in fat, with plenty of healthy carbohydrates, in keeping with the most widely endorsed national guidelines. Others achieve success with our Moderate Carbohydrate Plan, which offers a lower percentage of carbs and a higher proportion of protein and healthy fats. We'll explain the differences between the plans and give you some tips on selecting the one that's best for you. And down the road you're welcome to switch plans if you'd like to try something new. We offer you choice, flexibility, and a customized approach to weight loss.

Eating healthfully will certainly help you lose weight, but it's just as important to build regular exercise into your life. We'll help you become more active by recommending a range of fitness routines, so you can find one that you'll actually enjoy, *not* just have to suffer through, whatever your current fitness level.

Finally, the Duke Plan will help you develop a healthier mind-set, so you'll maintain the self-care habits to keep the weight off. We'll teach you not only to become more skilled at resisting temptation, but to avoid being tempted in the first place. Once you develop new, more positive thinking and living habits, you will begin to overcome your weight problem once and for all, without the constant restraint and deprivation required by trendy diets. You will approach food—at home, at work, in restaurants, on vacation, virtually everywhere—in a different and healthier way.

Maybe you're drawn to this book for health reasons. Studies have shown that losing only 5 to 10 percent of your total weight can lower your blood pressure, blood lipids (cholesterol and triglycerides), and blood sugar, to name just a few advantages. Often, patients find that they can reduce their medications (with their doctor's participation), as long as they stick with their new, healthier habits of eating and exercising. Even a simple regimen of regular exercise can lead to striking improvements in your endurance, flexibility, and strength. Fatigue, impaired sleep, and even chronic pain often improve—sometimes fairly quickly—when you revamp your self-care habits.

It's clear that many people struggle with weight today, but why? Of course, there are myriad reasons. For some, it's a constellation of medical conditions, medications, and social or psychological factors. Others may be predisposed to being overweight because of genetic or biological tendencies. We all find ourselves in an environment where food is abundant and the need—indeed, the opportunity—to be physically active is less than ever. For our ancestors, finding enough food to support life was a regular challenge, so it's likely that, with evolution, we developed an affinity for good energy sources like sweets or fat, as well as the ability to eat quickly and heartily when food was available and to store fat efficiently and burn it sparingly.

The genetic endowment that may well have enhanced survival in times past may not be serving us so well in today's food-focused, increasingly automated world, where portions are supersized and the TV remote rules. Indeed, if we do what comes most naturally in the modern world, most of us will gain unhealthy weight (and we have!). But that doesn't have to be our destiny. Armed with sound information about the challenges we face, and how to overcome them, we *can* choose a different path and realize a different outcome.

As we often tell our patients at Duke, if you are overweight, you're at higher risk of developing such serious medical conditions as high blood pressure, abnormal cholesterol and triglycerides, diabetes or prediabetes, arthritis, and breathing difficulties, or even dying prematurely from certain kinds of cancer, heart disease, or stroke. You can find a wealth of information on these conditions at our website, www.dukediet.com. The Duke program's comprehensive, multifaceted approach—a realistic eating and exercise plan, combined with a psychological/behavioral component and sound medical advice—can help you not only address these weight-related issues but improve your quality of life.

Our residential program clients are people just like you, and the plan they follow to regain their health and confidence uses the same information and skills that you will follow and incorporate into your own life. Even without the protective cocoon of our residential setting just off the Duke University campus, you will find that you can re-create elements of the Duke Diet & Fitness Center experience in your own home and reap its life-enhancing and health-promoting benefits. That's not to say you won't stumble at times or feel a bit stuck or frustrated. Maintaining a steady and healthy pace of weight

What Is Metabolic Syndrome?

Metabolic syndrome is a condition defined as a cluster of three or more of the following risk factors in adults:

- Increased abdominal fat: waist circumference in a woman of at least 35 inches, or 40 inches or greater in a man
- Elevated blood pressure on several measurements: 130 or greater systolic (top number) or 85 or greater diastolic (bottom number)
- Elevated level of triglycerides (blood fats): greater than 150 after a twelve-hour fast
- Low level of high-density lipoprotein (HDL)—the "good" cholesterol: under 40 for a man or less than 50 for a woman
- Elevated blood sugar: 110 or greater after a twelve-hour fast—for instance, first thing in the morning, before breakfast; this includes blood sugars in the prediabetes range

If you have metabolic syndrome, you face an increased chance of developing cholesterol deposits in the arterial walls (*atherosclerosis*), which causes most heart attacks and strokes, and also an increased risk for developing diabetes.

Metabolic syndrome occurs in only 5 percent of adults of normal weight, but in 22 percent of those who are overweight, and in 60 percent of those who are obese! For these people, the most important interventions are weight loss and exercise.

loss requires a degree of patience and perseverance. Keep in mind that it takes time for old, destructive habits to be replaced by new ones—but it can be done!

As Dr. Binks so often tells patients in our goal-setting class, your weight control program is very much like a business plan. In business, you do your best to set achievable goals and to prepare action plans for dealing with potential bumps in the road. Inevitably, glitches will come along that you couldn't anticipate, but that doesn't mean that you have to scrap your whole plan. You can simply tweak it to address the new challenge. That's exactly what you'll do when setting your health goals on the Duke Diet: Develop a plan, based on what you know about yourself and your life, and then adjust it, as needed, to cope with the unexpected. We'll offer you concrete strategies to combat diet fatigue and to help you stay motivated. We will help you identify early warning signs that you may be slipping and develop strategies to respond quickly and effectively to stop a potential relapse in its tracks.

The Duke Plan will not only help you shed pounds, it will also give you a renewed sense of pride and satisfaction at seeing and feeling your health improve. We're here to guide you every step of the way, both in this book and on our website, www.dukediet.com, where you'll find helpful Q&As; articles from Duke experts on nutrition, fitness, behavioral health, and medical topics; interactive tools to help you chart your progress, including a Weight Tracker and a Lifestyle Journal; hundreds of appealing recipes to vary your menus, along with your own Recipe Box to store your favorites; message boards, where you can get useful tips and advice from your fellow dieters; and much more. It often takes a community to help people make life-changing breakthroughs, and you'll find a vibrant one at www.dukediet.com.

WHAT IS THE DUKE PLAN?

The Duke Plan begins with a core four-week program designed to help you eat well and enjoyably, exercise regularly, and develop new habits of thinking and action that will promote steady weight loss, improve your health, and give you the satisfaction that comes with taking control of your life. Here are the basic elements of the program.

- **The Duke Diet Nutrition Plan.** Unlike trendy diets, you won't have to turn your life inside out on the Duke Plan. As one of our clients has said, "It's about evolution, not revolution!" You will eat generously from all six food groups—proteins, healthy fats, healthy starches, dairy products, vegetables, and fruits. Specified servings of each will make it clear how to regulate your intake of calories and balance your nutrition plan. To get you started, we offer four complete weeks' worth of meals—breakfast, lunch, dinner, and one or two snacks (if desired) each day.

We'll also help you tune back in to your body's natural ability to tell whether you're hungry or full. If you're like many of our clients, you've been on so many different diets that sent you bouncing back and forth between deprivation and overeating that you may no longer trust your ability to read your body's cues. You'll recover that innate ability and also learn to distinguish between the hunger that's a call for food and hunger for other reasons, such as the sight and smell of food, boredom, celebration, stress, or other emotions. We will teach you to identify the true needs associated with this faux hunger and show you alternative, safe, healthy ways to deal with these eating triggers.

• **The Duke Diet Exercise Plan.** Weight control is a matter of balancing energy intake (food) and output (physical exertion). That's one of many important reasons to build regular exercise and other physical activity into your life. We know that this isn't exactly news to you, and we know that it might make you groan. We can sympathize—today, we all lead such overcommitted lives that the mere thought of any extra claim on our time can seem overwhelming—even if that extra activity didn't have other downsides like making us sweat and strain, look awkward, or feel clumsy.

But the fact is that exercise is anything but an extra. Our bodies are designed to *move*. Being a couch or computer potato is like having a gleaming, powerful, finely tuned car and always leaving it parked in the garage. In time, the tires will deflate, the oil will gunk up, the shine will be dimmed by dust—and that's analogous to what happens in our own bodies. We need regular use to run smoothly.

We'll help you develop a fitness program that works for *you,* whatever your fitness level—even if you've been inactive for some time or think you hate exercise. You won't have to perform heroic feats of strength or endurance, but simply find ways to make moderate activity—some aerobic, some strength building, and some flexibility promoting—part of your weekly routine. If you want to expand your fitness repertoire, you'll find instructional videos on our website, too.

Here's the best part: Once you get moving, you may notice benefits right away. You may feel stronger and more energetic, sleep better, and have more endurance and flexibility. The hustle and flow of daily life may agitate you less because exercise can ease stress. And if you keep the exercise going on a regular basis, you are very likely to notice additional health benefits. For instance, if you're being treated for hypertension or diabetes, you will probably experience improved control of those conditions and might end up reducing, or even eliminating, your need for medication. Fitness works!

• **The Duke Diet Behavioral Plan.** Since many of our clients are real diet veterans, at first they're dubious that the Duke Plan will help them shed weight without deprivation and keep it off for good. But the critical element of the program—and a major Duke difference—is that we work to help them change not just their diets, but also the way they think about food and about themselves.

All diets encourage you to control what you eat, and some also step up your exercise regimen. However, white-knuckled willpower is no match for the unhealthy habits of a lifetime. We'll show you how to uproot those habits by teaching you new skills, new approaches to food, and a new understanding of what makes *you* tick when it comes to managing your health.

We'll help you recognize self-defeating patterns, such as all-or-nothing thinking—the "I blew it, so I'm a failure" mantra that sends you spiraling off your plan—and perfectionism, which makes you set such lofty goals (*I'll do two hundred push-ups and sit-ups a day!*) that you have little hope of attaining them anytime soon. We'll show how to set smaller, interim goals that you can actually achieve and enjoy the satisfaction when you do. As you make gradual, sustainable progress toward your desired weight or health goals, we will teach you how to truly appreciate every success and stay positive and focused—not only on your day-to-day achievements, but also looking toward your long-term goals.

Finally, we'll show you that you don't have to work alone to launch your new, healthy lifestyle. We will teach you how to maximize the value of your existing support troops—your family, friends, and coworkers—and give you the tools to recruit new ones. Remember, you can also tap into the resources of the virtual community at www.dukediet.com.

Let's face it—over the course of our lives, we *learn* any number of behaviors that are not so healthy. The good news is that anything that is learned can be *unlearned.* The way to do so is to make positive, incremental changes that both are healthy and feel right. Ripples of change will gradually build to a current of progress that will ultimately sweep you to success.

WHAT CAN YOU EXPECT?

Now for the big question: How fast will that current of progress be for me? Here at Duke, we gauge progress by a variety of measures. Pounds lost, of course, is a major one. Our patients lose, on average, 1 to 1.5 percent of their body weight each week, and after a year, on average four out of five have maintained their weight loss or continued to lose. In addition, more than 80 percent report substantial improvements in overall quality of life.

Early in the program, virtually all our clients lose weight at a pretty fast rate—often several pounds in the first week. In fact, you may already know how much "water weight" you tend to lose when you first start to diet and that you shouldn't pay too much attention to that initial weight loss. After the first week of dieting, weight loss often levels off at a steady pace of one pound to two pounds a week. Some people lose more quickly than others (and generally speaking, the higher your starting weight, the more quickly you will lose). The key word here is *steady.*

So, while we know you want to be thin or trim tomorrow, we urge you not to jump the gun by eating less than is specified in our meal plans. You didn't gain those pounds and inches in a matter of days or weeks, and to take them off, you'll have to grant yourself a reasonable window of time. After all, even a pound or two per week can really add up!

You should also know that it's quite normal for weight to fluctuate from day to day. Salt intake/water retention and hormone shifts (in women) are among the many variables that can influence your weight. Men tend to lose weight more rapidly than women, and young people lose it more quickly than those at midlife and beyond. Certain medications and health conditions may also influence the rate of weight loss. We encourage you to mark your weight loss progress on a graph or on the Weight Tracker at www.dukediet.com. The visual record of your progress will help you better understand your body's natural weight loss rhythms.

Frustrating as temporary plateaus, or pauses, in your weight loss can be, they don't mean that the program isn't working. Long-term weight loss requires long-view thinking and keeping your eye on all the positive changes you are making for your health each day as well as your ultimate weight loss goals. So, whenever the needle on your scale seems stuck, the last thing you should do is panic and get discouraged. Big payoffs—lost pounds and inches, improved health and vitality—come to those who stick with the program and recognize that weight loss success is a long-term proposition.

Here are some encouraging benchmarks to keep in mind. Say, as an example, that you begin the program on April 1 and steadily drop a pound or two per week. By Memorial Day, you'll have shed ten to fifteen pounds— enough to make you want a new outfit for a graduation or a (healthy) holiday barbecue. By the Fourth of July, you'll have dropped another five to ten pounds, for a probable overall loss of fifteen to twenty-five pounds—which may be enough to finally let you feel comfortable in a bathing suit.

And if your weight loss goals are higher? Remember that by steadily losing just a pound or two per week, you can take off fifty, maybe one hundred pounds in a single year. Imagine how different you'll look by September, by New Year's Day, and by springtime—and how encouraged you'll feel when you see your body change, and when your friends and family compliment you.

Pounds lost and clothing sizes dropped are just two of our measures of success at the Duke Diet & Fitness Center. Others include how much better our clients feel, both physically and emotionally. Nearly all of them report improvements in their agility, breathing, and endurance—as well as in their overall sense of well-being.

Let's look at those benchmarks again. If you begin the plan on April 1, by Memorial Day, you may be sleeping more soundly, suffering less from stress and fewer aches and pains, and possibly finding it a lot easier to keep up with your kids. By the Fourth of July, you'll be so invested in your exercise routine that you may even hate skipping a single workout (really!). Later in this book, we'll discuss in greater detail how to evaluate your progress in these areas—and how very rewarding these changes can be.

Finally, at the Duke Diet & Fitness Center we measure success in terms of health restoration. All our clients begin the program with a medical workup to check baseline blood pressure, blood sugar, cholesterol, and other lab values. If you haven't had a medical evaluation recently, you may wish to ask your doctor to perform the same tests. If your initial results fall outside the normal range, your doctor will recommend repeating the battery of tests at an appropriate interval. Chances are, if you have completed the core four-week program and are maintaining your new, healthier habits, you'll see positive changes in some of these gauges of health, even in a relatively short period of time. That objective evidence of your body's renewal can be potent—and powerfully motivating—proof that you're making real progress.

START WHERE YOU ARE

How many pounds do you think you want to lose? And what exactly do we mean by *overweight*? Medically speaking, the term is not as vague as it sounds. *Overweight* means having a degree of body fat that is usually not consistent with good health. *Obese* is a more advanced degree of *overweight,* implying a percentage of body fat high enough to pose a serious threat to one's health. It's worth noting that these terms apply to some 65 percent of American adults.

To determine an individual's degree of overweight, we use an indicator called *body mass index* (BMI), a measure of weight that takes height into account. This is calculated by multiplying your weight (in pounds) by 703, then dividing that number by your height (in inches) twice. You can use a calculator or, if you prefer, try the interactive BMI Calculator at www.dukediet.com.

Here's an example of how it works for someone who is five feet, seven inches tall, weighing 175 pounds:

175 pounds times 703 divided by 67 inches, then again divided by 67 = 27.4

The following chart illustrates what that number means:

BODY MASS INDEX	CLASSIFICATION	WHAT IT MEANS
Less than 18.5	Underweight	Increased risk of health problems associated with underweight, such as inadequate nutrition.
18.5–24.9	Normal	Healthy body weight for height.
25–29.9	Overweight	Heavier than optimal for height—carries an increased risk of weight-related health problems.
30–34.9	Obesity I	High risk of common medical problems associated with obesity, such as type 2 diabetes, high blood pressure, abnormal cholesterol, and breathing disorders. In most people, a BMI of 30 means they're about 30 to 40 pounds overweight.
35–39.9	Obesity II	Very high risk of common medical problems associated with obesity, such as type 2 diabetes, high blood pressure, abnormal cholesterol, and breathing disorders.
40 or greater	Obesity III (severe obesity; previously referred to as morbid obesity).	Extremely high risk of associated medical problems. People with a BMI of 40 or greater are typically 100 pounds overweight or more.

So the BMI in the preceding example—27.4—would fall squarely into the Overweight category. Our clients at the Duke Diet & Fitness Center have BMIs ranging from overweight to the upper stretches of the obesity spectrum. In most people, BMI does correspond fairly well with degree of body fatness. However, as useful as this measurement is in correlating excess weight and health problems, it's not foolproof. For example, a muscular, well-conditioned athlete (like a bodybuilder) might well chart in the Obesity range yet still have a healthy percentage of body fat and, in fact, be at low risk for health problems.

Where you carry your body fat also makes a difference. Excess abdominal fat (also called central or visceral fat), which tends to concentrate around your waist and on your upper trunk, is linked to a heightened risk of diabetes, heart disease, and other serious conditions, while the fat that tends to accumulate under the skin in ample hips and thighs (subcutaneous fat) poses a less significant health risk. How much abdominal fat is considered excessive? In men, a waist circumference greater than 40 inches or in women, greater than 35 inches, can be cause for concern.

READY TO GET STARTED?

Here's one of our favorite stories from a patient to encourage you!

A New Lease on Life

I started the program in September 2003 at the urging of a friend. My marriage had just ended and I'd reached my highest weight ever. I was miserable. I knew that I needed to do something and I made up my mind to change. I knew that to alter my behavior I would have to set clear, specific goals and develop a strategy for achieving them. And I would have to take total responsibility for my plan.

This program literally saved my life. The whole mind-body emphasis is so all-encompassing. It treats the whole person. It's not just about eating and exercise—it's about learning why we eat, what our trigger foods are, and how to handle cravings. It's also about getting active in a way you can live with.

In the last year and a half, my life has changed drastically. My confidence level, my agility, my health, not to mention the fun of shopping for attractive clothes—everything has changed. I've battled weight for ages, and being overweight had consumed my life. Now I've gotten back to where I knew I needed to be.

With the help of this program, I've realized that I deserve to be healthy and happy. I'm worthy of being thin and feeling good, and I owe that to myself. The Duke Diet has given me a new lease on life, and I know that it can do that for others, too!

—Susan, age 44

Just to give you an overview, part one will introduce you to the nutrition, fitness, and behavioral health components of the Duke Plan—the way the eating plans work, how to choose the right one for you, how to determine your fitness profile and establish a realistic plan, and how certain tools and strategies can help you achieve lasting weight loss. We will also supply helpful medical information throughout.

Part two will zoom in on the core four-week program, with meal plans and recipes from the famous Duke residential program (as well as information on how to cope if you don't cook!), step-by-step fitness routines (illustrated with photographs), and specific behavioral exercises that will help you develop new habits, clear action plans, and skills for effective eating control, stress reduction, and reducing emotional eating, as well as how to rally your support team.

Part three will look to the future: maintaining and improving your weight loss beyond the four-week program, upholding your fitness goals, shoring up your support systems, and sustaining your own morale.

As you've undoubtedly noticed, we're quite proud of our new website, www.dukediet.com. Our robust and interactive Web community is another part of the Duke difference!

So take the time to read this book fully—not necessarily in one sitting but all the way through—and to turn to www.dukediet.com to get the complete package of nutrition, fitness, and behavioral strategies, and valuable medical information that we have to offer. We believe that they constitute the most comprehensive and effective plan available today for losing weight and keeping it off.

Meet Howard Eisenson, M.D.

After 20 years as a practicing family physician, I was looking for something different. I was trained to address the whole person in my work—to see patients not as cases but as unique individuals. But as our health care system has evolved, connecting with patients while addressing their most challenging medical problems has become increasingly difficult. The rapid-fire pace of medical practice gave me less time with my patients. Thus, I sought a place where collaboration with a multidisciplinary team of skilled professionals was encouraged, where we'd have the time and resources to do our best work, where we could address our patients' needs as individuals while empowering them with the knowledge and the skills to enhance their health—in short, to make a lasting difference in their lives. In 1999, I was recruited to join the staff at the Duke Diet & Fitness Center, and I'm pleased to report that I found everything I was looking for. My work here affords me the opportunity to practice the style of medicine that I believe in. Most of our patients come to us with a host of health concerns, and they are delighted to find out that our staff will actually take the time to help address those issues. Obesity may have been their admission ticket but they value, and are delighted with, our "whole person" approach to care. As we do with our own patients, we will try to set you on a path toward better health and meaningful life change.

Meet Martin Binks, Ph.D.

Before joining the Duke Diet & Fitness Center as director of behavioral health and research director several years ago, I was at the Medical University of South Carolina Weight Management Center, where I combined patient care with education, research, and program development in an outpatient weight loss setting. Prior to that, I first began working with people who struggle with their weight through the development of a research program at Fairleigh Dickinson University where we studied the benefits of resistance exercise (weight training) in addition to aerobic exercise in women undergoing weight loss treatment.

In my years working in the field, I have always been concerned that the overall belief in the general public seems to be that if someone can just design the right diet, develop the perfect diet pill, or come up with some other magic bullet, then the obesity problem will be solved. It's just not that easy, because it's a complex problem that requires a multidisciplinary approach and change at both the individual and the societal levels. When I came to the Duke Diet & Fitness Center, I joined a team of physicians, behavioral health specialists, dietitians, exercise physiologists, and others who understand what their clients are going through and who work together to help people take a realistic approach to the lifestyle changes we recommend. We help people make small but fundamental shifts in their lives, not only in the areas of eating and activity but also in the emotional or interpersonal patterns that may lead to overeating or underexercising. What intrigues me about our work at the center is that despite its being a four-week core program, the focus is squarely on the long-term view of weight control. We focus on how people can make changes that fit into their lives. I like to remind people: You are more than the sum of the pounds you weigh. If you are happier and healthier in your world, then you have achieved true success.

Can you sense our enthusiasm? We're passionate about what we do and delighted to have the opportunity to work with you. So let's get started!

CHAPTER TWO

The Duke Diet Nutrition Plan: What You Will Eat

The first question everyone who comes to the Duke Diet & Fitness Center asks is, "What can I eat?" What the new client often really means is, "What *can't* I eat? Do I have to give up . . ." Insert your own favorites: Bread? Pasta? An occasional cocktail? Barbecue? Dessert?

The answer is a resounding No! On the Duke Plan, you don't have to give up anything completely. No food groups or categories (even dessert) are off-limits. In fact, "All things in moderation" is one of our mantras. As we discussed in chapter 1, the Duke program is not just a diet but a *lifestyle*.

We're going to give you the tools to change your eating habits, not for a couple of weeks or a month, but for the rest of your life. We will teach you how to handle hard-to-control foods, not avoid them, and encourage you to incorporate your favorite foods into your meal plan in a healthy way. We'll help you stop viewing food as the enemy and see it as what it truly is—part of a healthy and fulfilling life.

You probably already know from firsthand experience that very restrictive white-knuckle diets usually backfire, leading you to feel deprived, which later can lead to overindulgence. As we often tell our clients, you don't need to go hungry or deny that food is a pleasurable part of life to be *very* successful with weight loss. There is no prize for doing it the hard way. In fact, our experience suggests that the people who do best at keeping weight off long term are those who learn to include many of their favorite foods in moderation.

So we can't help but smile when we see new arrivals at Duke stare in disbelief at the amount of food on their trays. Elisabetta Politi, our nutrition manager, and her staff often have to work very hard to convince skeptical clients that, yes, you can in fact lose weight eating "all that food." You'd be surprised how full and fulfilling 1,200 or 1,500 calories a day can be—if you make the right choices. That's what lies ahead for you—plenty of delicious, healthy food, laid out in a clear-cut, four-week plan featuring easy-to-make recipes direct from Duke's world-renowned kitchen (plus many all-new recipes at www.dukediet.com). To stoke your motivation, keep in mind that on the Duke Diet Nutrition Plan, you will:

- Choose from two different meal plans, with plenty of flexibility in both.
- Fuel your body with healthy and delicious foods, including many not allowed on most popular diets.
- Avoid the constant hunger and nagging cravings that come with deprivation dieting.
- Develop a new, healthier relationship with food, so it will no longer feel like "the enemy."
- Lose that "I can't—I'm on a diet" mentality.
- Look better and feel more energetic and alive!

How is all this possible? The Duke Diet Nutrition Plan is based not on gimmicks but on well-researched scientific principles, notably, on hunger management, calorie management, and healthy, balanced food choices. It is a sensible approach that has helped thousands of clients who have come to Duke to learn to manage food and control their weight in a whole new way. It's a program that works—and it can work for you.

OUTSMARTING HUNGER

Hunger management, or what we like to call "outsmarting hunger," is one cornerstone of the Duke Diet Nutrition Plan. Hunger is a protective mechanism, ensuring that we consume enough calories and nutrients to stay alive. The trouble is, in our modern world, food is abundant, servings are supersized, the media bombards us with "eat this" messages, and food is associated with everything from family bonding and celebration to shared sadness. Our ability to recognize true hunger, to be in tune with our bodies' natural signals, has been all but stifled. It has become very difficult to tease apart how all these situational and emotional influences affect our desire to eat.

In chapter 5 we will give you a useful tool, the Hunger-Fullness Scale, that can help you learn to reconnect with your body's true appetite and distinguish that signal from the many other eating triggers—stress, boredom, challenging emotions, mouthwatering ads, and just plain old habits—that can masquerade as hunger. Strategies to cope with these triggers are woven throughout this book and on www.dukediet.com.

But what makes you *think* or *feel* you're hungry or full? Research shows that certain foods tend to fill you up more than others, and it's no surprise that these play a big role in weight loss. We call them low-energy-density foods, which means that they are high in water and fiber but low in calories. Generally, the more water a food contains (think fruits and vegetables), the lower its calorie count, while denser foods with less water pack more calories into the same volume.

Picture six Hershey's Kisses (a total of 150 calories) and then guess how much raw broccoli would constitute 150 calories. The answer: three cups, probably more than you could ever eat at one sitting. Obviously, for the same calories, the broccoli would take up much more space in your stomach than the chocolate and fill you up much more. So one of the keys to outsmarting hunger is incorporating low-energy-density foods wherever you can into your meals.

Here's an example. You want pasta for dinner? Fine. But instead of having the usual heaping bowl containing at least two cups of pasta (320 calories, even before you add the sauce and cheese), try having one cup of pasta (160 calories), tossed with a cup of cooked broccoli and some sauce and reduced-fat cheese. You'll feel just as full (and probably not as sleepy) and wind up 110 calories ahead of the game.

What if you made similar substitutions at every meal? At breakfast, instead of having a three-egg cheese omelet cooked in a tablespoon of butter (about 550 calories, without the hash browns and toast), you could use one whole egg beaten with two whites as your base and fill the omelet with a quarter cup each of spinach and mushrooms or tomatoes, sautéed with cooking spray, onions, and/or garlic and sprinkled with a tablespoon of grated Parmesan or your favorite reduced-fat cheese. That would seem like just as much food but add up to less than 150 calories.

For lunch, instead of getting a Double Quarter Pounder with Cheese (740 calories) and a large side of fries (570 calories), what if you had a salad with two cups of lettuce and an ounce each of lean roast beef and turkey breast, with a tablespoon of dressing and a small baked potato on the side, dabbed with low-fat sour cream? This whole meal totals roughly 400 calories— much less than even a single serving of those fast-food fries!

Let's add up the number of calories you could eliminate by making the adjustments in the preceding examples: $110 + 400 + 910 = 1,420$. And that's just in one day! Since you lose approximately a pound for every 3,500 calories you cut, you could lose a pound and a half each week at that rate—or more than sixty pounds in a year.

Soups and other low-energy-density foods, such as fruits and vegetables, fill you up because of their high water content. It is very easy to calculate the energy density of a food: You simply divide the number of calories per serving by the serving's weight in grams. You can find this information on the Nutrition Facts panel of most food labels or in food count books or computer programs. Very-low-energy-density foods are those that calculate to less than .6. They include peaches (.43), oranges (.47), strawberries (.3), broccoli (.28), cucumbers (.13), and lettuce (.18). Low-energy-density foods range from .6 to 1.5; they include oatmeal (.62), plain low-fat yogurt (.63), black beans (.78), and baked potato with skin (1.1). Medium-energy-density foods range from 1.5 to 4.0, and include frozen yogurt (1.6), lean sirloin steak (1.9), bread (2.6), and pretzels (3.9). High-energy-density foods calculate at or above 4.0, including onion rings (4.1), cheddar cheese (4.1), milk chocolate (5.4), and regular mayonnaise (7.2)—don't go overboard on these.

Slim Down with Soup

Here's another practical hunger-fighting strategy that comes from a Pennsylvania State University study. Two hundred overweight men and women were all placed on a calorie-controlled diet and randomly assigned to one of four groups. Group I included one mugful (10.5 fluid ounces) of soup in their daily diets, Group II included two mugfuls, Group III skipped the soup and instead got two servings of a dry snack food per day eaten just before lunch and dinner, and Group IV were not provided with any specific foods.

Guess who lost the most weight? One year from the start of the study, the subjects in Group II, who'd had two servings of soup a day (the less calorie dense option) had lost 50 percent more weight than the other groups.

The conclusion: Soup fills you up enough to help you hold down your calorie consumption over the rest of the meal. In this study, the participants chose from among 18 different commercially available soups. Of course, not all soups are created equal—we're not talking about rich ones laced with butter and cream, which would undermine weight loss by adding rather than replacing calories. So be sure to follow our nutrition guidelines when making your selections.

Some low-energy-density foods may also be rich in fiber. Fiber leaves you more satisfied after a meal because it slows digestion. In addition to many fruits and vegetables, other fiber-rich foods include whole grains like brown rice, wild rice, whole wheat, oatmeal, and multigrain cereals. Although these foods are relatively low in calorie density, you still need to watch how much you eat.

Researchers have also observed that for managing hunger, protein and adequate amounts of healthier fats can be great allies. One reason may be that it takes you longer to digest protein and fat than carbohydrates, so you don't get hungry again as fast. Another may be that people feel more satisfied when they eat protein and so are less likely to overdo it with the rest of the meal. The same is true of fats—they contribute to that sense of "I've had

Friendly Fiber

Fiber, which is found only in plants, cannot be fully digested by the body, so it fills you up for fewer calories. In addition, many higher-fiber foods take a little longer to chew, which can give your brain more time to register that you have eaten. But in addition to these important benefits for improving hunger management, fiber provides some wonderful health benefits as well. There are two kinds of fiber:

- Insoluble fiber (also called *roughage*), which doesn't dissolve in water, so it passes straight through the body. On the way, it helps clear out the digestive tract, so it may reduce constipation.
- Soluble fiber, which does dissolve in water and, as it passes, can bind to cholesterol molecules so the body can flush them away. When you see those claims on oatmeal boxes that daily use can reduce your cholesterol within a month, you can believe them. They're true!

Most fiber-rich foods have a mixture of insoluble and soluble fiber, and both are helpful, so you should aim for a blend of high-fiber foods every day. The American Dietetic Association recommends that we consume 25 to 35 grams of fiber a day, but most of us get only about 11—less than half of what we need. So step up the fiber, but do it gradually to avoid increasing intestinal gas (which will subside as your body gets used to more fiber). If you need it, you can try a dietary aid like Beano (which comes in liquid and pill form). Drinking six 8-ounce glasses of water a day should also help.

Good sources of fiber include:

- Whole grains like brown rice and whole- and multigrain breads (about 3 grams of fiber per serving)
- Pastas made with whole wheat (about 3 grams of fiber per ½-cup serving)
- Oatmeal and other whole- and multigrain breakfast cereals (3 or more grams of fiber per ½-cup serving)
- Dried or canned legumes—black, red, and white beans, chickpeas, black-eyed peas, lentils, and others (about 3 grams per ⅓-cup serving)
- Fruits and vegetables (2 to 3 grams per serving)

enough," or satiety, which is why we don't encourage clients to go ultra–low fat or fat free at the Duke Diet & Fitness Center. Our bodies need a certain amount of the good fats (you'll find a box on them later in this chapter) to function well.

There's more to hunger management than just the sensation of fullness. There are also some psychological influences. Many of our clients talk about the "full-plate effect"—the impact that just seeing a plate heaped with food has on their appetites. When salad and vegetables are piled high on their plates, alongside reasonable servings of lean protein and carbohydrates, our clients start to doubt that they'll have room to finish all that food. By the same token, when they use a larger plate and see extra space on a plate—even if that plate contains the same portions of the same foods or their caloric equivalent—they believe that the meal will leave them hungry. So don't underestimate the power of your mind when it comes to hunger management.

CALORIES IN, CALORIES OUT

In the preceding section, you saw many references to calories. A calorie is a unit of energy produced when food is broken down. The calories you consume power you through your day, help your cells regenerate, and keep your mind and body sharp. For the most part, only four kinds of food supply calories: protein and carbohydrates (4 calories per gram), alcohol (7 calories per gram), and fats (9 calories per gram).

Many of the popular diets sidestep the issue of calories by focusing on eliminating one food group or another. The news flash is that no matter what those trendy diets claim, weight loss involves reducing the number of calories you eat and increasing the number you burn. A calorie is a calorie, whatever its source. We will help simplify things by showing you how to monitor your caloric intake by controlling portions and counting servings of various food groups, but we will also remind you that monitoring your calories is an important part of a healthy weight loss plan. In providing both our Traditional and Moderate Carbohydrate Meal Plans, we give you choices that match your preferred eating style without all the smoke and mirrors that accompany so many popular diets.

Get Down with the Count

So you will be counting calories. Does this mean that you'll have to live with a calculator at the ready, so you can compute the value of every mouthful? Don't worry! The Duke meal plans already include the calculations to ensure that you get just the right number of calories every day. But what if you're making substitutions or, down the road, just living your life—going out to lunch and parties, having dinner at friends' houses, or grabbing a bite on the run? We want to make life easy for you by giving you the knowledge (or perhaps reinforcing the know-how you already have) to estimate the number of calories in many foods at a glance.

We use a system drawn from the time-tested one of the American Dietetic Association, which allows you to choose foods in the six basic groups, based on servings. The six groups are:

- Starches (about 80 calories per serving)
- Vegetables (25 calories per serving)
- Fruits (about 60 calories per serving)
- Fats (35 to 45 calories per serving)
- Dairy (90 to 100 calories per serving)
- Protein (35 to 100 calories per serving)

The Duke Diet Nutrition Plan will show you the number of servings from each group to include in every meal, based on which meal plan you choose (Traditional or Moderate Carbohydrate), so you can calculate calories easily. We will stress the healthier options within each category (for example, we will emphasize leaner, lower-calorie protein choices over the higher-calorie options). Of course, you can also use our Nutrition Lookup on www.dukediet.com.

Note that servings listed on nutrition labels should not be confused with portions. Portions are the actual amounts that you'll put on your plate or consume. For example, if you look at the Nutrition Facts panel on a 10-ounce bag of potato chips, you might see that one serving equals 110 calories. But how is "serving" defined? Examine the label more closely—you might be surprised to see that the chip maker's idea of a serving is 1 ounce, or one-tenth of the bag. If you eat half the bag, you'll consume not one but five servings, for a much higher total of 550 calories.

Over the last decade, steps have been taken by the Food and Drug Administration (FDA) to make labels less misleading, but confusion is still all too common. However, once you learn to pay attention to serving size, you'll be well on your way to a lifetime of healthy eating.

We also have helpful ways to estimate the number of servings without measuring everything, which is handy whether you are eating out or cooking at home. For example, one cup of ice cream is about the size of a baseball, while large cereal and soup bowls hold a cup and a half of food (two cups if they're filled to the brim). Two tablespoons of liquid is just about the amount you could hold in your cupped hand, and one ounce of nuts is one small handful. Of course, hand sizes vary, so we recommend that you do a little testing for yourself. Measure different foods and see how they compare with your hand size, or come up with your own helpful visuals. The following table offers more helpful visual guidelines for estimating serving sizes.

EYEBALL GUIDE TO SERVINGS PER PORTION

PORTION	VISUAL REFERENCE	NUMBER OF SERVINGS	CALORIES (APPROXIMATE)
The Bread, Cereal, Rice, and Pasta Group			
1 cup of potatoes, cooked rice, cooked pasta, cold cereal	a baseball	2 starches	160
1 pancake	a compact disc	1 starch	80
1 piece of corn bread	a bar of soap	2 starches	160
1 baked potato	a computer mouse	2 starches	160
The Vegetable Group			
½ cup of cooked broccoli	½ a baseball	1 vegetable	25
½ cup cooked asparagus	6 asparagus spears	1 vegetable	25

PORTION	VISUAL REFERENCE	NUMBER OF SERVINGS	CALORIES (APPROXIMATE)
1/2 cup cooked carrots	7 or 8 baby carrots or sticks	1 vegetable	25
1/2 cup cooked corn	1 6-inch ear of corn	1 starch	80
The Fruit Group			
1/2 cup grapes (15 grapes)	a lightbulb	1 fruit	60
1/2 cup stewed or canned fruit (unsweetened)	a small individual applesauce container	1 fruit	60
1 medium-sized piece of fruit	a baseball	1 fruit	60
1 cup cut-up fruit	a baseball	1 fruit	60
The Meat, Poultry, Fish, Dry Beans, Eggs, Cheese, and Nuts Group			
1 ounce cheese	an individually wrapped single cheese slice, 2 dominoes, or 4 stacked dice	1 dairy or protein	110
1 teaspoon peanut butter	a bottle cap	1/6 protein, 1/6 fat	30
1 tablespoon peanut butter	3 bottle caps	1/2 protein, 1/2 fat	90
3 ounces cooked meat	a deck of cards, a cassette tape, or a checkbook (for a fillet)	3 protein	240–300
3 ounces cooked fish	a deck of cards, a cassette tape, or a checkbook (for a fillet)	3 protein	75–165

PORTION	VISUAL REFERENCE	NUMBER OF SERVINGS	CALORIES (APPROXIMATE)
3 ounces cooked poultry	a deck of cards, a cassette tape, or a checkbook (for a fillet)	3 protein	150–180
Fats and Oils			
1 teaspoon butter or full-fat margarine	a bottle cap or the tip of your thumb	1 fat	35–45
2 teaspoons light margarine	2 bottle caps	1 fat	35–45
2 tablespoons reduced-calorie salad dressing	a Ping-Pong ball	2 fats	70–90
Snack Foods and Sweets			
1 ounce small candies	1 small handful	miscellaneous	100–150
1 ounce chips or pretzels	2 small handfuls	miscellaneous	100–150
½ cup ice cream	half a baseball	miscellaneous	100–150

THE REAL DEAL

Now let's talk about the key elements of the Duke Diet Nutrition Plan. We'll provide you with an outline of how the plan works, the core strategies you'll need, the techniques you will use to develop a meal plan—and then we'll teach you to how take the plan and make it work for you, for life.

First, the meal plans. By using the recipes in chapter 9 of this book (and you'll find many more great ones on www.dukediet.com), you'll be introduced to the principles of healthy, weight-conscious meal planning and preparation. You'll be able to hit the ground running and start shedding pounds right away simply by following the week-to-week plans that we have already created for you. However, as the saying goes, not *only* do we want to give you a fish, we also want to *teach* you to fish on your own—to build your own foundation for a healthy life!

CHOOSE HOW YOU LOSE!

We recognize that there are many different ways to lose weight, ranging from very-low-carbohydrate diets (which often make up the difference by being higher in fat and, typically, higher in protein) through more traditional lower-fat, higher-carbohydrate options. We believe that the Duke Diet Nutrition Plan is among the healthiest, most satisfying, and most effective diet strategies available today, based on the current medical science of weight control.

The Duke Diet offers a choice of two different plans, based on your food preferences, and, just as important, on what might have worked best for you in the past. Remember that regardless of which plan you are on, we want you to find what is comfortable and works for you. Also remember that these meal plans are a general guide. You've been on diets, and you know your own body better than anyone. You'll want to use what you know and, when you are comfortable, tailor your plan to meet your own needs.

The Traditional Meal Plan is ideal for people who enjoy carbohydrates (we know there are lots of you out there)—who are willing to forgo a little dietary fat to enjoy their starches. There are other reasons someone might choose this plan:

- It most resembles the traditional approach of the Duke Diet & Fitness Center and has been used very successfully throughout much of the center's four-decade history.
- It may help keep you from feeling deprived and help you avoid cravings by letting you eat a little more of the carbohydrate foods you love.
- Since the slightly higher amounts of carbohydrates in this plan are closer to what many families tend to eat, this plan may be more suitable to people cooking for a family.

The Moderate Carbohydrate Meal Plan is popular with our clients also. We introduced it in 2003, as accumulating research suggested that lowering carbohydrates can be a helpful and safe way to lose weight. Here are some advantages of this plan:

- It includes all food groups, but is lighter on the starchy carbs.
- People often report feeling more satisfied (and are better able to control hunger) when they eat more protein.
- For some people, this plan may help subdue cravings more effectively than a reduced-fat, higher-carbohydrate diet.

Our experience has shown that both plans, moderate and traditional, are of comparable effectiveness in helping people lose weight. Both plans let you eat plenty of food, including many of the foods you most enjoy. Both are low in saturated fat and encourage the use of heart-healthy fats. Both have plenty of fiber and provide a complete balance of essential nutrients. So choose the one that's most comfortable for you—or feel free to try both. In fact, many of our clients switch plans when they want a change. When they get comfortable with the program, some of our clients use what they've learned about the two plans to create a customized version just for themselves.

FOOD, GLORIOUS FOOD

Let's look at each of the six food groups—starches, vegetables, fruits, fats, dairy products, and protein—in turn. Bear in mind that just because a food appears in one group (such as dairy), that doesn't mean it contains nothing from one or more of the other categories (say, protein or fat). In fact, some foods actually can fit into more than one category. When you're in doubt about how to categorize a certain food, don't stress out (or worse yet, neglect to count it in your daily calories). Simply make your best guess as to which food group it belongs to, and then when you get a chance, be sure to look up the calories on our website or use one of the free calorie calculators available, such as the one at www.usda.gov. Even if you make a few miscalculations, you'll still achieve the main goals of keeping nutrition in balance and calories in check. What we're working for here is progress, not perfection.

Starches

Starches (also known as carbohydrates) have gotten a bum rap in recent years. For many people, this is a much-loved group—after all, who doesn't like bread, baked goods, pancakes, and pasta? This group also includes cereal, grains, and starchy vegetables like potatoes and yams. Starches are a good source of many minerals, including iron, as well as B vitamins and dietary fiber. When it comes to weight control and health, it pays to concentrate on the more complete starches, like whole grains, high-fiber cereals, brown rice, whole-wheat bread and flour, and sweet potatoes or yams. These choices are among the more filling and nutritious starches, in comparison with white rice, potatoes, and white bread. However, while more complete options are the better carbohydrate choices, we don't consider them the only ones you can eat. We want you to feel free to enjoy the starches that you prefer on occasion. Sometimes there's nothing that hits the spot better than a good old baked potato with low-fat sour cream or a little dab of butter. Just pay attention to portion sizes and calories and make these choices part of an overall plan that favors more complete carbohydrates and the right amount of protein and heart-healthy fat to keep you from feeling hungry.

Vegetables

It's certainly no secret that vegetables are good for you. They provide vital nutrients such as folic acid, vitamin C, iron, potassium, and magnesium. Many are packed with vitamin A, and all contain fiber and are low in calories. They are low-energy-density foods—often so low (as in the case of leafy greens) as to make a negligible impact on your overall count in a given day, yet they really fill you up. Studies over decades show that people who eat a diet rich in vegetables can reduce their risk for everything from diabetes and high blood pressure to cancer and heart disease. Many vegetables contain *phytochemicals,* naturally occurring plant compounds that help us stay healthy, fight disease, and live longer.

When selecting vegetables, think of yourself as a painter filling your palette with a full spectrum of rich colors—the broader your range of hues, the more beautiful your painting will be. Similarly, the broader the range of colors in the vegetables you choose, the better the effect they'll have on your health.

Some people—you know who you are!—aren't huge fans of vegetables unless they're smothered under melted cheese and creamy sauces, deep fried in batter, or overpowered by the flavors of butter or bacon. Too often, when people with such preferences go on a diet, they steam all their vegetables and hold their noses while eating them plain or try to replace them with such heroic amounts of salad that they start to feel like rabbits. Obviously, these unappealing strategies can't last, so they're soon abandoned. And, of course, vegetables are so very important when it comes to controlling hunger. That's

A Vegetable a Day . . .

Eating several servings of vegetables and fruits every day can improve your health and reduce the risk of certain cancers and illnesses. The reason is simple: Both are good sources of fiber and contain many beneficial phytonutrients including vitamins, minerals, and antioxidants. In choosing vegetables and fruits, it's good to go for variety because each provides different nutrients. Here is a list of potential health benefits you'll reap from eating your veggies and fruits, according to the latest research:

- A lower risk of many cancers
- A reduced risk of heart disease and stroke
- Better blood sugar control and prevention/management of diabetes
- Fewer gastrointestinal disorders
- Lower cholesterol
- Improved blood pressure
- A reduced risk of blindness due to macular degeneration, which is a deterioration of the retina, especially if spinach and other leafy green vegetables are plentiful on your plate
- Protection against cataracts
- A strengthened immune system
- Better preservation of mental alertness with aging
- Increased longevity

Fresh, Frozen, or Canned?

It may surprise you to find out that in some cases, *cooked vegetables are healthier than raw* and that frozen or even canned vegetables may be more nutritious than fresh. Processing vegetables (either by freezing or by canning) straight from the field preserves their vitamins and antioxidants, which may be lost when fresh vegetables sit around waiting to be packed and trucked to your grocery store. A few days there in the bins and then another couple days in your refrigerator will diminish their nutrient value even more.

If you have a nearby farmers' market, as many communities do, you'll find much fresher, though more season dependent, vegetables to choose from. But be sure the vegetables are fresh picked. All too often—especially in large urban centers—farmers' markets sell the same trucked-in produce your local supermarket provides.

Fresh vegetables often taste better than canned and frozen, which might make you more likely to eat them. If you use canned goods, be sure to check the labels for the sodium content. Many food manufacturers now offer reduced-sodium or even salt-free options.

As for the raw-versus-cooked debate, your body may actually be able to use more of the nutrients and phytochemicals in certain vegetables if they've been cooked as opposed to eating them raw. Spinach and carrots, for example, release more beta-carotene and free up other nutrients when they are exposed to heat. This may be because certain nutrients are sealed in plant cell walls, which heat helps to break down.

But the bottom line for maximizing your health is this: Eat your vegetables—fresh, frozen, or canned; raw or cooked—and the more, the better.

why at Duke we spend considerable time and effort helping clients explore new types of vegetables and tasty ways to prepare them. But if you aren't convinced you will find vegetables you like by themselves, we will show you how to include vegetables within recipes for bean and tomato soups, healthy lasagna, light casseroles, and stews.

Steaming rather than boiling vegetables may give them an enjoyable texture you've missed before. If you like, you can take vegetables right out of the steamer and sauté them in a pan with a spritz of cooking spray, a dash of fat-free broth, minced garlic, and your favorite herb to make them an aromatic and delectable focus of your meal. Or, if you think cooked vegetables are mushy and slimy, you might find that you enjoy them raw. Here's a testimonial.

I've never been a fan of carrots. I just found them boring. But one day, when I was leading a group of clients in an exercise on eating with heightened awareness of flavors and textures (a.k.a. "mindful eating"), I brought baby carrots and decided to use them instead of my usual Hershey's Kisses. (Granted, that didn't make me too popular because everyone had heard we gave out chocolate in that class.) I was amazed to discover how sweet and even complex the baby carrots tasted, with just the right amount of crunch—and so was my whole group. To this day, one of the clients from that group uses baby carrots when what used to be his late-afternoon candy craving strikes. And they've really helped him keep the weight off. (Don't worry, we did the exercise a second time with the Kisses so everyone was happy.)

—*Martin Binks, Ph.D.*

Baby carrots might not be your thing, so it pays to try all sorts of unfamiliar vegetables—such as snowpeas, snap beans (these are very sweet and healthy!), artichoke hearts, okra (the quintessential Southern love-it-or-loathe-it vegetable, which is great with tomatoes, onions, garlic, and spices like curry), bok choy (a healthy member of the cabbage family, which you can use in a stir-fry without adding much green vegetable taste), spaghetti squash (which you can sauce and substitute for real pasta, adding negligible calories), tomatillos, and zucchini. These are just some of the many often-neglected vegetables that can really make a meal memorable. And be creative about slipping vegetables into meals wherever you can—whether you're adding peppery watercress and juicy tomato to a sandwich or broiling a portobello mushroom instead of a burger.

Be adventurous. Try new things. Don't give up on vegetables. They're well worth the effort. You'll find lots of interesting ways to prepare them in this book and even more on www.dukediet.com.

Fruits

Like vegetables, fruits can be real lend-a-hand friends when it comes to weight loss. Because most fruits contain fiber, they can help you feel full on fewer calories; for many of us, they are healthy and satisfying substitutes for sugary desserts.

What's more, fruits are rich in nutrients. Some are an excellent source of vitamin C, especially citrus fruits. Just don't be fooled into thinking that because fruit is so good for you, you can eat as much as you like—the calories do count. Our plans recommend two to three servings of fruit a day, for enjoyment and health.

You may be tempted to fulfill your daily fruit allotment with juice—no washing, no slicing or scooping, no peeling; just a quick gulp and you're done. An occasional glass of juice can be tasty, but if you choose juice over actual fruits, you'll be depriving yourself of fiber, which is filling. And often, you'll be consuming extra calories, since it's easy to overdo it with juice. But whatever you choose, be sure to include a variety of fruits in your diet.

Fruit and Diabetes

Many people with diabetes believe that they must avoid fruit. Not true! Though fruit is high in fructose, a simple sugar, it can and should be included in a healthy eating plan for those with diabetes. The key to effective blood sugar control is balancing your consumption of *all* the essential nutrients. If you have diabetes, you can certainly eat a limited amount of fruit—two to three servings, regardless of which meal plan or calorie level you are on—without having a significant negative effect on blood sugar.

Fats

For a while, fats had such a bad reputation that some authorities seemed to suggest that we should severely limit fat intake (to less than 10 percent of total calories on some plans). Some advocates of high-protein diets took the opposite view: that, for weight loss, it was more important to restrict and all but eliminate carbohydrates, with no concern about the amount of fats (both saturated and unsaturated) consumed. For the majority of our patients, we subscribe to the view that both carbohydrates and fats are important parts of a balanced diet and should be included in moderation, with the emphasis on the healthier options. Many of our clients—and, no doubt, a lot of you— spent a decade diligently searching for nonfat versions of every conceivable snack, including ice cream, baked goods, and chips, and proceeded to eat them as if they could do no harm. Did any of us really believe that eating half a box of fat-free cookies was healthy?

In some respects, though, the low-fat revolution was helpful. It gave us products like low-fat yogurt and sour cream, which are good options for people who are trying to control their weight. In fact, our nutrition staff favor the lower-fat options, provided clients consume those they find to be satisfying in taste. But the marketing frenzy that led to labeling things like candy as nonfat (as if it ever had fat or as if this made it healthy) has proven confusing. So let us be the voice of reason.

We have already been clear that calories count, and lowering the fat will usually reduce them. We also recognize the difference between unhealthy (except in small amounts) saturated and trans fats (best to avoid) and health-promoting mono- and polyunsaturated fats (including omega-3 fatty acids). These healthier fats are necessary for normal functioning of the body. They are important vehicles for fat-soluble vitamins, they add flavor and texture to foods, they appear to have a protective effect on our arteries, and (of special interest to people controlling their weight) they may make us feel not just full but fully satisfied.

How can you tell which fats are undesirable? Saturated fats are usually solid at room temperature. They are found mostly in animal foods, including beef, pork, poultry, butter, cream, cheese, milk, and ice cream. We should definitely limit our consumption of this kind of fat. While fats from vegetable sources are generally less saturated and healthier, certain ones, in-

Healthy and Unhealthy Fats

All fats are not created equal. Some are health promoting, but others increase our risk of heart disease. The key is to replace most of the saturated fats in our diets with healthier options.

HEALTHY FATS	LESS HEALTHY OR UNHEALTHY FATS
Monounsaturated Fats Olive oil Peanut oil Sesame oil Variety of nut and seed oils: peanut, almond, macadamia nut, sesame Avocados, olives Full-fat ice cream	**Saturated Fats** Butter Lard Tropical oils such as coconut, palm, palm kernel, cocoa butter Fatty meats Whole milk
Polyunsaturated Fats Corn oil Soybean oil Sunflower oil Safflower oil Oil found in fish: salmon, tuna, mackerel, sardines, herring, anchovies Variety of nut and seed oils: walnut, pumpkin, flax Heart-healthy spreads, such as Benecol and Take Control (if used two to three times a day in place of regular margarine or butter, these products may lower cholesterol by up to 14 percent)	**Trans (Hydrogenated) Fats** Shortening Hard stick margarine (check labels) Many baked goods, especially processed ones (check labels): croissants, doughnuts, muffins, biscuits, chips, crackers, cookies, cakes Many fried foods, such as French fries, chicken nuggets, fish sticks

cluding cocoa butter and tropical (palm and coconut) oils, are highly saturated.

Unsaturated fats are generally liquid at room temperature. They come from plants, such as olives, corn, nuts, and seeds, as well as certain fish.

We encourage you to choose healthy fats over others whenever possible. That being said, saturated fats are present in meat (especially in red meat) and in dairy products, and are fine in moderation. The current American Heart Association recommendation is to limit consumption of saturated fats to 10 percent of your daily calorie allotment. To figure out how many grams of saturated fat that is, take 10 percent of your daily calorie allotment and divide it by 9 (the number of calories in a gram of fat). For example, if you eat 1,500 calories a day, you should limit your daily saturated fat intake to roughly 16 grams.

Just remember that fats must fit into your overall calorie profile and be part of a balanced diet in which most fats come from the healthy group. For instance, butter, which is mostly saturated fat, is acceptable in the Duke Diet Nutrition Plan in moderation—you might be surprised to see how little you actually need to get a satisfying flavor boost. Your baked potato doesn't have to swim in butter; a teaspoon (paired with a dab of low-fat sour cream) will give you the lift and taste you want. Or say you love garlic bread. If you rub a cut clove of garlic over a piece of toast, then brush it with less than a tea-

Cholesterol and Heart Health

What is cholesterol, exactly, and how does it lead to heart disease?
Cholesterol is a fatlike substance that our bodies manufacture. It is also present in animal products like eggs and meat. Cholesterol can be very beneficial—it plays a host of essential roles in our bodies, from maintaining cell structure to helping the nervous system function. There are two types of blood cholesterol: high-density lipoprotein, or HDL (the good kind), and low-density lipoprotein, or LDL (the harmful kind).

HDL cholesterol is considered good because it helps remove excess LDL cholesterol from the blood. (When you're trying to remember which type of cholesterol is which, think "heart healthy" for HDL and "lousy" for LDL.)

LDL cholesterol is considered bad because when there's too much of it circulating in the blood, it clogs the arteries, forming fatty deposits called plaques. Plaque buildup within the walls of our arteries is called atherosclerosis. It interferes with the flow of blood through the arteries and with other aspects of normal circulatory function, which raises the risk of heart attack and stroke.

spoon of butter (or olive oil, if you prefer), you'll have a flavorful—and much healthier—treat.

Trans fats are a different story. They're formed when vegetable oil is hardened to become margarine or shortening through a process called *hydrogenation*. At one time, hydrogenated fats were thought to be a healthy alternative to saturated fats, and since they improve the texture of some foods (like piecrust) and also prolong the shelf life of processed baked goods, crackers, and other snack foods, they started cropping up everywhere. But studies show that the initial belief in the health promise of trans fats was unfounded. They raise the level of bad, or LDL, cholesterol, lower the level of good, or HDL, cholesterol, and appear to be even worse for us than saturated fats.

The evidence against trans fats is so compelling that the federal government has legislated that all food labels must now list trans fat content. Certain municipalities (including New York City) have passed legislation that bans restaurants from using trans fats in cooking entirely. Even the fast-food chains are beginning to phase them out.

Some big food companies are jumping out ahead of the law and starting to promote their products as trans fat free. Those are the labels you want to look for (and watch out for the mention of "hydrogenated" anything in the ingredient lists). But bear in mind that just because trans fats are the "evil du jour," their mere absence does not guarantee that any given food is actually good for you. In fact, when they reduce fats, companies often bump up other undesirable additions, like sugar and salt, in their products to improve the taste.

Let's turn our attention to the healthier fats. Monounsaturated and polyunsaturated fats are both heart healthy—they can even help lower overall cholesterol levels—and provide significant health benefits. Among them are such kitchen staples as olive and sesame oils (real flavor boosters), corn and safflower oils (to use when you don't want to add oil flavor), peanut oil (great for stir-frys), and everybody's favorite vegetable, the avocado. Don't forget that although these fats are healthy, they are still fats, meaning that they're high in calories (9 calories per gram as opposed to 4 calories per gram found in carbohydrates or protein). So by all means, incorporate them into your diet, but exercise restraint. Remember, it's calories in versus calories out.

Nuts also have their place in a balanced diet. While they do contain about 200 calories and about 13 to 20 grams of fat per ounce, that fat is mostly of the good, unsaturated kind, which helps lower cholesterol. So practice moderation and enjoy them. Another important fat category is the omega-3 fatty acids. These come from fish and also from walnuts, flaxseeds, pumpkin seeds, and sunflower seeds. The omega-3s have been found to benefit us in many ways, such as reducing abnormal blood clotting, regulating heart rhythm, stimulating the immune system, and minimizing wrinkles.

Dairy

When we were kids, most of us were told to drink our milk. Dairy products contain an impressive variety of minerals, particularly bone-building calcium, as well as protein, vitamin A, vitamin D (usually added to milk), and many of the B vitamins. Recently, dairy foods have been getting a lot of media play for their possible role in weight management. In April 2004, a study suggested that people who got additional calcium in their diets lost more weight than people who didn't. Both calcium from dairy sources and calcium from supplements increased weight loss, but the benefits were greater when the calcium came from dairy sources. These findings are interesting; however, researchers continue to explore the science behind calcium's role in the body's fat-burning mechanisms. The jury is still out on whether calcium supplements or dairy products (or both) help you lose weight, but there are nevertheless plenty of good reasons to include them in your diet.

Because certain dairy foods like cream, half-and-half, and sour cream are high in calories and also in saturated fat, we recommend that you stick to low-fat alternatives, replacing sour cream with low-fat sour cream or yogurt, for example. You don't have to go fat free—nonfat products often are less satisfying, and in some cases they're bulked up with unwanted flavor enhancers such as sugar. Flavored low-fat yogurts and milks, for example, can be just as high in calories as their full-fat counterparts. When it comes to dairy products, it really pays to read labels.

Protein

This category may, at first glance, be the most confusing, in that it features foods that might well be thought to belong in other groups (for example, cheese is a protein food that's often thought of as a dairy food). In fact, as we have noted earlier, some foods actually fit into more than one category. The principle here is functional, not literal, classification—we've assigned foods to categories according to the role they play in your overall nutrition plan. Protein derives from a wide range of sources, from the ones you expect like meat and fish to nuts, beans, and, yes, cheese. It is the body's major construction material, and it's needed to produce hormones and enzymes essential to normal growth, development, and function and to build, maintain, protect, and repair body tissue. It can also serve as a source of energy when needed. Protein is also an important source of most B-complex vitamins and several minerals, including iron.

You may have noticed earlier that the calories for one serving (1 ounce) of protein ranges widely (from 35 calories for shellfish to 100 for cheese). This variability is mostly due to varying fat content. To save calories, we encourage you to choose leaner options for the majority of your protein servings. Good lean protein options include skinless poultry, fish, and (sparingly) lean cuts of meat. But remember that no foods are off-limits—just use the higher-fat versions very sparingly. Eggs are another rich source of protein and nutrients; they contain no less than thirteen vitamins and minerals, including vitamins D and E, folic acid, some omega-3 fatty acids, and antioxidants—all this in a tidy package of less than 100 calories!

According to the American Heart Association's current guidelines, you can include as much as one egg (213 milligrams of cholesterol) per day in your diet, provided you control the overall level of cholesterol (keeping it to less than 300 milligrams per day). However, if you have high cholesterol, our nutrition staff recommend eating less than four eggs a week. If you enjoy eggs, you can limit other cholesterol-containing protein sources, such as meats, poultry, and dairy products. Keep in mind that egg whites contain only traces of cholesterol, so adding these to your diet is a great way to get protein.

Egg whites come in pint containers at your grocery store—simply follow the measuring instructions on the carton. There are also great gadgets available for separating yolks from whites, and egg substitutes, though not equal in nutritional value to real eggs, are good, too.

A word on fish: Particularly beneficial are oilier varieties that are higher in omega-3 fatty acids, such as salmon, tuna, mackerel, sardines, and herring. If you're eating fish more than once a week—as we recommend you do—

you'll want to choose those less likely to be high in mercury and other unhealthy pollutants. Some good choices are salmon, tilapia, snapper, and shrimp. Species such as shark, swordfish, king mackerel, and tilefish may contain higher levels of mercury and other contaminants. To avoid excessive levels of these contaminants, you shouldn't eat these types of fish more than twice a week. The Food and Drug Administration (FDA) and Environmental Protection Agency (EPA) warn that for women who are or may become pregnant, for breast-feeding women, and for young children under the age of twelve, it's probably safest to avoid the types of fish and shellfish that have higher levels of mercury and eat only those that have lower levels. Information about the levels of mercury in various types of fish you eat can be found on the FDA food safety website: www.cfsan.fda.gov/~frf/sea-mehg.html or on the EPA website at www.epa.gov/ost/fish.

PUTTING IT ALL INTO ACTION

That's the end of our core nutrition information. Now it's time to put the pedal to the metal—to take what you've learned and use it to build a plan for lasting weight loss. The key to success is having a clear plan that provides for adequate nutrition balance and healthy choices, yet also keeps your meal options interesting and delicious and gives you confidence that you won't feel deprived.

Each week of the Duke core nutrition plan provides menus to guide you in preparing the meals and snacks for that week. If a suggested meal or snack contains an ingredient that you don't like or can't eat, we suggest that you look over the other recipes in chapter 9, find a substitute that appeals to you, and plug it into your plan. If you want even more tools to help you tailor your plan, you can use the Meal Planner at www.dukediet.com to choose from hundreds of recipes.

Planning your meals ahead takes the guesswork out of the trip to the grocery store. Imagine now much harder it would be if you went without planning and wound up roaming some of the most challenging aisles of the store—for example, the baked goods and ice cream sections. There might be samples on offer, which you'd probably try, and who knows what less-than-ideal items might find their way into your cart?

You're only human. Why expose yourself to that level of uncertainty and temptation? There are no prizes for doing this the hard way.

We know from decades of experience that thinking before you eat is an important part of the battle for lasting weight loss. We wouldn't urge you to do it if we didn't consider it *essential*. In part 2, you'll find a new plan for each week of the core program. Now that we've convinced you (we hope!) of the importance of meal planning, let's go step by step through the process of choosing between the two plans, selecting your calorie level, and transforming the Duke Plan into action.

Step 1

Decide which eating plan you'll follow, at least to start—either the Traditional or the Moderate Carbohydrate Meal Plan. You've probably already made up your mind about this, but if not, now's the time. Consider what you like to eat: Are you a fan of carbohydrates? Do you like protein and tend to have fewer cravings at a lower-carb level? What kind of diet has worked for you before? It might help to flip ahead to part 2 to review the meal plans and determine which choices look the most appealing. But don't feel too much stress—you can try both and switch back and forth at the end of any week. What matters most for weight control is—yes—calories in versus calories out.

Step 2

Determine the calorie range that is likely to help you lose weight at a safe and effective rate of one to two pounds per week. In general, if you're a woman, you'll likely accomplish that if you eat between 1,200 and 1,500 calories daily; if you're a man, a good range is between about 1,500 and 2,000 calories (for men of smaller stature, fewer than 1,500 calories may be appropriate). Your calorie levels may be higher if you're more than moderately overweight when you're starting out. We suggest starting at the lower end of these calorie ranges, and we'll provide meal plans to match. These plans form a basis you can build upon to meet your individual needs. Once you follow this calorie level for some time and see how you feel, you can simply adjust by adding or removing some foods. For example, if you find that you are overly hungry, unusually tired, or irritable up to a week after you start your plan, you add

50 to 100 calories a day. You could add these calories by eating additional servings from any food group or combination of food groups you choose, either as part of your meals or as a snack.

Remember, the idea is not to be overly rigid in your approach. You can and should use your own judgment. If you find yourself losing weight too quickly (more than 2 to 3 pounds a week), add 50 to 100 calories a day. If you are losing a little too slowly for your liking, subtract 50 to 100 calories. Whatever you do, just never go below 1,200 calories, whether you are a man or a woman, since it's unsafe to do so without medical supervision. Above all, keep in mind that your diet should not be uncomfortable or overly depriving. Of course, it may take a few days to adjust to your new plan, since you are probably making quite a change from the amount of calories you were eating before you began.

Step 3

Look over the following charts and decide how many servings from each food group you will have daily, based on your calorie range and the eating plan you've chosen. (You can also go to www.dukediet.com, where we have meal plans for a wider range of calorie levels: 1,200 to 1,400; 1,400 to 1,600; 1,600 to 1,800; and 1,800 to 2,000.)

TRADITIONAL MEAL PLAN (DAILY)

	1,200–1,400 WOMEN	1,400–1,600 MEN
Fats	2–3 servings	3 servings
Dairy	1–2 servings	2–3 servings
Protein	6–7 servings	6–7 servings
Vegetables	3 servings	3–4 servings
Fruits	3–4 servings	2–3 servings
Starches	6 servings	8 servings

MODERATE CARBOHYDRATE MEAL PLAN (DAILY)

	1,200–1,400 WOMEN	1,400–1,600 MEN
Fats	1–2 servings	2–3 servings
Dairy	1–2 servings	1–2 servings
Protein	11–12 servings	14 servings
Vegetables	4–5 servings	4 servings
Fruits	3 servings	3–4 servings
Starches	2–3 servings	3 servings

Become very familiar with the number of servings you need each day. You may want to post your personal serving information on your refrigerator door or put a little card in your wallet. Meanwhile, record your plan overview here:

My eating plan is the _____.

My calorie range is _____.

MY DAILY SERVINGS

FOOD GROUP	SERVINGS (BREAKFAST)	BREAKFAST	SERVINGS (LUNCH)	LUNCH	SERVINGS (DINNER)	DINNER	SERVINGS (SNACK)	SNACK
Starch								
Fruit								
Vegetable								
Dairy								
Protein								
Fat								

Step 4

Look over the foods listed in the preceding food group sections, flip through the weekly meal plans in chapters 5 through 8, and check out the recipes in chapter 9—they'll really give you something to look forward to! At least in the first couple weeks of the core four-week program, when you're just learning to live with the Duke Plan, it might be helpful to stick to the menus as closely as you can and make substitutions only when necessary. Later on, when you gain more confidence in working the system, you can choose your own foods more freely.

Step 5

Keep track of not just what you're supposed to eat, but what you *actually do eat* every day. Be sure to watch—and log—your serving sizes and calories carefully. We provide you with a simple and easy monitoring card in Week 1 to do just that, or you can use the handy Food Log at www.dukediet.com. As we always say to our patients, be careful to approach your Food Log as a tool for success rather than self-judgment and reproach. Remember, progress, not perfection, is the key.

LITTLE BY LITTLE

As we've said—and we can't emphasize it enough—on the Duke Plan, you don't have to overhaul your life completely or trade in your taste buds for new ones that respond only to brown rice and greens. We've gone into considerable detail about nutrition to show you how to work with the diet to incorporate the foods you enjoy. After the first couple of weeks, once you get familiar with your chosen plan, you'll be more comfortable customizing your menus. The range of recipes you'll find in chapter 9, and the even broader selection on www.dukediet.com, will inspire you to be creative in your cooking and give you the variety to eat what you like.

Remember that the Duke Plan is not about deprivation. You'll be developing eating habits that will sustain you—and help keep your weight under control—for the rest of your life. For the long run, think "evolution, not revolution," for evolutionary, rather than all-at-once, changes are the ones that tend to stick with us and become ingrained as habits. The small, incremental changes you make in the course of each week—not just in your diet but also in your activity level and your thinking, as you'll see in the next two chapters—will yield enormous dividends over time.

CHAPTER THREE

The Duke Diet Exercise Plan: Why You Will Get Fit

We can tell you a lot of great success stories from our years at the Duke Diet & Fitness Center, and many of our favorites involve exercise. Why exercise? Because so often we see people who fear or avoid activity for many different reasons. They may arrive at Duke secretly hoping to dodge physical exertion and achieve success through calorie reduction alone. Then we get to see them transform themselves into exercise devotees. This is one of the most immediately rewarding aspects of the Duke program.

Why is getting active so difficult for so many of us? At the heart of the matter is the fact that, in our modern, technology-dominated world, we have less *need* to move than ever before in history. We don't walk anymore; we drive—right up to the cash machine and the dry cleaner's pickup window, and through the express take-out line at the nearby fast-food restaurant. Once there, we don't have to roll down our windows by hand; we simply push a button. If we're coming from work, chances are that we've been sitting in front of a computer all day moving nothing but our fingers, rather than literally performing manual labor. Back home, we pull into the driveway—power steering makes it a cinch—hit a button, and the garage door opens. We head inside, watch TV, surfing with the remote for our favorite shows, and then we turn in, exhausted. Sure, we're tired, and rightfully so, since we do work hard and expend so much mental energy dealing with life—energy that, unfortunately, burns very few calories, compared to physical exertion.

Today, we're so overconnected and overcommitted that it is hard to find time to be physically active. Often the day never really seems to end. You may have a spouse and kids who need your attention. You make lunches and log on to the computer to coordinate their schedules and help them with their homework—and there you find a work question that needs to be answered tonight. Or perhaps you are married to your job, multitasking, talking to someone on the cell phone as other callers beep in—a problem at work, a friend who needs advice. We rarely have actual *downtime*, as we used to when quiet relaxation was as simple as picking up a book and unplugging the phone. We're forced to choose between exercising and relaxing.

Even those of us who make exercise a priority are sometimes too overwhelmed to get any. According to a recent report from the U.S. Surgeon General, 60 percent of American adults get less than the minimum recommendation of thirty minutes of moderate-intensity exercise (like brisk walking) per day that is recommended for maintaining health. What's more, 25 percent of all adults are not active at all!

During the first week of the Duke Diet & Fitness Center program, we talk with our clients about potential consequences of inadequate physical activity, which range from a few extra pounds to serious health problems that can include obesity, high blood pressure, high cholesterol, diabetes, heart disease, osteoporosis, arthritis, and certain cancers (notably breast and colon cancer). Indeed, numerous studies show that physical inactivity is associated with an increased risk of death. As these clients acquire new information and begin to experience physical improvements associated with exercise, they start to get it—exercise really matters! And it's not just about dress and pants sizes; it's about life.

If you've been inactive for a long time, you may feel intimidated by the very idea of exercise. You might already have aches and pains or a medical condition that you're afraid will worsen. Maybe you find rigorous exercise so exhausting that you can't even think about the payoff. You may be self-conscious about your abilities, or you may simply not like to sweat. We hear these reasons all the time. You're certainly not alone—and we can help you.

Confessions of a Powerlifter

I was once a competitive powerlifter and a bodybuilder. As it has for most of us, my life has become very busy and I can no longer approach exercise with that level of time—or mental—commitment. At the end of a difficult day, I sometimes have trouble getting "up" for exercise and give in to the urge to skip it, even though the gym is only ten steps from my office. I get buried in my work, and it's hard to shut off my mind and focus on my body, even though I know how good a workout will make me feel. So I recognize that I have to be flexible—to sneak in exercise when I can during the day. Sometimes I exercise at home before work. Other times, when I get an unexpected opportunity (such as a canceled appointment), I walk or run along the wall of Duke's beautiful East Campus.

I'm a fairly goal-oriented guy, so the idea of exercising because it's good for my health sometimes seems too abstract (and far off) to get me going. So I deliberately build tasks into my life, things that need doing anyway, that let me work up a sweat. I don't have a riding lawn mower or a leaf blower. That way I know that I'll be dedicating a couple hours a week for most of the year to physically demanding yard work (which I enjoy, and which destresses me). I'm out in the fresh air, I get satisfaction when I admire my freshly cut or raked lawn, and I get all the benefits of exercise. I also try to make activity-building choices, such as parking farther away from the building at the office and walking in the airport as opposed to sitting—using all the tips we teach our clients. Of course, my optimal goal is always to do more planned exercise, but when life gets in the way, I still have an active baseline to fall back on. The key for me was getting out of my old "regimented exerciser" mind-set and adopting an open-minded and flexible approach to activity.

—*Martin Binks, Ph.D.*

Early experiences with exercise can shape the way we see ourselves. All too often we hear decades-old horror stories from clients who were chastised for being unable to climb the rope or do the right number of push-ups in gym class, or later in life, literally throwing in the towel when they can't master

Health Benefits of Exercise

- Lowers your risk of heart disease
- Reduces your risk of certain cancers—notably, colon and breast cancer—and may improve outcomes in those being treated for cancer
- Lowers blood pressure
- Improves your lipid profile (cholesterol and triglycerides)
- Helps you lose weight and keep it off, and thus prevents obesity
- Helps you burn fat without losing muscle
- Helps prevent and control diabetes
- Builds and maintains healthy bones
- Enhances immunity
- Improves stamina, strength, and mobility
- Helps older people maintain independence and reduces risks of falls
- Relieves stress and improves mood
- May help preserve cognitive function as you age
- Enhances emotional well-being

the fancy footwork in an aerobics class full of skinny people in spandex. For these folks, fitness comes to mean failure or embarrassment.

Society and the media tend to reinforce unrealistic attitudes about exercise with stories about celebrity workouts and size-zero clothes. So many of our patients believe that in order to get fit they have to spend countless hours in the gym on some heroic and rigorous course of training. Not true! Even if you had that much time, wouldn't it be better—and healthier—to spend it enjoying your family and friends or engaging in hobbies? Remember this mantra: *moderate and sustainable*. It applies to fitness as well as to dietary changes.

At Duke, our answer to the question "What is fitness?" follows the guidelines of the American College of Sports Medicine (ACSM), one of the nation's foremost fitness organizations: Fitness is "the ability to perform moderate to vigorous levels of physical activity without undue fatigue—

Moves and Mood

Exercise is good for your body, but it can also raise your spirits. This is not just an effort to motivate you—there's real, hard-scientific evidence that exercise brightens moods.

In fact, Duke researcher Dr. James Blumenthal has shown that exercise can be helpful in combating depression. While it is often speculated that exercise helps by stimulating the release of certain substances in the brain that influence mood, this has not yet been proven. However, it does seem that exercise can improve mood in both depressed and non-depressed people. We see people feeling better about themselves all the time at the Duke Diet & Fitness Center. Typically, and often within just a few days, people start to experience a sense of accomplishment and a heightened sense of well-being if they manage to do even a little more exercise—especially when they didn't feel like doing it. So try your best to do something active each day. Your mind and body will thank you.

and the capability to maintain this capacity throughout life." Sounds reasonable, doesn't it? And yes, we can tell you from experience, it *is* achievable!

So don't worry—we're not about to crack the whip to get you in shape through some punishing, one-size-fits-all regimen. We don't believe in pain for gain, but just the opposite: finding what *you* can do, enjoyably, to build activity into your routine. Remember, you're trying to lose weight and keep it off for life. Maintaining an active lifestyle (and a good fitness routine) is one of the core strategies for maintaining long-term weight loss. That's not going to happen if you hate what you're doing every day.

We're going to start by focusing on the principles of exercise and what you stand to gain from each type. We will help you identify—and overcome—your barriers to exercise. Then we will show you how to determine your personal fitness level and develop a workout program that works for you.

It may be wise to consult your doctor for a preworkout checkup before starting any new fitness program. We especially recommend this for men over forty-five and for women over fifty-five. It's particularly important to do so if you already have heart disease or heart disease risk factors such as smoking, high blood pressure, diabetes, abnormal cholesterol, or a worrisome family history (for instance, heart attack or coronary artery disease in a

From Cringing to Confident

I had never really embraced the need to exercise. To be honest, I hated the very idea. Moving my body vigorously had always made me feel clumsy and inadequate, in part because I had never been able to stop focusing on how I might look to other people. But now I have a new attitude about it.

To increase the chance that I'd actually make it to the gym, I joined the one closest to my home. For the first little while I had to push myself to attend, but now, for the first time, I feel happy and charged up when I exercise—and as if something is missing when I skip it. I look forward not so much to the exercise itself as to the feeling of accomplishment I get after completing thirty minutes on the stationary bike or treadmill or my forty-five-minute workout with weights. Sometimes when I'm tired and really don't feel like going, I make a deal with myself to just "suit up" and try to work out for five minutes. Almost invariably, after five minutes I am "over the hump" and feeling energized and motivated to complete my usual workout.

I still worry that I could backslide and find myself a couch potato with aching joints again. But I take it one day at a time and trust myself to catch those sneaky negative thoughts before they get a chance to undermine my new self-confidence.

—*Joanne, age 37*

parent or sibling at a young age—less than forty-five for your father or a brother and less than fifty-five for your mother or a sister). Then, if your doctor agrees, we will help you start small and think in terms of gradual, incremental steps toward putting more movement into your days. Perhaps you will be surprised to learn that while there may be some truth to the idea that more is better when it comes to exercise, the greatest health gains are realized by those who progress from an inactive lifestyle to a moderately active lifestyle. In a study of nearly 10,000 men, Dr. Stephen Blair and colleagues at the Cooper Clinic demonstrated that those who went from "unfit" to "fit" over a five-year period reduced their relative risk of death by 44 percent, compared to people who remained unfit!

Believe it or not, many clients tell us that finding the right routine was all it took to help them overcome their dislike of exercise, and a lot of them have come to look forward to their daily workouts. They tell us that exercise makes them feel more energetic and alive.

THE ELEMENTS OF FITNESS

At Duke, we teach our clients that there are four elements of fitness. The first element is activities of daily living, or as we call them, ADLs. These include everything from waking up, getting out of bed, combing your hair, putting on your robe, and stepping out to get the newspaper to doing household chores, taking care of the yard, and walking your dog. The good thing about ADLs is that as they accumulate throughout the day, they burn calories with little or no conscious effort on your part. Remember, every little bit counts: If you burn 100 calories more than you take in each day, in a year you can lose ten pounds. Think about that the next time you have just a little extra time to add some steps, take the stairs, or do something active. It *all* adds up!

The next element is fitness-building activities, which fall into three groups: cardio (also called *aerobic* exercise, which strengthens your cardio-vascular system), strength training, and flexibility training. The third element is mind-body activities like yoga and Pilates, and the fourth is recreational activities like dancing and sports. If you experiment with recreational activities, which include everything from shooting pool to shooting hoops, you're bound to find a few that you truly enjoy enough to make them part of your routine.

Let's look at how to incorporate each of these elements into your life.

Activities of Daily Living (ADLs)

The first step toward becoming more active is finding opportunities to build extra movements into your day. You're probably already doing a lot of the activities listed here, and you might want to check off ones that you can easily add or do more often. Do a little brainstorming and come up with your own list of ADLs. Jot them down in a notebook or record them in your Lifestyle Journal on www.dukediet.com.

At Home

- During TV commercial breaks, do a few sit-to-stand exercises (great for quadriceps strengthening), sit-ups, push-ups, stretches, marching in place, or exercise ball routines.
- Stand or, better, pace while talking on the phone.
- Climb stairs.
- Do moderate housework like vacuuming or heavy chores like scrubbing floors.
- Take the dog for brisk walks instead of letting Pokey out in the yard.
- Play actively with your kids.
- Work in the yard—garden, mow the lawn, or rake leaves.
- Wash and vacuum your car instead of taking it to the drive-through car wash or detailer.
- Get off the bus or subway one stop earlier.
- Before and after shopping, take a few laps around the store or mall; use a handbasket, when possible, instead of a cart.
- Give your business to those neighborhood stores or services that you can safely access by foot or on your bike.

At Work

- Move the trash can to the opposite side of your office.
- Instead of keeping a coffeepot or a jug of water at your desk, consider the health benefits of taking periodic walks to the break room.
- Eat a healthy lunch that you brought from home, then walk for the rest of your lunch break.
- Get up to talk directly to colleagues on occasion, rather than always e-mailing them.
- Stand up to stretch a few times a day, and stand or pace during some of your phone calls.
- Get off the elevator a few floors early and take the stairs.
- Park as far as you can from the front door and walk (you may take pleasure in realizing that your new, preferred parking space is always reserved for you!).
- Conduct at least some of your work meetings while walking—either with a colleague or while talking on your cell phone.

At Play

- Window-shop at the mall. Brisk mall walking can be a good option when darkness or inclement weather prevent you from walking outdoors.
- Become a regular at your local museum or botanical garden.
- At the playground with your kids, play! Swing on the swings, teeter on the seesaw, or play Frisbee, tag, or catch.
- Hit some balls at the driving range.
- Go bowling or skating.
- Take a ballroom dance or salsa class with your spouse or friends, or go by yourself and make new friends!
- When playing golf, walk instead of using a cart and carry or drag your own clubs.
- Take up Ping-Pong or tennis.
- At a picnic, play badminton or volleyball.
- At the lake, rent a canoe, kayak, or rowboat.
- On vacation, sightsee on foot or bicycle instead of taking a bus tour—or if you take a bus tour, select the kind that allows you to get off and on when you wish.
- Walk instead of sitting in airports during layovers; avoid the moving walkways and escalators unless you really need them (if you do use them, walk while you're on them).

These are just a few of the calorie burners you can sneak into your day, and you can no doubt think of more. But can things like vacuuming more often really help you lose weight and get healthier? Some very convincing research says yes. A study conducted at the Cooper Institute in Dallas, Texas, compared the effects, over twenty-four months, on sedentary adults who were asked to accumulate thirty minutes of moderate-intensity physical activity (in part by increasing their ADLs) on most, if not all, days of the week with those who adopted a traditional structured aerobic fitness program at a fitness facility. The researchers found that both groups experienced significant improvements in physical activity, cardiovascular fitness, blood pressure, and percentage of body fat. Therefore, a program that includes an increase in ADLs might be just what is needed to get you started on the road

One Step at a Time

I was in my early fifties when I came to Duke and so sedentary that I was afraid to "walk the wall," the 1½-mile scenic pathway around Duke's East Campus. It just sounded so far, and I doubted that I could keep up with other walkers. Luckily, I found a pal with the same worries, so we teamed up to try walking it at our own comfortable pace. We made it! That was a major victory for me.

So we did it again—and again. Each time, the distance seemed to shrink, and instead of viewing the walk as an ordeal, we started to enjoy it. It was setting our own comfortable pace that made the difference, and I keep that in mind now that I've taken up hiking. I like the idea that you don't have to sprint or jog to burn some serious calories—that just walking at your own speed can do it. I never would have guessed that you could wear the tread off walking shoes. Now I do it all the time!

As far as ADLs go, I confess that, at first, the idea of parking farther from my destination annoyed me—it even seemed silly. I'd grumble, "What a waste of time—that's not exercise!" Then I shifted my focus from the negative and started looking for good reasons to do it. I started telling myself that some poor soul would come along—maybe an elderly person with a walker—who really needed that closer parking space. With those pictures in my head, I began parking at a distance, feeling that I was doing a good turn while getting exercise.

I've lost twenty-seven pounds altogether and am more active than ever. Sure, I have slips—who doesn't?—but I don't stress about them anymore. I just start each day fresh and ready to try to be active, which gets me back on track.

—*Greg, age 57*

to fitness and better health. This may be especially true if your barriers to physical activity include lack of time, dislike of vigorous exercise, or lack of access to facilities.

The chart on page 59 shows how many calories you can burn and how much weight you can lose just by increasing your daily activities. It's based on calories expended by someone who weighs 150 pounds. If you weigh more

ADL	LENGTH OF TIME	CALORIES BURNED PER WEEK	POUNDS LOST IN ONE YEAR
Using stairs instead of the elevator or escalator	5 minutes, 5 times a week	225 calories	3 pounds
Playing actively with kids	1 hour, 3 times a week	612 calories	9 pounds
Taking a walk on your lunch break	10 minutes, 5 times a week	170 calories	2.5 pounds
Parking your car farther away from the entrance and walking the extra distance.	5 minutes, 7 times a week	119 calories	2 pounds
Mowing the lawn	1 hour a week	374 calories	5 pounds
Doing housework	2 hours a week	408 calories	6 pounds
Energetic dancing	2 hours a week	816 calories	12 pounds
Tossing a Frisbee with your dog	30 minutes, twice a week	204 calories	3 pounds
Working in your yard or garden	2 hours a week	712 calories	10 pounds

than that, you will burn even more. You will find a personalized Activity Calculator for own your weight and even more ADLs on www.dukediet.com.

Fitness-Building Activities

As we've said, these activities are grouped into three categories, according to their benefits: aerobic conditioning or cardio, muscular strength and endurance, and flexibility.

Aerobic Conditioning

This term refers to how well your heart, lungs, and arteries deliver oxygen to your muscles, and to how well muscles use it. That's why we think of aerobic

Body and Mind Renewal

There's an old proverb: *It is solved by walking.* Walking, my primary exercise, requires no special training, coordination, skills, or gear (except for a good, comfortable pair of shoes). I like to take a brisk walk as many days during the week as I can, preferably outdoors, and whenever possible I love to take those walks with my wife, Beth. Our lives are so busy that it's hard to find enough time for each other, so our walks are an important time of togetherness for us. We make them such a priority that if it's dark outside or uncomfortably cold and wet, we go to a well-lit parking lot near our home or to a mall that stays open late.

Sometimes, when I'm meeting with someone on business, I invite him or her to join me for a walk around the Duke campus. You'd be surprised how often people accept my invitation—and how productive those meetings can be.

I'm fortunate (well, actually, I kind of planned it that way) that I live close enough to work that on nice days I can ride my bike to my office along a former railway bed, now converted to a walking and biking trail. I wear biking shorts, with my clothes in a knapsack. I shower and change at the office, and start my day feeling wonderfully invigorated, physically and mentally.

I also try to get some strength training into my routine. I have a set of weights at home, and I combine free-weight exercises with body-weight exercises a few times a week. There is a mental boost and feeling of self-satisfaction I receive from my exercise routine: I feel better, and I have more energy and concentration to devote to my work.

—*Howard Eisenson, M.D.*

exercise as the kind that makes you breathe a little harder. Examples of aerobic activities are walking, jogging, aerobics classes, swimming, running, cycling, and dancing. For most of us, the easiest and best aerobic activity is walking—yes, simple walking, not jogging or sprinting. For starters, it's one of the safest do-anywhere exercises you can perform—it's much easier on your knees than running and it's fine on level surfaces, even for most folks with joint pain or arthritis of the knees (swimming is also a superb alterna-

Every Step Counts

Need extra motivation to move? Try wearing a pedometer! Our patients find pedometers very useful. Setting and achieving daily and weekly step goals provides a great way to gradually increase your activity.

It is recommended that people aim for about 10,000 steps per day to maintain health. But it is important not to be overwhelmed by that goal—instead, start where you are. Put on a pedometer and go about your daily business. At the end of the day, check how many steps you've done and write the number down. Once you know how many steps you average daily (say, 2,500, for example), you're ready to set some targets. Next week, start by adding 500 steps to your daily average, so now you are getting about 3,000 steps each day of the week. Once you are able to do that somewhat consistently, gradually increase your steps until you've reached your optimal goal of averaging 10,000 steps per day (which equals roughly five miles). Does five miles sound impossible? Don't worry, it has seemed so to many of our patients, too. But by setting reasonable short-term goals, you'll get there. Walking five miles doesn't take anywhere near as much time as you might suspect when you focus on increasing your ADLs.

tive in that case). You can heighten the pleasure it gives you by walking outdoors in pleasant surroundings and bringing along your iPod or, even better, a companion. Multiple scientific studies have demonstrated the health benefits of walking. One of the most impressive studies looked at people with diabetes and demonstrated that walking at least two hours per week reduced their risk of premature death by 39 to 54 percent!

The benefits of aerobic exercise don't end with your workout session. The metabolic boost or increased energy expenditure you get from it can last for a couple of hours after you stop, and possibly longer.

Muscular Strength and Endurance

How strong are you? Muscular strength is the ability of your muscles to lift weight or work against resistance; muscular endurance refers to how quickly your muscles tire. Both are enhanced through strength training exercises: lifting weights, using resistance tubes and stability or medicine balls, and doing activities using your own body weight such as push-ups or sit-ups. Strengthening exercises can help us function better in our daily lives.

Strength training can decrease the loss of lean muscle tissue, slow the bone loss that comes with age, ease the pain of arthritis, improve diabetic control, and help us maintain good balance and prevent falls. It can also help prevent sports injuries because strong muscles absorb shock during movement. Think about riding in a car with worn-out shocks. Every time you hit a bump, you get a huge jolt, which hurts! The same thing happens if your muscles are weak. Strength training is very popular with our patients at the Duke Diet & Fitness Center. It can be tailored to match your abilities and conditioning level and, as with any activity, can lead to a sense of accomplishment. Try it and you'll see!

Flexibility

Flexibility, which refers to how well you can move your joints without pain through their natural range of movement, is often pushed to the back burner. But lack of flexibility suggests that your muscles may be in an overly contracted state, which can not only cause you discomfort but also increase your risk for injury when you perform quick movements. Activities that help you improve flexibility include stretching, yoga, tai chi, and Pilates, which also offer stress reduction and relaxation benefits.

Balance

As we grow older, our sense of balance may decline. We've all heard about elderly people falling and breaking bones, which is one reason to maintain our balance skills. But another is that people whose balance is poor often feel afraid to move freely, are less likely to enjoy a range of physical activities, and are less likely to maintain their independence as they age. Fortunately, balance can be improved. Remember learning to ride a bike when you were a kid? You thought you might never be able to ride without the training wheels, but you eventually did.

Our clients tell us that many of the exercises we recommend in this book and on www.dukediet.com have helped them regain and improve not only their balance but also their coordination, stability, motor skills, stamina, and comfort and confidence while exercising.

Mind-Body Activities

Mind-body exercises are especially popular among our patients because they not only give you a good workout but also stretch your muscles, release tension, and help calm your mind, while promoting fitness and health. Many gyms, health spas, and hospital wellness centers offer classes on mind-body exercise, which are well worth investigating.

Yoga

The best-known form of mind-body exercise, yoga is a 5,000-year-old practice that puts you through a series of standing, sitting, and lying-down postures, as well as breathing, relaxation, and meditation techniques. It may be difficult to choose from the many styles of yoga, so take some time to explore before committing to one. Keep in mind that yoga at your local gym will most likely be geared toward the physical benefits, while classes at a yoga center will have a more spiritual focus, emphasizing breathing and meditation. Either will help increase your strength and flexibility. Yoga DVDs and videos that let you try out the moves at home are widely available.

Tai Chi

Tai chi, which has been practiced for centuries by Chinese monks, is a system of slow, gentle body movements that foster relaxation. Tai chi may also help you to improve your sense of balance.

Pilates

Pilates, developed in the 1920s, is the relative newcomer among the mind-body systems. Like the others, it involves concentration on breathing while strengthening the body's core, or midsection, muscles. One of the early proponents of Pilates was the ballet choreographer George Balanchine, and it has long been a favorite among ballet dancers. We recommend that you take at least one formal Pilates class with a qualified instructor to learn the proper form and breathing techniques before you try an at-home routine.

Meditation

While not an exercise per se, meditation can help reduce stress and improve your quality of life. It involves breathing and focusing your mind, much as you do in many of the other mind-body techniques.

How Much Time Do I Have to Spend Exercising?

For general health purposes, most guidelines recommend that you aim for thirty minutes of aerobic exercise on most days of the week. However, if your goal is to lose weight and keep it off, we recommend that you aim for more like forty-five minutes to an hour nearly every day. Of course, this amount might be unrealistic for you at first, especially if you've been inactive for a while. At the end of this chapter, we will help you evaluate your personal fitness level and set appropriate goals.

Meanwhile, we're sure that lots of you are thinking, "No way! I can't free up an entire hour or even half that—especially not during the week!"

You can let go of the panic button. There's no need to cram all your exercise into one big push. A twenty-week study done at the University of Pittsburgh School of Medicine compared two groups of overweight women. The women in one group were instructed to break their exercise up into ten-minute bouts throughout the day, and the other women were told to do their exercise as one session. Both groups were instructed to exercise five days a week, and the amount of exercise they were asked to get progressed from twenty to forty minutes per day over the course of the study. All the participants followed a diet of 1,200 to 1,500 calories a day. The study found that short bouts of activity produced similar weight loss and similar changes in cardiorespiratory fitness and improved the likelihood that people would complete the total amount of time that was recommended. Another study, done here at Duke, suggests that the total amount of exercise is more important than the intensity—for a host of health benefits. So the key is to find activities that you will perform regularly and add up those minutes.

Let's say you want to start by doing thirty minutes of exercise a day, in three stints.

- Morning: Walk your dog at a brisk pace for ten minutes, park farther from the office, and get off the elevator a few floors early and take the stairs.
- Midday: Go outside and walk around the building for ten minutes on your lunch hour and then repeat the elevator trick when you return to the office.
- Evening: Take a stroll (or a brisk walk if you are up to it) after dinner, or walk the dog. Or perhaps handle some light household chores for ten minutes.

That's thirty-plus minutes right there! And every minute is taking you closer to your weight loss goal. For maximum effectiveness, walk with a purpose, as if you were trying to avoid being late for an appointment. Once you get comfortable at thirty minutes, it's a simple matter to add a few more mini–exercise sessions or five more minutes to each session. Before you know it, you'll be doing an hour of exercise a day! And as you reach these reasonable, very achievable goals, think of the confidence it will give you, not to mention the health benefits. Chapter 4 will provide you with in-depth guidance on setting and achieving all your health and wellness goals, as well as on planning to avoid slips.

Recreational Activities

Participating in recreational sports such as tennis, golf, hiking, and cycling is another great way to get fit and healthy. The good thing about sports is that you focus on the fun of doing them, not necessarily on the calories you're burning or the health benefits. As with other forms of activity, start with sports gradually. As you build your level of fitness, you can challenge yourself more. Don't take up squash if you've been sedentary for years or sign on for a ten-mile hike until you've logged time in other fitness-building activities. You'll find information on the calorie-burning potential of various sports in chapter 10 of this book and on www.dukediet.com.

WHAT'S STOPPING YOU?

"I just don't have time."

"I'm too tired to exercise on top of work and running my household."

"I don't have an exercise companion, so it's hard to stick to my routine."

"I travel on business too much to get regular exercise."

These are just some of the reasons mentioned by clients at the Duke Diet & Fitness Center that prevent them from getting or staying active!

That's why we believe that it is so important to look ahead and try to see just what might get in the way of your best-laid exercise plans *before* you start to slip, and ensure that you have a plan to deal with those obstacles. Identifying and overcoming barriers to exercise is so very important. What are your barriers to exercise? The instrument we use to help clients identify theirs was created by the U.S. Centers for Disease Control and Prevention (CDC) and is reproduced for you here. Please circle your responses, and be honest and thoughtful. You'll learn a lot!

HOW LIKELY ARE YOU TO SAY?	VERY LIKELY	SOMEWHAT LIKELY	SOMEWHAT UNLIKELY	VERY UNLIKELY
1. My day is so busy now; I just don't think I can make the time to include physical activity in my regular schedule.	3	2	1	0

HOW LIKELY ARE YOU TO SAY?	VERY LIKELY	SOMEWHAT LIKELY	SOMEWHAT UNLIKELY	VERY UNLIKELY
2. None of my friends or family members likes to do anything active, so I don't have a chance to exercise.	3	2	1	0
3. I'm just too tired after work to get any exercise.	3	2	1	0
4. I've been thinking about getting more exercise, but I just can't seem to get started.	3	2	1	0
5. I'm getting older, so exercise can be risky.	3	2	1	0
6. I don't get enough exercise because I have never learned the skills for any sport.	3	2	1	0
7. I don't have access to jogging trails, swimming pools, bike paths, and so forth.	3	2	1	0
8. Physical activity takes too much time away from other commitments—work, family, and so forth.	3	2	1	0
9. I'm embarrassed about how I will look when I exercise with others.	3	2	1	0
10. I don't get enough sleep as it is; I just couldn't get up early or stay up late enough to exercise.	3	2	1	0
11. It's easier for me to find excuses not to exercise than to go out to do something.	3	2	1	0
12. I know too many people who have hurt themselves by overdoing it with exercise.	3	2	1	0
13. I really can't see learning a new sport at my age.	3	2	1	0
14. It's just too expensive. You have to take a class, join a club, or buy the right equipment.	3	2	1	0

HOW LIKELY ARE YOU TO SAY?	VERY LIKELY	SOMEWHAT LIKELY	SOMEWHAT UNLIKELY	VERY UNLIKELY
15. My free times during the day are too short to include exercise.	3	2	1	0
16. My usual social activities with family or friends do not include physical activity.	3	2	1	0
17. I'm too tired during the week, and I need the weekend to catch up on my rest.	3	2	1	0
18. I want to get more exercise, but I just can't seem to make myself stick to anything.	3	2	1	0
19. I'm afraid I might injure myself or have a heart attack.	3	2	1	0
20. I'm not good enough at any physical activity to make it fun.	3	2	1	0
21. If we had exercise facilities and showers at work, then I would be more likely to exercise.	3	2	1	0

Scoring: Enter the circled number in the spaces provided, putting the number for statement 1 on line 1, statement 2 on line 2, and so on.

Enter your scores for questions 1 to 3 on the first line below and then total the scores for that line, enter your scores for questions 4 to 6 on the second line below and then total the scores for that line, and so forth. Your barriers to physical activity fall into one or more of seven categories: lack of time, social influences, lack of energy, lack of willpower, fear of injury, lack of skill, and lack of resources. A score of 5 or more in any category shows that this is an important barrier for you to overcome.

_____ + _____ + _____ = _____
  1   2   3

Lack of Time

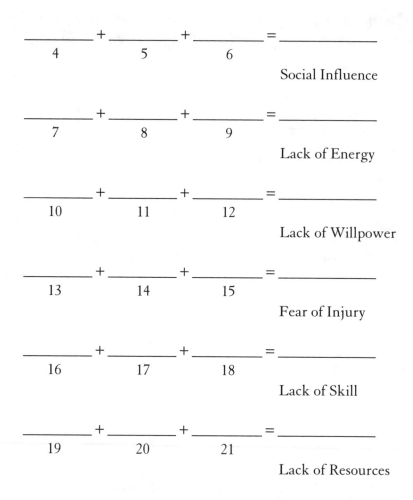

_____ + _____ + _____ = _____
   4   5   6

                                   Social Influence

_____ + _____ + _____ = _____
   7   8   9

                                   Lack of Energy

_____ + _____ + _____ = _____
   10   11   12

                                   Lack of Willpower

_____ + _____ + _____ = _____
   13   14   15

                                   Fear of Injury

_____ + _____ + _____ = _____
   16   17   18

                                   Lack of Skill

_____ + _____ + _____ = _____
   19   20   21

                                   Lack of Resources

Source: Physical Activity for Everyone: Making Physical Activity Part of Your Life: Overcoming Barriers to Physical Activity. Centers for Disease Control and Prevention website: www.cdc.gov/nccdphp/dnpa/physical/life/barriers_quiz.pdf

STRATEGIES FOR CHANGE

Look over the barriers you've identified in the questionnaire, and then review the following list of solutions. Many of them come from actual brainstorming done by clients at the Duke Diet & Fitness Center. Then do a little brainstorming of your own to come up with a few more. We will talk more about setting achievable goals and planning for obstacles in chapter 4.

Find the Time

- At the beginning of each week, plan out your exercise sessions. Record them in your Lifestyle Journal at www.dukediet.com, in a notebook, or on the calendar on your PDA. You are more likely to exercise if you view each session as an appointment.
- Try waking half an hour earlier so you can exercise in the morning before other obligations kick in, schedule lunch-hour workouts, or hold walking meetings.
- Do you watch TV every day? If you get up and move during the commercials, in three hours of viewing you'll accumulate fifty minutes of exercise!
- Build more activity into your routine chores. Raking the yard, washing the car, and doing energetic housework are all great workouts.

Find Some "Fast" Friends

- Take a group exercise class and make friends while you get fit, or sign up for salsa or ballroom dancing class.
- Meet a friend for workouts. That way, you can keep each other accountable for showing up.
- Do something physically active with your family that you all enjoy. Toss around a Frisbee or a volleyball, go skating or biking, or walk through the zoo. You'll have fun, and you'll be modeling healthy habits for the rest of the family.

Find the Energy and Motivation

- Exercise when your energy levels are high. If evening workouts are not for you, then try a bike ride before breakfast.
- Fire up your iPod or turn on your stereo. Music is energizing!
- Lay out your tracksuit and sneakers at night, then as soon as you awaken put them on. You're less likely to skip exercise if you're suited up.

Do Well by Doing Good!

One of our clients organized her social life around volunteering for, and participating in, charity athletic events. She and her husband trained for 5K runs and mini-marathons, which they found to be great motivators as well as truly uplifting experiences because they were helping to raise money for good causes. Charity athletic events give you the chance to push yourself physically while gaining the satisfaction of making a difference. Don't worry—you don't have to be a triathlon star. There are events for people at every degree of ability. Pick one that suits your level of conditioning and interests you.

Charities that sponsor fitness-related fund-raising events include the American Heart Association, the Arthritis Foundation, the American Cancer Society (which hosts some events especially for dog owners), Susan G. Komen for the Cure, and the Leukemia & Lymphoma Society, among many others.

- List the benefits of exercise that are important to you, then post them on your refrigerator door or bathroom mirror to keep them in your awareness.
- Don't feel like working out? Contract with yourself to exercise for *just five minutes* and then see if you want to continue. If you're still dragging afterward, give yourself permission to take the day off. Sometimes you do, in fact, need to rest or skip a day. But much of the time, you will simply be having a motivation lapse. Five minutes and the good feeling that goes with it will fuel your resolve, and you'll want to keep going. Often, getting started is the hardest part.
- Record your exercise progress in your notebook or your Lifestyle Journal on www.dukediet.com. Seeing what you've already accomplished can be powerfully motivating.
- Keep your body guessing. If you vary your workout type and intensity, you won't get bored with the same old routine.
- If lack of energy is a persistent problem, check with your doctor for help in finding the cause.

Be Wise and Be Safe

- If you're concerned about injury from exercise, get a thorough checkup to put your health risks in perspective. If you suffer from conditions that affect your ability to exercise, such as heart or lung problems, or if you have significant risk factors for heart disease (among them, smoking, diabetes, high cholesterol, or high blood pressure), your doctor can advise you about the kind and level of exercise you can do safely. If you have problems like joint or muscle pain or stiffness, a history of recurring injuries, or trouble with balance, a consultation with a physical therapist can be very helpful in developing an appropriate exercise plan that encompasses not only the activities to avoid but also the ones to emphasize.

- Start slowly and see how you feel before trying more challenging workouts. Make sure you warm up properly before exercise, and that you stretch afterward. We'll tell you more about that in your fitness routines. Stop or slow down if you feel out of breath. If you experience dizziness, faintness, nausea, or pain with exercise (especially pain in the chest, neck, arm, or jaw), stop exercising and seek medical advice.

- Choose low- to moderate-intensity physical activities to start. You are not likely to harm yourself by starting slowly and working up to walking twenty to thirty minutes per day. And remember, moderate-intensity activity has been shown to be great for weight loss—there is little advantage to pushing yourself harder, and there may well be some risks.

- Try pool exercises like water aerobics or swimming laps. Working out in water burns calories without putting much stress on your joints—perfect if you have arthritis or other types of joint pain.

- Work with a qualified coach or a certified personal trainer, either on your own or in a class, especially when you are starting out, to make sure you're exercising with proper form to avoid injury. The American College of Sports Medicine is an excellent source for information on physical fitness and appropriate qualifications for personal trainers.

Build the Skill

- Find a physical activity that you really enjoy, take your time to get used to it, and chances are that you will get comfortable and feel more skilled as time goes on. There are so many options—from recreational activities like dancing and playing golf or tennis to more formal types of exercise like running and group exercise classes.

- Check out your local recreation or community center, YMCA, hospital wellness center, or any place that offers fun activities to try. These centers may cost less than other gyms or health clubs.

FITNESS THAT FITS YOU

Ready to get started? By now, you know that we don't expect you to zoom from zero to sixty in the blink of an eye. Some of you may be regular exercisers, others may be occasional "weekend warriors," and some of you may not have exercised in years, or perhaps very little in your whole lives. Wherever you fall on the fitness spectrum, it's fine. We will meet you where you are.

We have designated three entry points—call them *levels*—for the Duke Diet Exercise Plan. We will help you determine your personal fitness level and then give you a complete workout program, including the types of exercises you should do, how often to do them, how hard you should work, and for how long. No matter where you begin, you're going to see improvements, possibly in as little as a week or two. We will show you how to progress from one level to the next, so that you continue to challenge your body in order to lose weight and keep it off. You can also get a personalized fitness plan with many additional workouts and videos demonstrating each exercise on www.dukediet.com.

While we recommend working up to forty-five to sixty minutes of physical activity a day, there is some evidence to suggest that your ultimate activity goal for weight loss—especially lasting weight loss—should be sixty to seventy-five minutes a day of moderate-intensity activity such as brisk walking or thirty minutes a day of vigorous activity such as aerobics, cycling, or jogging, on most days of the week. Remember that you don't need to work at this level right now. Even down the road, it isn't likely you will need to block out a full, daily sixty- to seventy-five-minute period for exercise. Remember, if you work toward being more active in the wide variety of ways we have shown you here and build several short activity sessions into your day, you will rapidly accrue minutes and hardly miss the time. At Duke, we always stress that moving more is the ultimate goal—one step at a time.

Many of our clients could not even imagine working out at all when they came to us, but after taking it a step at a time, they now consider themselves exercisers. So don't get hung up on the numbers—just focus on progress!

Whatever your fitness level, remember that exercise is easier if it is fun (or at least not unenjoyable). Plan your program around activities you find appealing. Ask yourself, "Would I rather work out alone, with a close friend, or in a large group? Would I prefer to be outside on a sunny day or in the focused atmosphere of a dance studio or a weight room? Is competition what really gets my blood going? Am I a morning person, or would I rather work off my stress at the end of the day?"—and so on. The answers to these questions are all good clues as to which types of activities and support you need. We will talk more about building your support network in chapter 4.

Before answering the following questions, review the "Health Conditions and Exercise" box to see if you need to get clearance from your doctor before embarking on a fitness plan. Then read over the following exercise-level profiles and decide which one best fits you.

Health Conditions and Exercise

Common sense is your best guide when you answer these questions. Please read them carefully and answer each one honestly, yes or no.

1. Has your doctor ever said that you have a heart condition and that you should be careful about exertion?
2. Do you get pain in your chest when you exercise?
3. In the past month, have you had chest pain when you were at rest?
4. Do you lose your balance, get dizzy, or lose consciousness?
5. Were you ever told that you have a bone or joint problem that exercise could make worse?
6. Are you currently taking medication for your blood pressure or a heart condition?
7. Do you know of any other reason why you should not exercise?

If you said yes to any of these questions, consult your doctor before starting on any fitness plan.

Fitness Prep Level

- Your personal slogan is "Why walk when we have cars?" and your most frequently asked question is "Do you deliver?"
- You have become or perhaps have always been inactive.
- You spend most of your day sitting—in the car, at your desk, at the computer, on the couch.
- You tend to avoid ordinary activities that demand some exertion, like stretching for items on high shelves or walking to the bus stop.
- You can't really walk very far—say, at the mall—without having to sit down at intervals to rest.
- You get winded (short of breath) easily and do your best to avoid going up and down stairs.
- You're probably very out of shape, or deconditioned, to use the technical term.

Our Recommendation for Fitness Prep Level Exercisers

Take it slow! For now, don't worry about strength training, although you may want to try a beginners' class in yoga, tai chi, or shallow-water aerobics. Focus on working toward getting your 10,000 steps from ADLs or comfortably paced walking each day. That's the number many experts recommend for good health. It helps to wear a pedometer, a device that counts your steps automatically, available at any sporting goods store.

For many people, it takes only a couple of weeks to feel at ease with the goal of 10,000 steps. In fact, once you are getting around 8,000 to 10,000 steps nearly every day for a week or two, and doing so at a comfortable pace, then go ahead and give Level 1 a try. Once you get comfortable with the new additions to your fitness routine in Level 1, you can keep working on increasing your number of steps and keeping them steady at 10,000 per day.

Level 1

- You're not a professional couch potato, but you have your moments (or days or weeks).
- In the past year, you've undertaken some form of *moderately intense*

aerobic exercise, meaning twenty-minute or longer stretches of *continuous activity* that makes *you sweat and breathe a little harder,* one to four times per week.

- You do not currently participate in any form of strength training.

Our Recommendation for Level 1 Exercisers

You have a nice base to build on. Try to increase the duration and/or intensity of the exercise you are already doing, especially if it's one you like. For each week of the core program, we'll give you cardio, strength training, and stretching workouts, tailored to Level 1. Keep aiming for 10,000 steps total from ADLs and walking, but try to include some cardio activities that are of slightly higher intensity to challenge yourself.

- **Cardio.** If you're not already walking briskly or doing other aerobic exercise (like swimming, cycling, or playing tennis) for thirty minutes three times a week, start and build from there. Exercising for a longer period of time may mean that you slow your pace, so that your session is less intense. As you begin the Level 1 workout, we're going to encourage you to try to bring your pace to a solid moderate-intensity level before you add more minutes.

  Keep in mind that "moderate intensity" is a moving target that spans low-moderate and high-moderate levels. One good way to check your intensity level is the talk test. If you're working at moderate intensity, you should be able to carry on a conversation while exercising. If you can not only talk but sing, your intensity level is too low; if you're too winded to talk comfortably (for example, you need to gasp for breath with every word), your intensity level is too high. If you can say a short phrase of several words comfortably—that's the target!

  At Duke, the primary yardstick we use to gauge workout intensity is the Rating of Perceived Exertion, or RPE, which was developed by Swedish psychologist Gunnar Borg and is also favored by such institutions as the American College of Sports Medicine. It is a subjective measure that records, literally, just how difficult or easy you perceive a given exercise to be.

How to Measure the Intensity of Exercise

We recommend that you use the following scale to gauge the intensity of your workout. We encourage you to aim for the moderate-intensity level, which lies in the shaded area between 11 and 14 on the RPE scale.

Rating of Perceived Exertion Scale

6   No exertion at all

7

   Extremely light (7.5)

8

9   Very light

10

11   Light

12

13   Somewhat hard

14

15   Hard (heavy)

16

17   Very hard

18

19   Extremely hard

20   Maximal exertion

How to interpret:

9 corresponds to *very light* exercise. For a healthy person, this is like walking slowly at your own pace for some minutes.

13 on the scale is *somewhat hard* exercise, but it still feels okay to continue.

17, *very hard,* is very strenuous. If you are a healthy person, you can continue, but you are very tired and really have to push yourself.

19 on the scale is *extremely strenuous.* For most people this is the most strenuous exercise they have ever experienced.

The value of the RPE is that it helps you focus on how you feel as you exercise. The intensity level you should strive for is one that makes you feel good but still challenged. If you're going a little light on yourself, you can visualize the RPE and pick up the pace. But it's just as critical to recognize when you're really knocking yourself out. For one thing, your body can handle only so much, and for another, if you overdo it, you'll be far less likely to work out again soon. We're intelligent beings, which means that we (or at least, most of us) know better than to repeatedly subject ourselves to pain.

Overdoing it is especially tempting when you're beginning a new fitness program. You get all gung ho and eager to test your mettle. Resist! The key is to find an intensity range where you feel comfortable (while not slacking off) and stay within it. If you stay in your mid-moderate zone (11 to 14 on the RPE scale), you'll exercise longer and not be too sore and miserable to fulfill your weekly goals. Moderate-intensity exercise can provide the same benefit as more intense exercise for weight loss, and probably close to the same benefits for overall health.

With many exercises, you might experience some discomfort that's tolerable. However, there is a big difference between discomfort and pain. We can all handle discomfort; we can't handle pain as well. If you are experiencing significant or persistent pain, stop immediately and talk to your health care professional.

• **Strength.** Another important aspect of the Level 1 workout plan is strength training. Try to add two sessions a week to your schedule, but not on back-to-back days because your muscles need time to recover. The key here is efficiency—just get your strength training done and get going. If you belong to a gym, you'll probably see people sitting on weight machines, reading the paper while they rest between sets. Bad idea! Not only does that work against maintaining a reasonably intense workout, but it makes strength training seem onerous and time consuming—and if you feel that way about it, you'll be disinclined to keep it up.

You don't have to join a gym to get the benefits of strength training. Chapter 10 of this book and www.dukediet.com will give you exercises that you can easily do at home. All you'll need is a sturdy chair, some dumbbells and exercise tubing, and a few other inexpensive tools that you can find in any sporting goods store or purchase at www.dukediet.com.

- **Flexibility.** We'll give you a series of stretches to end your workout.

Level 2

- You've got a rhythm going, more or less.
- In the past year, you've done some form of aerobic exercise—meaning twenty minutes or more of continuous, perspiration-promoting activity five or more times per week.
- You also do some form of strength training, on at least a semiregular basis.
- You're ready to enliven your routine with some new, interesting twists. Good for you!

Our Recommendation for Level 2 Exercisers

If you are exercising at Level 2, we're guessing that you recognize how good working out can make you feel. You probably also have a sense of the kind of exercises you like. Keep doing those, of course, but perhaps think about throwing a few new ones into the mix, just to keep yourself interested. You'll find plenty of suggestions in this book and even more on www.dukediet.com.

- **Cardio.** As you begin Level 2, keep up those ADLs and aim for those 10,000 steps. Increase the duration of your aerobic exercise sessions to forty-five to sixty minutes a day five days a week. You might want to cross train, which simply means incorporating different types of aerobic activities to keep your weekly program fresh. You might go cycling or swimming one day, take an aerobic dance class the next, and on the third, simply walk briskly (aiming for that moderate-intensity RPE of 11 to 14).

- **Strength.** Up your sessions to three per week, on nonconsecutive days. Here, too, you should try new things—say, the free weights, if you've been working on the machines in the gym, or vice versa, just to mix things up.

- **Flexibility.** We'll give you a new series of stretches to end your workout. Whatever your fitness level, you can benefit by working yoga, tai chi, or Pilates into your weekly routine. These practices will help you develop a strong, flexible body that will power you through your life—whether you're a homemaker chasing energetic little ones, a weekend dancer, or a sports enthusiast. You will be ready for anything!

GIVE YOURSELF CREDIT

We know from our clients that being overweight can make even the thought of exercise seem overwhelming, but take heart. We have seen so many dramatic breakthroughs when it comes to getting more active that we know that it's possible for you to achieve one, too! So give the fitness program a try, and remember these watchwords: *Progress, not perfection.* All we ask is that you try, every day, to include at least a little more physical activity in your life.

CHAPTER FOUR

The Duke Diet Behavioral Plan: How You Will Change

Losing weight and keeping it off for life involves more than just calorie consciousness and regular exercise. Lasting change comes with examining and altering habits of mind and behavior that prompt us to overeat in the first place. That's why behavioral health is such an integral part of the Duke Diet & Fitness Center program. We help you focus on you as a whole person and how you interact with the world you live in. We help you consider your personal experiences and how they influence weight control and health as well as the social influences in your life. We want you to be able to understand and change the long-standing behavior, thought, and emotional patterns that may influence your ability to control your weight.

For many, unhealthy habits such as overeating or underexercising develop over a lifetime and are likely the result of a combination of factors, including an environment where food is abundant and it's hard to be active. We will show you new and healthier ways to deal with each of these challenges to weight control and help you improve your relationship with food and exercise, thereby enhancing your quality of life. Your good health and overall well-being are the ultimate goals of the Duke Plan.

The Business of Life

One of my first patients at the Duke Diet & Fitness Center was Mark, a successful businessman who had a long history of losing and regaining large amounts of weight. He had tried plenty of diets and was already well versed in many of the behavioral strategies we use at Duke. At first, it seemed there wasn't a lot that I could teach him, but then I got an idea. I asked him, "So, what haven't you done yet?"

He thought for a moment and then replied. "I've never written out a comprehensive, long-term plan."

For years, I'd been telling patients that setting an agenda for lifestyle change was very much like developing a business plan. But in talking to Mark, I realized that the idea was more than a metaphor—that it would really help patients if we mapped out behavioral health strategies, just as a business planner would chart a company's course for its fiscal year. We could show them how to set a range of goals from worst case to best case, help them anticipate obstacles that might keep them from reaching those goals, offer them action plans to overcome obstacles, suggest correctives to get them back on track when they weren't hitting their targets, and more. Thus, the Duke behavioral health goal-setting and action-planning curriculum was born—thanks to one stuck patient!

—*Martin Binks, Ph.D.*

We will start this journey by looking at the core areas of a healthy and balanced life that we call the Pillars of Lifestyle Change.

THE PILLARS OF LIFESTYLE CHANGE

We're all wound so tightly into the fabric of our own lives that at first it can seem hard to tease out the patterns that interfere with our health goals. To simplify the process, we help clients review their lives systematically, in terms of six key areas we call *pillars*: environment, stress management, body image and self-image, professional life and social life, emotional well-being, and support system. Few, if any, of us exist in such perfect harmony and balance that all of our pillars are equally sound. In addition, our lives shift constantly and, at different times, make one pillar or another stronger or less strong in relation to the next. We teach patients to periodically rate the strength of their pillars to highlight the areas of their lives that most need attention at that given time. This provides a useful structure to help you set goals that are about more than just eating a certain way or exercising a certain amount— goals that help you achieve a balanced and healthy lifestyle.

We will look briefly at each of these pillars, tell you what each one means, then ask you to rate them on a scale of 1 to 10 (a 1 means that this pillar is in need of significant attention, and a 10 indicates a pillar that is relatively strong). To help you start thinking, we'll ask you a few key questions for each pillar, or if you prefer, you can log on to www.dukediet.com, where we provide a self-assessment tool for the pillars.

If you rate any pillar below a 5, or if any pillar is much lower than the others, we suggest you focus your attention there to start. We will offer you strategies for strengthening the pillars throughout this book, as well as on our website, and we encourage you to brainstorm some fresh approaches of your own.

As you begin to work with the pillars, keep in mind that the goals you set should be realistic: Work on making incremental changes, taking small steps to strengthen areas that need it. Rather than trying to turn a 1 into a 10 right away, try to improve each pillar by just one point. You will be amazed at how quickly the smaller goals you've reached will add up to significant progress. Let's look at each pillar.

Environment

Do your physical surroundings promote health and self-care? If you're trying to lose weight while living in a gingerbread house with icing on the roof, the answer is no! Joking aside, you should ask yourself whether you keep your cupboards stocked with chips and cookies that never stop "speaking to you"; if it's really necessary to park near the doughnut shop or, when dining out, to get your meal from the all-you-can-eat buffet rather than ordering a finite meal from the menu; and if it's wise to have a bag of candy on hand "in case friends come over," which you end up nibbling while you watch TV. Is your gym halfway across town or right next door to your office, and do you have exercise equipment at home for the days when you just don't feel like heading out to aerobics class? Many aspects of your environment are within your control. When you set the stage to support good choices, you are more likely to make those choices.

Tips for Strengthening Your Environment Pillar

Start eliminating tempting but unhealthy foods from your cupboards. Purchase some new culinary tools that will inspire you to prepare healthy meals. You'll find a wealth of recipes in chapter 9 of this book and many more on www.dukediet.com. If dining out is your downfall, try to eat in more frequently or choose more health-friendly restaurants (in chapter 7 of this book and on the website you will also find helpful strategies for dining out).

Do you have to work hard to avoid temptations in your office, such as the doughnuts by the coffee machine? Perhaps you could find somewhere else to take a break, or you could bring your own coffee in a Thermos and your own healthy snack and avoid that area altogether. To make exercise easier, you could join a gym close to your home or office and also make sure you have equipment and exercise videos at home so you don't have to leave the house to work out. These are just a few ways to start improving your environment. Stay tuned for more as you go through the weekly program!

Stress Management

Short-term stress, in small doses, is what makes life interesting. It can motivate us to succeed, and it's a lifesaver when it mobilizes us to take fast action in an emergency or in threatening situations. However, in our modern, fast-paced society, most of us endure a constant and, at times, harmful level of stress. Our world and our schedules seem so demanding that our bodies and minds are sometimes overwhelmed and overtaxed. With cell phones, handheld devices, and e-mail, our time is rarely our own, and because of this technology we're expected to be more productive than ever before.

Gone are the days of the leisurely *Leave It to Beaver* American lifestyle. We work all day and well into the evening, and on weekends, too. What little free time we have, we tend to schedule beyond reason. Even our kids have demands on their time that were inconceivable to most people just a generation ago.

Chronic stress can have serious physical and emotional fallout. Without good mechanisms in place to manage it, many of us resort to unhealthy coping strategies, including overeating and skipping exercise. If you can both reduce your sources of stress and develop better skills for unloading stress, you will improve your chances for achieving balance in your life.

Tips for Strengthening Your Stress Management Pillar

Change your thinking: To disrupt the cycle of stress and reduce its impact, consider readjusting your thinking about it. Sometimes it's the way we view or approach stressful situations that makes them more stressful than they have to be. For example, if you have a tight deadline at work, rather than focus on the pressure and how impossible the task seems, think about what you *can* do.

Take positive action: Find one small section that looks easy to handle and start there. Even if it means simply organizing your paperwork or making a list of what you need to do, every small step helps to reduce the pressure and may lead you to accomplishing more.

Set limits: As much as you might try, no one can do *everything*! Identifying the stressors in your life and deciding which ones you could reduce or eliminate altogether is an effective stress-busting strategy. For example, if you have difficulty saying no, you might set yourself the goal of turning down at least one nonessential request per week. The church bake sale will still go on if you don't volunteer when you are already overcommitted.

Obviously there are things we can't say no to, but think about whether you can delegate at least some of those duties. If you spend all day Saturday chauffeuring your kids, maybe you could create a carpool with other parents so each of you can make fewer trips, or try sharing share the load with your spouse or significant other. The section on effective communication later in this chapter can help you learn to articulate your needs and set appropriate boundaries, which can go a long way toward reducing stress.

Learn to unload stress. You have already seen that exercise and mind-body practices like yoga and tai chi can be very helpful in reducing stress. Relaxation techniques such as deep breathing exercises, progressive muscle relaxation, and meditation are also useful. See chapter 8 for more information on unloading stress, and visit www.dukediet.com, where you can purchase a relaxation CD featuring members of the Duke Diet & Fitness Center's behavioral health staff.

Body Image and Self-Image

When you struggle to control your weight—and perhaps you have been doing so for a long time—the number on the scale and your belt or dress size can take on too broad a meaning in your life and start to define who you are.

Judging yourself very critically in relation to your weight can sap your self-esteem and have a negative impact on the quality of your life. For example, we see so many clients who decide that they have to postpone realizing certain dreams—taking a special trip, finding a soul mate, or pushing for a new job or a promotion—until they get to some ideal weight. Yes, a healthy weight is something, but it's not *everything*. Dr. Eisenson notes sadly that some of our patients are so focused on weight it can seem as if they only want to be remembered for being thin. Surely, a good life is measured by things other than weight!

To get started assessing this pillar, ask yourself a few questions: *Do I say a lot of negative things about myself or my appearance? Do I postpone or avoid doing things out of fear of not being good enough or of being judged? Do I have trouble accepting compliments, whether about my appearance or more generally?*

Tips for Strengthening Your Body Image and Self-Image Pillar

If you rate this pillar as low, you may struggle with a self-critical voice. This negative dialogue can come from many sources. Perhaps there have been important people in your life whose criticisms influenced how you view yourself. Or perhaps you've succumbed to the media bombardment of messages that suggest that thin is the only acceptable body type. Wherever that critical voice came from, you have the power to change it—the power to reconsider and reinvent the standards by which you judge yourself. Positive self-talk techniques like those outlined in the "Changing Destructive Thinking" section in chapter 11 can help you counteract that critical voice and adopt a healthier self-perception.

Another great exercise is to look in the mirror and pick out something you like about what you see (good hair, good skin, a winning smile—we all have good qualities). Think about your accomplishments, too. Are you well read? A mainstay of a community group? A devoted and beloved friend, parent, child, aunt, or uncle? A loving spouse? Do you have a great sense of humor?

Practice appreciating *all* of your good qualities. They mean a lot! It may feel a little awkward at first to praise yourself, but if you do, in time the critical voice can give way to a more realistic and accepting one. These are just some steps to get you started. Of course, the support of mental health professionals can also be very helpful for many people who struggle with these issues.

Professional Life and Social Life

Whether it's raising kids and running a household, working outdoors, or toiling away in a store or office, work consumes the lion's share of our time. Our professional life influences our health and overall well-being on many levels. At the surface there are the day-to-day interactions with coworkers, customers, and, of course, your boss. Taking stock of these interactions and how they might be improved is an important part of this pillar. For example, the coworker with the candy bowl on her desk, the friend who asks you out for happy hour (during your usual workout time), the possibly well-meaning but hurtful friend who tracks everything you eat—all these people influence your weight control efforts. In addition, our work lives are a part of our overall identity, and the satisfaction we get from our jobs is an important part of a balanced lifestyle. Are you doing work that you consider meaningful, that stimulates you, or that utilizes your talents and abilities? Do you take pride in your work accomplishments? Do you get the recognition you deserve or the satisfaction you need? It is important when rating this pillar to consider both of these elements of your work or professional life.

Your social life is similar to your professional life in having components that skim the surface but also reach deeper. Do you have meaningful social interactions? What do you do for fun? Are your interests broad and varied? Do you enjoy seeking new and exciting experiences—or are you reluctant to do so for lack of time or, perhaps, fear of the unknown? Have you become stuck in the habit of socializing around food? Throughout this program, we encourage you to seek a wide range of social and recreational experiences.

Tips for Strengthening Your Professional Life and Social Life Pillar

How satisfied are you with your professional and social life? Do your office-mates represent a particular challenge or are they potential sources of strength? Do you have trouble communicating your needs or coping with confrontation, either at work or with friends?

For example, if your boss chews you out for not having something done yesterday, can you reasonably explain the delay, without defensiveness, and negotiate a new deadline? Do you need to speak with your boss about setting aside some time for yourself? Do you need to negotiate for a promotion? When a friend asks you out, are you comfortable suggesting that it might be better to meet at a museum or a movie than to go out for dinner or drinks? Effective communication provides a healthy foundation for getting your needs met in all interpersonal relationships and is an excellent tool for creating a healthy professional and social life.

Perhaps this pillar presents a larger challenge for you than simply improving your interpersonal skills. Maybe you feel that you need a major shift in your focus, either in terms of your career or the overall focus of your life. It is very important to know that there are many resources out there to help people explore new directions and make meaningful shifts in their lives. The behavioral health staff at the Duke Diet & Fitness Center often work with people to help them expand their horizons and find new direction in their lives. While we can't address these issues fully in this book, we encourage you to seek the support of career counselors, therapists, and other qualified professionals in the community if you wish. Remember, a healthy lifestyle is about more than diet and exercise!

Emotional Well-Being

When we're coping with uncomfortable emotions of any kind, like anger, sadness, or insecurity, or even when we are experiencing positive emotions, many of us reach for our favorite foods (which are, all too often, not the healthiest choices) to either comfort or celebrate. It's likely that we started developing this habit very early in life, when our parent(s) realized that the best response to crying or fussing was to pop something into our mouths and that ice cream made a very welcome reward. Eating just feels so good that almost

Effective Communication

As you can see, many of the adjustments you'll want to make in your six Pillars of Lifestyle Change will come through communicating your needs effectively to others. Here are some tips on how to do it:

- **Practice active listening.** Silently hear out the other person and try to understand the feelings underlying his or her words. Don't merely appear to be listening while you're really formulating your response—really listen! Reflect quietly for a moment before responding, so the other person feels acknowledged.
- **Build a bridge.** Demonstrate that you understand what the other person has just said by paraphrasing the content. You could start by saying say something like, "If I understand you correctly" or "It sounds like you are saying..." This is the beginning of the bridge.

  It can be hard to build a bridge in a heated conversation, when all you want to do is defend yourself or fight back, but it's worth it. Bridge building can diffuse tension and move an argument to a constructive plane. It is often helpful to acknowledge the emotion behind the other person's statement. For example, if your boss said, "You really blew that presentation," you'd be tempted to get defensive and try to convince him or her that your approach was the right one. But it would be better to bite your tongue and offer a bridge-building response like "I know you are not pleased with the way I handled the presentation. I hope it didn't leave you in a bind."
- **Cross the bridge.** Once you've built a bridge, you can cross it by respectfully stating your thoughts and feelings about the situation. You can use personal language like "I think...," "I feel...," or "I'm upset too, but I need you to...." Or you can use more general terms like "It seems that...." Avoid making absolute, defensive, or accusatory statements that can easily be argued with or denied. Using the presentation example, you might say, "I'm upset about how the presentation went, too. I'd like to share my thinking with you, though, if this is a good time."
- **Make requests and set limits.** After you've engaged in a constructive conversation with the other person, suggest measures that will lead to resolution. In the discussion about the presentation, you could add, "What can I do to resolve the bind you're in?"

  To use a more personal example, let's say you're out to dinner with your spouse and he or she scolds, "How can you order dessert? What about your diet?" You could angrily insist that your spouse mind his or her own business, but it would be more effective to build a bridge by acknowledging that the reprimand might be well meant. You could start by saying, "I know that you're trying to help me" (the bridge), and then cross the bridge by calmly articulating your feelings, "but when you criticize my food choices in public, I feel embarrassed." Clinch the exchange by making your request or setting your limit: "I'd prefer that you discuss your feelings with me when we're alone."

You can find more information about effective communication on our website, www .dukediet.com.

everyone, at one time or another, looks to food not just to allay hunger but also for any number of emotional reasons.

We approach this pillar in two ways. First, look at your overall emotional well-being. Ask yourself: "Am I often sad or down, anxious or worried, or do I find it difficult to manage my emotions?" If the answer is yes, then we strongly recommend that you speak to your doctor or seek guidance from a mental health professional. Then ask yourself how you cope with your emotions: "Do I often eat when I am upset, bored, lonely, or distressed? Do I find that food is often the most important part of a celebration—as opposed to the event itself?" If so, the following tips and other strategies in this book will help you start to control emotional eating.

Tips for Strengthening Your Emotional Well-Being Pillar

If your score for this pillar is low, you're not alone! We all find it challenging, from time to time, to cope with uncomfortable emotions, which often arise

Notes of a Former Feeling Stuffer

Until I got to Duke, I didn't really make the connection between overeating and negative emotions. I often felt that my family was "nowhere" when I needed their support, and knew that this feeling always sent me straight to the refrigerator. But what I didn't recognize were the emotions that their dismissive attitude aroused in me. Working with the Duke staff, I came to see that, when people acted like I didn't matter, I felt powerless and I got angry. Since I didn't know how to stick up for myself, I turned to food to cope.

The communication skills training I received has made a big difference. Now I ask for what I need in an effective way, so I'm more likely to get it and feel much less powerless. And instead of denying my anger and smothering it with food, I acknowledge it and accept the fact that negative emotions are just a part of life. What we have to do is manage them, and now I can, in healthier ways.

—*Gail, age 54*

when we're frustrated in our efforts to get what we truly need from others. Understanding your emotional needs and how to get them met is a core skill we teach at the Duke Diet & Fitness Center.

Time after time, our patients report that learning to reconnect with and embrace their emotions, rather than running to food to help stuff feelings down, is a life-changing experience. Of course, emotions are part of what makes the human experience unique and fulfilling. Using the Emotional

Emotional Awareness Exercise

When you're experiencing an uncomfortable emotion, try these steps, which can help you understand where the feelings are coming from, and how to manage them.

1. **Connect with the emotion.**
   • Take a deep breath, close your eyes, and continue to breathe comfortably and fully with nice, gentle, full breaths.
   • Focus on your bodily sensations. Recognize how your body feels "in the moment" without judging or interpreting. Notice how your chest rises with each breath and how the air flows through your nose and into your lungs.
2. **Observe the emotion.**
   • Ask yourself, "What am I sensing? What am I feeling? What am I *thinking?*" Resist the urge to figure out *why* you are feeling a certain way—just experience the emotion.
3. **Evaluate the emotion.**
   • Practice recognizing your true needs. Perhaps you are bored? Then your need might be for activity. However, if you are lonely, the answer may be quite different— activity involving friends or at least other people. Now ask yourself, "What do I need right now? What is missing?"
4. **Choose an action.**
   • Understand that there is no right or wrong here—individual needs vary. We'll offer some ideas, but the best actions are the ones you come up with yourself—the ones that meet your needs in the moment. For example, you may need to:
   Express the feeling in private (cry, write in your journal, etc.).
   Release the feeling through action. For example, you might find release through movement, such as taking a walk or dancing.
   Use relaxation techniques like deep breathing or meditation.
   Express the feeling to others you trust and seek their support.

Awareness Exercise on page 91, you can begin to find new ways to experience your emotions—even the negative ones. It can make a big difference.

Support System

A strong support system is an important element in weight control and long-term success. The word *support* connotes something different to each of us. Some of us thrive on praise and recognition for our efforts, while others prefer not to have attention focused on our progress when we're trying to lose weight. Some find that sharing meals with others helps them keep a grip on what they eat; others may feel judged by their dining companions or resent seeing them freely enjoy the foods that they're trying to limit.

We want to help you recognize what is or is not supportive for you and show you how to get the help you need from your support squad. Your potential sources of support include your family and friends, a church or other faith-based organization, community groups or clubs, self-help groups, fitness clubs, and professionals such as dietitians, personal trainers, and health care providers. And don't forget the new allies you can find online on the message boards of www.dukediet.com.

When you assess your support system pillar, there are two important questions to ask yourself: "How many supporters do I currently have? and "How helpful are they?" It is important to really think about both of these factors when rating this pillar. Despite the fact that your supporters are well-meaning, some of them may not be very good at meeting your needs.

Tips for Strengthening Your Support System Pillar

Many of our more successful clients tell us that good support systems are essential. So as you begin the core program, it will be important for you to rally the troops around you. Who will be your staunchest allies? Your spouse or partner? Your best friend? Friends at your community center or a trainer at your health club? Or maybe the virtual army of support troops who are experiencing the same challenges and changes that you are, whom you can meet at www.dukediet.com.

It's important to consider this question carefully. Some people who may be very supportive in other areas may not be the right ones for weight loss. Many people don't understand the complexity of the weight loss process and

Network for Success

The better you are at rallying your troops, the more likely you are to achieve lasting change. That's been our experience in working with clients at the Duke Diet & Fitness Center. The people in your life may all have different kinds of support to offer. Consider the types of support listed here, and for each one, write down the name of someone in your life who might be a good choice.

1. **Listening and guiding** (someone who can lend a supportive ear and when appropriate give you advice without being judgmental):

2. **Sharing experience** (a like-minded person with experiences similar to yours):

3. **Practical help** (people who make it easier for you to succeed, for example, a spouse who helps out with extra chores or a grandparent who watches the kids while you go to the gym):

4. **Partnering** (buddies who might exercise or diet with you):

5. **Motivating** (cheerleaders, people who will encourage and inspire you and help you maintain your focus):

6. **Emotional help** (someone who knows you, understands you, and has your physical and emotional well-being at heart):

7. **Technical help** (people with expertise such as a personal trainer, dietitian, or health care provider):

When you approach your support team, try to keep your requests for help as specific as possible. Instead of saying, "I need your support while I'm dieting," ask, "Could you commit to watching the kids for an hour on Tuesday and Thursday nights so I can take an exercise class?" Or "Do you think we could try eating out less than twice a week? Maybe it would be fun to try cooking together." People often want very much to be helpful, but it is not clear how—they may need you to tell them.

can be unhelpful despite their best intentions. There are the self-proclaimed weight loss gurus, always ready to offer unsolicited advice like "I lost ten pounds by cutting carbs and didn't exercise one bit." (But how long will they keep those pounds off? And is dieting without exercise really a path to optimal health?) There are sympathizers who believe that dieting is all about painful deprivation and feel sorry for you. "Here," they say, "you've had a rough day. You deserve a piece of this pie, and a little ice cream on top couldn't hurt."

Needless to say, these folks are not helpful, but how do we let them know? We see many patients who have trouble asking for the right kind of support because they're embarrassed, because they feel that it's weak to reach out to others, or even because they don't feel entitled to receive help. Some believe that their loved ones should be automatically supportive—but what people don't always realize is that perhaps these folks just don't know how yet. We've created a tool for you, a letter that you can use as a guide in developing a letter of your own to present to your supporters. Following is a model, and you will find a downloadable version that you can customize on www.dukediet.com.

Letter to Supporters

Dear Supporter,

I am currently participating in the Duke Diet & Fitness Center program for weight loss. This program is a comprehensive approach to weight loss that focuses on nutrition, fitness, behavioral health, and medical information. The Duke program has been helping me learn how to eat healthfully, maintain a proper exercise regimen, and make other healthy choices for my overall well-being.

I have learned that, in addition to my own commitment, I need support from others, like you. My work with the Duke program has taught me that "support" may be broadly defined as "the respectful demonstration of caring and concern for another person."

Support can take a variety of forms, and what is supportive for one individual may not necessarily be so for another. For example, some individuals find praise, approval, and recognition for their accomplishments to be extremely motivating, whereas others prefer not to have their weight management efforts be a focus of attention.

I know it may be difficult for family and friends to fully comprehend what kind of support I need now. We will talk about that along the way, but I hope with this letter I will be able to give you a better understanding of the types of things that tend not to be helpful to people trying to lose weight, so we can spend our time focusing on the positive and strategizing together about the ways you can help me succeed in following my plan.

Here are some things that tend to be less helpful:

- **Freely offering unsolicited advice.** Unsolicited advice can, in fact, make me feel bad about myself and lower my self-esteem. Duke has taught me what I need to know, and receiving unsolicited advice can be confusing, especially if it does not match what I have learned. I know what to do to be successful, and it will be difficult to maintain my focus in the face of unwanted advice from others.
- **Having other people monitor my eating and exercise.** I know it is often done out of concern for me and a desire to see me succeed, but like most people, I tend to rebel against attempts to be controlled. I am afraid that your tracking my eating and exercise habits will backfire and lead to more eating and less exercise.
- **Equating my weight loss plan with deprivation.** I will be making my own educated choices. I do not need to be on a deprivation diet in order to succeed. In fact, I have learned that many successful people plan to eat their favorite higher-calorie foods on occasion as part of their overall healthy meal plan. There are no off-limits or bad foods in the Duke plan.
- **Pointing out past failures.** I realize you may have watched me start many plans in the past, only to slip up and regain the weight I lost, but it is not useful to be reminded of this, and it is worse yet to hear skepticism about the likelihood of my long-term success or my ability to recover from setbacks. This plan, unlike many others, has taught me how to deal with setbacks and get right back on track.

Please keep in mind that weight loss is a complicated process and is usually slow and irregular. You may feel that your questions about my weight or my progress are supportive, but they may be perceived as pressure or criticism and result in my feeling frustrated. The scale is not the only measure of progress, and I may prefer not to report the details of my weight loss for a variety of reasons. I ask that you simply encourage me when I share my successes with you, and know that I am taking care of my program—whether I am experiencing successes or setbacks.

I value your support, and I hope that you will try to do the best you can to help me. I appreciate your efforts. I'd be happy to talk to you about ways that you can help encourage me. I know I can make a success of my program with your help! Let's both work to keep the lines of communication open.

Yours in health,

WORKING WITH THE PILLARS

Life is always changing. Job demands shift, family situations come and go, and our needs change as a result. Maybe *you* change and your needs change right along with you. That is why reexamining your pillars, perhaps once a month, can help you see where you are and what you need to address to stay on track. Remember, adjustments don't have to be huge. As we explained before, the goal is to improve one point at a time—not go from a 1 to a 10 all at once! Your slogan is "Progress, not perfection." So set some goals and put the pillars to work for you!

GOALS AND ACTION PLANS FOR LASTING SUCCESS

This chapter is our last stop before we embark on the core four-week program, so it's time to start thinking about goals. Perhaps that means reaching your target weight, getting your blood pressure and cholesterol under control, or becoming more active. You may have some benchmarks along the way, such as dropping at least two dress sizes before your next birthday or getting into a new bathing suit by the Fourth of July.

But the goals we'd like to focus on now are the smaller, specific ones that you want to hit each day or each week. This is a cornerstone of the lifestyle-change approach. Success is an abstract concept unless you're shooting for targets that are attainable, measurable, and concrete. We will help you set your own personal goals in chapter 5, but here's an overview.

We want to work with you to set three levels of goals:

• **Optimal goal.** Your next-step goal, this is the goal you set to remind you that you want to keep moving ahead. It represents more than what you can do right now but is achievable in the near future. For example, you might want to make exercising five days a week for forty minutes each day an optimal goal.

• **Desirable goal.** This is your most-of-the-time goal, or the goal that you feel you can achieve 90 percent of the time, given your current circumstances. For instance, based on your level of conditioning, the time you spend at work, and the time you devote to your family, as well as your available free time, you might decide that your most-of-the-time goal should be to exercise five days a week for, say, twenty minutes. Then, as you get comfortable here, perhaps after a few weeks, you can set your sights on reaching your optimal goal. Eventually, your optimal goal becomes your desirable goal, and you can set a new optimal goal. Can you start to see how the system works to keep you progressing?

• **Minimal goal.** This is the backup plan, the goal you'll aim for when "life gets in the way"—for example, when unexpected houseguests show up, when the kids get sick, or when you get stuck on a big work project. This is not an ideal goal, but it is a good one to keep you on track in the short term until things return to normal and you can resume shooting for your desirable goal. An example might be exercising for twenty minutes three days a week.

By setting a backup, or minimal, goal, you'll stay on track and avoid the sense of failure people often tell us they feel when they can't quite hit their desirable one. You know that unexpected things come up, so you need to have a plan for dealing with them. The key is having a clear endpoint (for example, if the minimal goal occurs too frequently) and a specific plan to get back to the desirable goal as soon as possible. We will work through some examples of action plans shortly.

You'll notice that, in these examples, we've made our targets very specific. Rather than saying, "I'll add some yoga," we talk in terms of number of days exercised and actual minutes expended. Effective goal setting requires that we be very specific. We like to use the acronym SMART, which comes from business-speak, in defining goals.

• **Specific,** meaning that there can be no doubt about what you will do: *I'll eat no more than 1,200 calories a day. I'll walk four days a week for thirty minutes. I'll replace three negative thoughts per day with more posi-*

tive ones. I'll start with a five-minute deep breathing exercise once each day to learn how to reduce stress.

A good way to determine whether your goal is specific enough is to ask yourself, if someone else were to read it, would that person understand what it is you want to achieve?

• **Measurable**, meaning that your goals can be quantified. As in the preceding examples, you can measure goals in calories, servings, minutes, or the number of destructive thoughts you intercept and quash.

• **Achievable.** When setting goals, it is human nature to aim a little too high. When people's weight loss goals are unrealistic, they rarely achieve them. Maybe you'll never be a size 4 or 6 or recover your college waistline—and certainly not next week. Setting impossible goals only sets up a failure cycle, which we've seen sabotage so many patients. What's the point? Ask yourself honestly if you are willing to devote the time it will take to achieve the goals you've set. Are you physically capable of achieving them, given your other commitments? In other words, what are the goals you can rationally expect to reach?

• **Realistic and rewarding.** Remember that every goal you reach is helping to improve your quality of life—physically, socially, and psychologically. So along the way you should appreciate and even revel in all the little victories! You're less tired after a long day, your pants are getting looser, your blood pressure and cholesterol have improved, you've become better at saying no to stressful demands, and you feel more supported by your loved ones. These smaller milestones are very meaningful. Celebrate them!

• **Time-focused.** To keep yourself accountable for making improvements, set deadlines—daily, short term, and long term: Today I will get my shopping list written before 6 P.M. On Saturday I will boost my exercise regimen to thirty minutes three times a week. On the fifteenth, I will start working out with a personal trainer, and so on. Record these commitments on your calendar and stick to them.

ACTION PLANNING
FOR LASTING CHANGE

One of the keys to lasting change is planning. Planning is the mortar that binds the bricks of your program together, so as you get ready to embark on Week 1, it pays to strategize. You'll start by setting the full range of goals for yourself and then figure out a course of action to take in case you start to slip.

We've heard so many clients say, "I was going along fine, steadily losing pounds, and then I don't know what happened. Suddenly I was off track and gaining weight." It's important to stay on high alert for red flags, so you can check small slips before they become full-blown slides.

A helpful feature of our approach is that the red flags are built right into the goals. If you hit the minimal goal more frequently than you had planned, it's time to break out your action plan!

The key to successful action plans is mapping them out *before* any trouble starts. With every goal you set, you need to know exactly what you're going to do if you don't meet it. For the exercise example, you might have one or several potential plans in place, in case the first one you try doesn't quite fix the problem:

1. I'll get a friend to exercise with me.
2. I'll sign up for personal training on my lunch hour, so I will have to go.
3. Instead of walking, I will try a new activity, like riding my bike when I get home from work.

And so on. You can probably come up with a long list of similar solutions for any goal you set. Then, when you spot a red flag, all you have to do is choose a plan from your bag of tricks and get yourself back on course.

OVERCOMING BARRIERS

Every once in a while, even with careful planning and goal setting, something you did not plan for leads you to feeling stuck, as if you are facing an obstacle that you can't overcome. At Duke, we encourage patients to use the IDEA problem-solving method for tackling such barriers:

- **I**dentify the problem.
- **D**evelop a list of possible solutions.
- **E**valuate the list of possible solutions, pick one, and do it.
- **A**nalyze how well your plan worked.

Here's how the IDEA method looks in practice:

• **I**dentify the problem. What you should focus on here is one concrete problem—not an abstraction like "I hate exercise," but something specific like "I've skipped three sessions this week." What's behind the problem? Have you been unusually pressed at work and had trouble squeezing it in? Have you been too tired in the morning to get up early and too exhausted at night to work out? Do you worry that the more athletic people at your gym are looking at you or judging you? Do you feel like a klutz in aerobics class?

• **D**evelop solutions. In fifteen minutes or less, brainstorm as many tactics as you can for overcoming the barrier, even if some seem silly. Sometimes the most bizarre suggestion might stimulate your creative energy and lead to one you can use. For example, if you've been too tired to exercise mornings and evenings, you might come up with the following ideas: quit exercising and be happy with it, ride a bike to and from work, jump rope in the parking lot, and take a brisk walk during lunch hour at work.

• **E**valuate solutions. Once you have a list of ideas, you can reject the impossible ones and refine or accept the others. For example, perhaps working out at lunchtime seems okay. Give it a try!

• **Analyze solutions.** Remember that any plan, no matter how good, may not work perfectly the first time. Say, with the plan to walk at lunch, you've found that you get a little too sweaty and that this has stopped you from doing it on occasion. You might decide to adjust your plan further by bringing exercise clothes to the office and changing into them before taking your walk. Review your new plan on a regular basis to see how well it's working and consider ways to improve or, if need be, replace it.

THE JOURNEY BEGINS!

In the pages that follow, we'll introduce you to the four-week core Duke Plan. Each week will feature a complete meal plan with delicious recipes, an exercise schedule that you really can work with, and tools to help you keep honing the skills you need to lose weight steadily and keep it off for good. We hope these four weeks will change your life—inside and out! We'll leave you with an inspiring patient story.

The New Me!

I first started the Duke program in 2001, and I have lost weight and now have my blood pressure back under control!

The great thing about the program is how much I learned: what my goal weight should be, how many calories to eat each day, how to stay in nutritional balance, how to set achievable goals, and how to develop the life skills to sustain my weight loss. Now I pay attention to what I eat, ask for dressings and sauces on the side, and skip foods that are fried or laced with cream (I hardly miss them!). These are such simple steps, but they have helped me so much.

Exercise has made a difference, too. I gained the confidence I needed through the Duke fitness plan and started doing aerobics classes a couple of months after going home from the Diet & Fitness Center. I try to get to the gym four or five days a week. I love taking the classes because it's so easy just to let the instructor tell you what to do, how to do it, and for how long! Regular exercise is now so much a part of my routine that I just don't feel right when it's absent from my day.

My confidence level has improved 100 percent. I can shop at "regular-size" clothing stores. I can climb a flight of stairs without getting winded. I feel lighter, like there is less strain on my back and legs. And I'm just happier in general!

People tell me that I look so great. I love the reactions from people who haven't seen me in a couple of years. They can hardly conceal their amazement at the new me!

—Laura, age 25

PART TWO

A New Beginning:
The Four-Week Core Plan

CHAPTER FIVE

Week 1: Setting Goals

The big moment has come! You're ready to get started on the core Duke Plan. We hope that we've already convinced you that you won't feel deprived, but if you have any lingering doubts, a look at the Week 1 meal plan should reassure you. Did you ever think you'd be enjoying dishes like Banana Walnut Pancakes, Eggplant Sausage Lasagna, and Chicken with Ricotta and Pesto while were you trying to lose weight? That's a big Duke difference!

Each week of the core program has a theme and will teach you new strategies and skills. The theme of Week 1 is, of course, setting goals and developing action plans using the system we described in chapter 4. We'll help you track your progress, using either the self-monitoring card we provide here or the Food Log and Lifestyle Journal featured on our website. We'll help you make action plans to catch slips before they become backslides, offer you exercise pointers, inspire you with patient success stories—and more.

In Week 2, we will focus on eating and exercising with awareness, in Week 3 on staying motivated, and in Week 4 on managing stress.

So many clients have succeeded on the Duke Diet Nutrition Plan and they tell us it's because the plan is straightforward and personalized to fit *their* needs. Remember that what we call the Duke Plan is really a *lifestyle* that you're going to embrace. And unless all those clients are wrong—which we doubt!—you're actually going to enjoy it.

The more closely you stick to the program and the more intently you focus on learning the concepts and strategies, the more successful you will be in managing your weight. You are also likely to realize a host of other health benefits, including an improved feeling of vitality and a sense of confidence that you can continue the program for life. Some patients say that they start to see changes as early as Week 1, but don't be disappointed if you don't. People experience change to varying degrees and at varying rates. The important thing is that you try your best each day. If you make just a few small changes this week, you'll have begun the process of transforming your body, your health, and your life. Small changes can add up quickly. Remember that your goal is not instant results but steady progress. As far as your weight, that means losing on the order of one to two pounds a week.

But first, let us introduce you to the Week 1 Nutrition and Exercise Plans.

WEEK 1 MEAL PLANS

The Duke Diet Nutrition Plan gives you structured meal plans to help you get accustomed to eating in a healthy and balanced way. So we suggest that you try to stick closely to them during the four-week plan just as our patients at the Duke Diet & Fitness Center do.

If you want to make substitutions for foods you don't like or are unable to eat, that is fine. You can choose replacements from the same food groups to remain close to the plan's nutrient balance. We encourage flexibility and common sense in making substitutions. However, it is important, regardless of what you choose, to stay within a similar calorie count. You can feel free to repeat meals that you especially enjoy or switch the daily menus around, as long as you replace a breakfast with a breakfast, a lunch with a lunch, and so on. If on occasion you find yourself eating out unexpectedly, use the general nutrition strategies we outlined in chapter 2. Later, in chapter 7, we'll give you specific strategies for eating in restaurants. We recommend that you try to eat at home as much as possible, but if you're suddenly faced with dining out, remember that it is often safest to choose simple foods like grilled fish or chicken—as opposed to "combination foods" like lasagna and casseroles, which can vary a great deal in terms of ingredients and calorie content.

If you need additional help with determining the calorie and nutrient breakdown of foods—whether simple foods or combination foods that you aren't sure how to categorize—you can check them on www.dukediet.com. It is also important not to consume fewer calories than the plans provide in an effort to speed up your weight loss beyond what we recommend. Starving yourself will almost inevitably backfire—it may lead to binges, cause you to feel too tired to exercise, or simply convince you that change is too painful or difficult. Trust the plan you select, and if over a week or two your weight loss is not going as planned, then you can make adjustments using the guidelines here.

How many calories should you consume every day? The recommended range for women seeking weight loss is 1,200 to 1,500 calories and, for men, approximately 1,500 to 2,000 (for men of smaller stature, somewhat fewer than 1,500 calories is sometimes appropriate). Precisely how many calories you need will depend on your weight (heavier folks may need more calories), your age (older people tend to need relatively fewer calories), and your level of physical activity (more active folks tend to need more calories). We suggest you start out toward the lower end of the range (about 1,300 for women and 1,500 for men). Then make small adjustments to your calorie level as you notice certain things. If you're losing more than two pounds a week or you're very hungry, irritable, or fatigued, add another 50 to 100 calories a day to your plan; if you're not losing at least a pound per week, drop 50 to 100 calories a day. Do so by reducing from one or several food groups. If you prefer, you can also log on to our website and use the Calorie Calculator to get a personalized estimate of your calorie requirements, as well as a wider range of meal plans.

TRADITIONAL MEAL PLAN, WEEK 1
1,200–1,400 Calorie Level

DAY 1

BREAKFAST
Banana Walnut Pancakes (page 236)
½ tablespoon light pancake syrup
½ cup nonfat milk

LUNCH
3-ounce whole-grain bagel* with 1 tablespoon natural
peanut butter and 1 teaspoon all-natural fruit
spread
1 cup nonfat milk

SNACK
Choose any from snack list (page 344)

DINNER
Almond-Crusted Salmon (page 294)
¼ cup instant brown rice (measured dry; ½ cup
cooked)
8 medium spears steamed asparagus
1 small orange

DAY 2

BREAKFAST
Apricot-Cranberry Oatmeal (page 234)

LUNCH
Turkey sandwich (2 ounces lower-sodium deli turkey
on whole-wheat bread with 2 slices tomato and
1 tablespoon mustard)
1 small apple
6 ounces low-fat vanilla yogurt

SNACK
Choose any from snack list (page 344)

DINNER
Eggplant Sausage Lasagna (page 308)
1 cup steamed broccoli
1 cup fresh raspberries

DAY 3

BREAKFAST
2-ounce whole-grain bagel with 1-ounce slice of
low-fat cheese

LUNCH
Turkey chef salad (3 ounces lower-sodium deli
turkey, 2 cups spinach, 2 large chopped carrots
or 1 cup baby carrots, 1 ounce low-fat Cheddar
cheese, 2 tablespoons light ranch dressing)
Whole-wheat roll
1 medium orange

SNACK
Choose any from snack list (page 344)

DINNER
Asian Duck Salad (page 295)
¼ cup instant brown rice (measured dry; ½ cup
cooked)
1 cup steamed broccoli
6 ounces nonfat plain yogurt with 1 cup fresh or
frozen berries

DAY 4

BREAKFAST
Toasted whole-grain English muffin with 2 teaspoons
natural peanut butter and 1 teaspoon all-natural
fruit spread

* The bagels in these meal plans are smaller than the typical large bagels sold in bagel stores, which can sometimes top 4 ounces. A 2-ounce bagel is about 2½ to 3 inches in diameter, slightly larger than a "mini-bagel"—many packaged frozen bagels are 2 ounces. A 3-ounce bagel, often referred to as a "medium bagel," is about 3½ inches in diameter.

TRADITIONAL MEAL PLAN, WEEK 1
1,200–1,400 Calorie Level

LUNCH
Sloppy Turkey Joe (page 324) on whole-wheat hamburger/hot dog bun
1 medium red bell pepper, sliced
1 cup nonfat milk

SNACK
Choose any from snack list (page 344)

DINNER
Cranberry Pecan Salad (page 264) with Raspberry Vinaigrette (page 331)
3 ounces rotisserie chicken
1 small pear, sliced, with 6 ounces low-fat vanilla yogurt

DAY 5

BREAKFAST
Blueberry Bran Muffin (page 238) with ½ tablespoon trans-fat-free margarine
2 ounces cottage cheese, 2 percent fat

LUNCH
Jerk Shrimp Skewers with Tomato-Strawberry Salsa (page 314)
½ cup long-grain brown rice (measured dry; 1 cup cooked)
1 cup cherry tomatoes with 1 tablespoon vinaigrette

SNACK
Choose any from snack list (page 344)

DINNER
Salmon with Peanut Sauce (page 322)
Roasted Winter Vegetables (page 274)
¼ cup couscous (measured dry; ½ cup cooked)

DAY 6

BREAKFAST
Multigrain Pancakes (page 241)
2 tablespoons light pancake syrup
½ cup nonfat milk

LUNCH
Chicken Fajita Salad with Creamy Cilantro-Lime Sauce (page 261)
Fruit salad (1 medium orange, peeled and cubed, 1 tablespoon orange juice, ½ cup fresh raspberries)

SNACK
Choose any from snack list (page 344)

DINNER
Shrimp Jambalaya (page 323)
1 cup steamed broccoli
½ cup fresh raspberries

DAY 7

BREAKFAST
½ cup fiber- and protein-rich cereal (such as Kashi) with ¾ cup soy milk

LUNCH
Grilled chicken sandwich (2 slices whole-wheat bread, 2 ounces grilled chicken, 1 ounce low-fat Cheddar cheese)
2 large carrots (7½ inches long) or 1 cup baby carrots
1 medium apple

SNACK
Choose any from snack list (page 344)

DINNER
MahiMahi with Pineapple Salsa (page 315)
¼ cup instant brown rice (measured dry; ½ cup cooked)
4 cups fresh spinach sautéed in 2 teaspoons olive oil

TRADITIONAL MEAL PLAN, WEEK 1
1,400–1,600 Calorie Level

DAY 1

BREAKFAST
Banana Walnut Pancakes (page 236)
½ tablespoon light pancake syrup
1 cup nonfat milk

LUNCH
3-ounce whole-grain bagel with 1½ tablespoons
    natural peanut butter and 1 teaspoon all-natural
    fruit spread
1 cup nonfat milk

SNACK
Choose any from snack list (page 344)

DINNER
Almond-Crusted Salmon (page 294)
¼ cup instant brown rice (measured dry; ½ cup
    cooked)
1 cup steamed broccoli
1 medium orange

DAY 2

BREAKFAST
Apricot-Cranberry Oatmeal (page 234)
1 cup vanilla soy milk

LUNCH
Turkey sandwich (3 ounces lower-sodium deli turkey
    on whole-wheat bread with 2 slices tomato and
    1 tablespoon mustard)
1 small apple
8 ounces low-fat vanilla yogurt

SNACK
Choose any from snack list (page 344)

DINNER
Eggplant Sausage Lasagna (page 308)
1 cup steamed broccoli
1 cup fresh raspberries
½ large slice cracked-wheat bread

DAY 3

BREAKFAST
2-ounce whole-grain bagel with 2 ounces low-fat
    cheese

LUNCH
Turkey chef salad (3 ounces lower-sodium deli
    turkey, 2 cups spinach, 2 large chopped carrots
    or 1 cup baby carrots, 1 ounce low-fat Cheddar
    cheese, 2 tablespoons light ranch dressing)
Whole-wheat roll
1 large orange

SNACK
Choose any from snack list (page 344)

DINNER
Asian Duck Salad (page 295)
¼ cup instant brown rice (measured dry; ½ cup
    cooked)
1 cup steamed broccoli with ½ tablespoon
    garlic-flavored olive oil
6 ounces nonfat plain yogurt with fruit (1 cup fresh
    or frozen)

DAY 4

BREAKFAST
Toasted whole-grain English muffin with 2 teaspoons
    natural peanut butter, topped with banana slices
    (½ medium banana)
½ cup nonfat milk

LUNCH
Sloppy Turkey Joe (page 324) on whole-wheat
    hamburger/hot dog bun
1 medium red bell pepper, sliced
1 cup nonfat milk

TRADITIONAL MEAL PLAN, WEEK 1
1,400–1,600 Calorie Level

SNACK

Choose any from snack list (page 344)

DINNER

Cranberry Pecan Salad (page 264) with Raspberry
 Vinaigrette (page 331)

3 ounces rotisserie chicken

6 ounces low-fat vanilla yogurt with 1 cup fresh
 blueberries

DAY 5

BREAKFAST

Blueberry Bran Muffin (page 238) with
 ½ tablespoon trans-fat-free margarine

4 ounces cottage cheese, 2 percent fat

½ medium green apple

LUNCH

Jerk Shrimp Skewers with Tomato-Strawberry Salsa
 (page 314)

½ cup long-grain brown rice (measured dry; 1 cup
 cooked)

1 cup cherry tomatoes with 1 tablespoon vinaigrette

1 nectarine

SNACK

Choose any from snack list (page 344)

DINNER

Salmon with Peanut Sauce (page 322)

Roasted Winter Vegetables (page 274)

⅜ cup couscous (measured dry; ¾ cup cooked)

DAY 6

BREAKFAST

Multigrain Pancakes (page 241)

2 tablespoons light pancake syrup

1 cup nonfat milk

LUNCH

Chicken Fajita Salad with Creamy Cilantro-Lime
 Sauce (page 261)

Fruit salad (1 medium orange, peeled and cubed,
 1 tablespoon orange juice, ½ cup fresh raspberries)

SNACK

Choose any from snack list (page 344)

DINNER

Shrimp Jambalaya (page 323)

4 cups fresh spinach sautéed with 2 teaspoons
 olive oil

1 medium pear

DAY 7

BREAKFAST

1 cup fiber- and protein-rich cereal (such as Kashi)
 with 1 cup soy milk

LUNCH

Grilled chicken sandwich (2 slices whole-wheat
 bread, 2 ounces grilled chicken, 1 ounce low-fat
 Cheddar cheese)

2 large carrots, sliced, with 1 tablespoon vinaigrette

1 medium apple

SNACK

Choose any from snack list (page 344)

DINNER

MahiMahi with Pineapple Salsa (page 315)

¼ cup instant brown rice (measured dry; ½ cup
 cooked) with 2 teaspoons margarine

1 cup fresh cantaloupe

1 cup steamed broccoli

MODERATE CARBOHYDRATE MEAL PLAN, WEEK 1
1,200–1,400 Calorie Level

DAY 1

BREAKFAST
Broccoli and Cheese Quiche (page 239)
2 ounces low-fat vanilla yogurt

LUNCH
Butternut Squash Soup (page 251)
Turkey sandwich (1 slice whole-wheat bread,
   2 ounces roast turkey breast, and 2 tablespoons
   reduced-fat mayonnaise)
1 medium red bell pepper, sliced, with 1 tablespoon
   vinaigrette

SNACK
Choose any from snack list (page 344)

DINNER
Baked Salmon with Citrus Salsa (page 296)
Spinach Soy Nut Salad (page 277)

DAY 2

BREAKFAST
Yogurt, Nut, and Fruit Parfait (page 250)

LUNCH
Roast beef on a pita (3 ounces roast beef, 1 ounce
   low-fat cheese, 2 tomato slices, ½ cup shredded
   lettuce in ½ whole-wheat pita)
½ cup baby carrots with 2 tablespoons hummus

SNACK
Choose any from snack list (page 344)

DINNER
Turkey, Cheese, and Kale Panini (page 291)

DAY 3

BREAKFAST
Open-Faced Egg and Cheese Sandwich (page 242)

LUNCH
Peanut butter and banana sandwich (2 tablespoons
   natural peanut butter on 1 slice whole-wheat
   bread, topped with thin slices of ½ medium
   banana)
½ cup low-fat cottage cheese in a red pepper shell
   (1 medium red bell pepper, seeds removed)

SNACK
Choose any from snack list (page 344)

DINNER
Pomegranate, Steak, and Spinach Salad (page 271)
1 ounce low-fat Cheddar cheese
1 small apple

DAY 4

BREAKFAST
½ cup protein- and fiber-rich cold cereal (such as
   Kashi), ½ cup soy milk, topped with 1 tablespoon
   chopped walnuts

LUNCH
Grilled Cheese Sandwich (page 285)
½ cup baby carrots with 1 tablespoon vinaigrette

SNACK
Choose any from snack list (page 344)

DINNER
Blackened Fish (page 299)
1 cup green beans stir-fried in ½ tablespoon garlic-
   flavored olive oil
¼ cup quinoa (measured dry; ½ cup cooked)

MODERATE CARBOHYDRATE MEAL PLAN, WEEK 1
1,200–1,400 Calorie Level

DAY 5

BREAKFAST
¼ cup dry oatmeal cooked with ½ cup nonfat milk,
   ½ cup blueberries (fresh or frozen), and
   1½ tablespoons sliced almonds

LUNCH
Grilled Portobello (page 312)
2 ounces roasted chicken breast
½ cup baby carrots with 1 tablespoon hummus
1 medium apple

SNACK
Choose any from snack list (page 344)

DINNER
Thai Chicken Broccoli Salad (page 280)
1 medium red bell pepper, sliced, with 1 tablespoon
   vinaigrette

DAY 6

BREAKFAST
1 slice toasted whole-wheat bread, 1 tablespoon
   trans-fat-free margarine
4 ounces nonfat vanilla yogurt

LUNCH
Tortilla Soup (page 254)
2 ounces roast turkey breast
½ cup fresh pineapple (or canned pineapple in juice)
   with ½ cup low-fat cottage cheese

SNACK
Choose any from snack list (page 344)

DINNER
Chicken Breast with Ricotta and Pesto (page 301)
2 cups wilted spinach
¼ cup sticky white rice (measured dry; ½ cup
   cooked)

DAY 7

BREAKFAST
Toast with Egg Salad (page 248)
½ cup fresh raspberries

LUNCH
Chicken Salad in Whole-Wheat Pita (page 284)
1 cup cherry tomatoes with 1 tablespoon vinaigrette

SNACK
Choose any from snack list (page 344)

DINNER
Chicken Fromage with Sauce (page 303)
Roasted Pepper and Goat Cheese Polenta
   (page 337)
Cucumber–Red Onion Salad (page 265)
1 plum

MODERATE CARBOHYDRATE MEAL PLAN, WEEK 1
1,400–1,600 Calorie Level

DAY 1

BREAKFAST
Broccoli and Cheese Quiche (page 239)
1½ tablespoons sliced almonds with ½ cup fresh
    raspberries
½ cup nonfat plain yogurt

LUNCH
Butternut Squash Soup (page 251)
1 slice whole-wheat bread, 2 ounces roast turkey
    breast, and 2 tablespoons reduced-fat
    mayonnaise
1 medium red bell pepper, sliced, with 1 tablespoon
    vinaigrette

SNACK
Choose any from snack list (page 344)

DINNER
Baked Salmon with Citrus Salsa (page 296)
Spinach Soy Nut Salad (page 277, but with additional
    ¾ ounce soy nuts)

DAY 2

BREAKFAST
Yogurt, Nut, and Fruit Parfait (page 250)
Scrambled Egg with Peppers (page 246)

LUNCH
Roast Beef on a Pita (3 ounces roast beef, 1 ounce
    low-fat cheese, 2 tomato slices, and ½ cup
    shredded lettuce in ½ whole-wheat pita)
½ cup cottage cheese
½ cup fresh or canned pineapple

SNACK
Choose any from snack list (page 344)

DINNER
Turkey, Cheese, and Kale Panini with 1 tablespoon
    margarine (page 291)
1 plum

DAY 3

BREAKFAST
Open-Faced Egg and Cheese Sandwich (page 242,
    but use 2 ounces cheese, 1 egg, and 2 egg whites)
½ cup blueberries

LUNCH
Peanut butter and banana sandwich (2 tablespoons
    natural peanut butter on 1 slice whole-wheat
    bread, topped with thin slices of ½ medium
    banana)
½ cup low-fat cottage cheese in a red pepper shell
    (1 medium red bell pepper, seeds removed)

SNACK
Choose any from snack list (page 344)

DINNER
Pomegranate, Steak, and Spinach Salad (page 271)
Broccoli with Dijon Vinaigrette (page 259)
½ cup fresh raspberries with ½ cup low-fat cottage
    cheese

DAY 4

BREAKFAST
½ cup protein- and fiber-rich cold cereal (such as
    Kashi), ½ cup soy milk, 1 tablespoon chopped
    walnuts

LUNCH
Grilled Cheese Sandwich (page 285)
½ cup baby carrots with 1 tablespoon vinaigrette
½ cup nonfat milk

MODERATE CARBOHYDRATE MEAL PLAN, WEEK 1
1,400–1,600 Calorie Level

SNACK

Choose any from snack list (page 344)

DINNER

Blackened Fish (page 299)

1 cup green beans stir-fried in 1 tablespoon garlic-flavored olive oil

¼ cup quinoa (measured dry; ½ cup cooked)

DAY 5

BREAKFAST

¼ cup dry oatmeal cooked with ½ cup nonfat milk, ½ cup blueberries (fresh or frozen), and 3 tablespoons sliced almonds

1 cup nonfat milk

LUNCH

Grilled Portobello (page 312)

2 ounces roasted chicken breast

1 cup baby carrots with 2 tablespoons hummus

1 medium apple

SNACK

Choose any from snack list (page 344)

DINNER

Thai Chicken Broccoli Salad (page 280)

1 medium red bell pepper, sliced, with 1 tablespoon vinaigrette

---

DAY 6

BREAKFAST

1 slice toasted whole-wheat bread, 1 tablespoon trans-fat-free margarine

8 ounces nonfat vanilla yogurt

½ cup fresh raspberries

LUNCH

Tortilla Soup (page 254)

4 ounces roast turkey breast

½ cup fresh pineapple (or canned pineapple in juice)

1 medium red bell pepper, sliced, with 2 tablespoons hummus

SNACK

Choose any from snack list (page 344)

DINNER

Chicken Breast with Ricotta and Pesto (page 301)

2 cups wilted spinach, tossed with ½ tablespoon garlic-flavored olive oil

¼ cup sticky white rice (measured dry; ½ cup cooked)

DAY 7

BREAKFAST

Toast with Egg Salad (page 248, but use 2 eggs)

½ cup fresh strawberries

LUNCH

Chicken Salad in Whole-Wheat Pita (page 284, but use 4 ounces of chicken)

1 cup cherry tomatoes with 1 tablespoon vinaigrette

SNACK

Choose any from snack list (page 344)

DINNER

Chicken Fromage with Sauce (page 303)

Roasted Pepper and Goat Cheese Polenta (page 337)

Cucumber–Red Onion Salad (page 265; have 2 servings)

1 plum

How to Cope If You Don't Cook

We encourage you to use the recipes we've provided as much as possible because we know, from our experience with patients, that they'll awaken you to the pleasures of healthy eating. But even if you're already a five-star chef, you'll have periods when you don't have time to cook, and we've seen lots of people who don't cook at all make it successfully through the program. Here's how:

- **Stock your kitchen with healthy staples** that you can fall back on, with minimal effort: fresh fruits (blueberries have a fairly long life if kept refrigerated) and vegetables; plain, low-fat yogurt or sour cream; whole-grain cereal (with more than 4 grams of fiber and less than 12 grams of sugar per serving); instant oatmeal (but check the label; some have added sodium and sugar); reduced-fat cheese; whole-grain snack crackers; canned tuna or salmon packed in water (rather than high-calorie oil); and low-sodium soups (140 milligrams of sodium or less per serving). Keeping prepackaged or frozen dinners around can also be a convenient choice, but again, watch the calories and sodium. Remember, healthy does not always mean weight loss friendly—so you will need, as always, to attend to portion and calorie control.

- **Enjoy healthy soups and sandwiches.** All you need is whole-grain bread (read the label—the good stuff should have the word *whole* in the first ingredient, and the fiber content should be favorable, so compare several products), a lean protein like turkey, a slice of tomato, lettuce, and a low-calorie spread like mustard. Start with a bowl of vegetable soup, sprinkled with a little reduced-fat cheese, and you'll have a satisfying, balanced meal.

- **Check out the freezer case at your supermarket** for healthy, low-calorie prepackaged meal options, such as those from Healthy Choice, Health Valley, and Amy's. Be sure to read labels for calorie counts, sodium (remember, you want less than 500 milligrams per meal), and other nutritional values. Many national food chains offer fresh, nutritious, chef-prepared meals that you can simply reheat at home. However, it is often difficult to determine the calories and nutritional content of these in-store options—try asking the store for details.

- **Frequent the supermarket salad bar.** Stay away from the mayonnaise-based offerings (like tuna and chicken salad) and fill a container with lettuce, vegetables, lean meats, and fruits. Choose reduced-fat salad dressings. Try dipping your fork in the dressing rather than pouring it on, or if you prefer to pour, use modest amounts. (A drizzle of olive oil and a nice balsamic vinegar is healthy and hard to beat for taste.)

- **At fast-food restaurants, go for the healthy take-out options,** like grilled chicken sandwiches (hold or limit the mayo!) and entrée salads. Just remember to check what's in the salad and when you get it, "eyeball" the ingredients (as we teach in chapter 2) to estimate how many calories you are getting. If you like cheese on your salad, use it sparingly, as a garnish—a mound of cheese and a pile of croutons can turn an otherwise healthy salad into a high-calorie meal.

- **Try meal replacement bars or shakes** in place of one or two regular meals. This can be a simple and convenient way to help you adhere to your reduced-calorie eating plan. The brands we frequently recommend at Duke include Slim-Fast and Glucerna. Read the labels and simply count them as you would any other food in your plan.

SUPERMARKET SAVVY

Grocery shopping can be like running a gauntlet of tempting sample tables, ice cream freezers, fresh baked goods displays, and entire departments dedicated to high-calorie processed and convenience foods—a challenge when you're trying to lose weight. So at the Duke Diet & Fitness Center, we offer a popular class during which our nutrition staff takes a group of clients to the supermarket and shows them, aisle by aisle, how to make good choices and avoid being derailed from their healthy, well-thought-out plans by enticingly marketed alternatives. We can't shop with you in person, of course, but if you follow these guidelines, we'll be there in spirit—and help you make it home without countless unwanted consumed-in-store and take-home calories. You'll also find a host of supermarket shopping tips on www.dukediet.com.

1. Draw up your grocery list. Start by drawing up a grocery list at home, based on your meal plan for the week ahead. You can replace any items you don't want to eat with an appropriate substitution that has a similar calorie count. For example, if you hate spinach, go for zucchini, green beans, or another leafy green (the darker the greens, the higher the vitamin content). If you don't like fish, write down "skinless chicken breasts."

2. Shop the perimeter. Along the walls of the grocery store, you'll find the healthy foods that should be your mainstays: fresh fruits and vegetables, meats, fish, poultry, and low-fat dairy products. Beware of seasonal promotions: bags of caramels piled near the apples at Halloween, eggnog shelved next to the skim milk in December.

Load up your cart with nutritious, health-friendly options before you venture into the inner aisles, which are home not only to some staples of a healthy diet, but also to the high-fat chips and snacks, sugary confections, baked goods, and other more highly processed foods.

Restrict your shopping to only those aisles with foods included in your meal plan (on your shopping list); you do not have to walk up and down *every* aisle. Read labels to make sure that if you are opting for some of the more convenient processed or canned products, your choices are lower in calories and sodium and are trans fat free.

Good targets are:

- Dried and low-sodium canned beans, healthier varieties of baked beans and soups, low-sodium stewed tomatoes, and jarred *red* spaghetti sauce. Compare calorie counts of different brands.
- Water-packed salmon or chunk light tuna.
- Natural peanut butter (no sugar added).
- Whole-grain foods like whole-wheat pasta and breads, oat-

meal, and brown rice. Why not try a few new ones, like whole-wheat couscous and quinoa?

- Healthy snacks like rice or popcorn cakes and reduced-fat microwave popcorn (check the sodium).
- Flavor boosters like vinegars (red and white wine, with or without herbs, rice, and balsamic) are great calorie-free alternatives. When used sparingly, Dijon mustard, salsa, low-fat salad dressings, and hummus can all provide tasty enhancements.
- Low-fat deli meats like turkey and ham (watch sodium), as well as rotisserie chicken.
- Beverages like seltzer, calorie-free flavored water, and diet soda.

Label-Speak

Food labels have a language of their own, and the words on the labels often have very specific meanings according to the Food and Drug Administration (FDA) guidelines. Here are a few things to remember when you're decoding label-speak.

"Free" means that the food contains "physiologically inconsequential" amounts of that element. Other, similar terms include "without," "no," "zero," and for milk, "skim."

"Low" means that the food can be "eaten frequently without exceeding dietary guidelines" for one or more of these components: fat, saturated fat, cholesterol, sodium, and calories (specific examples below). Other terms meaning the same thing include "little," "few," "low source of," and "contains small amounts of."

When a label says that a nutrient is "reduced" (as in "reduced-fat" or "reduced-sodium") or that the food has "less" of a nutrient, it means that the food is at least 25 percent lower in that nutrient than the regular product.

If a food is said to be a "good source" of or "contains" or "provides" a nutrient, it contains from 10 to 19 percent of the Daily Value for that nutrient.

If a food is said to be "high," "rich in," or an "excellent source" of a nutrient, the food contains 20 percent or more of the Daily Value for that nutrient.

"Light" means either that a food has one-third the calories or one-half the fat of the original or that the food is low in calories and fat and the sodium content has been reduced by 50 percent.

In reference to meat, poultry, seafood, and game meats, "lean" means there's less than 10 grams of fat, 4.5 grams or less of saturated fat, and less than 95 milligrams of cholesterol per serving and per 100 grams (approximately 3 ounces). "Extra lean" means there's less than 5 grams of fat, 2 grams of saturated fat, and 95 milligrams of cholesterol per serving and per 100 grams.

Here are some more definitions:

Calorie free: Contains fewer than 5 calories per serving.
Low calorie: Contains 40 calories or fewer per serving.
Sugar free: Contains less than 0.5 gram of sugar per serving.
Low cholesterol: Contains less than 20 milligrams of cholesterol, and 2 grams or less of saturated fat per serving.
Fat free: Contains less than 0.5 gram of fat per serving.
Low saturated fat: Contains less than 1 gram of saturated fat per serving.
Sodium free: Contains less than 5 milligrams of sodium per serving.
Very low sodium: Contains 35 milligrams of sodium or less per serving.
Low sodium: Contains 140 milligrams of sodium or less per serving.

For a more in-depth understanding of food labels and terms, check out the following pages on the FDA website:

www.cfsan.fda.gov/~dms/foodlab.html
www.cfsan.fda.gov/~dms/fdnewlab.html

3. Eat before you shop. Otherwise, you might end up being tempted by all those impulse items spread throughout the store in eye-catching displays or positioned near the checkout line as a tempting target for the bored and hungry shopper. They can be quite a challenge. In addition, many stores offer samples: Half a brownie here, some barbecued wings there, a few tortilla chips dunked in salsa, some go-down-easy cubes of salami and cheese and, lo and behold, you've consumed an entire meal's worth of calories—and you're probably not even full!

4. If you buy in bulk, repackage at home. Use single-serving plastic bags or containers. That way, you won't have to measure before you cook and you'll be less likely to overshoot serving sizes.

Why Should I Check Labels for Sodium?

Sodium is necessary for good health and is naturally present in most foods in more than ample quantities, without adding any extra. Most of us consume far more than our bodies need, either because we add it to our food, because we eat in restaurants where it is liberally added, or because we buy processed foods high in sodium. Some folks may handle the excess better than others, but for many of us, a high intake of sodium may increase our risk of developing high blood pressure. It also increases the likelihood that we will retain water and experience bloating and swelling. For people who are overweight, many of whom already have or are at risk for high blood pressure, and many of whom already have problems with water retention, the typical American's high-sodium diet is particularly unhealthy.

The latest U.S. Department of Agriculture (USDA) recommendations suggest a daily allowance of 2,300 milligrams of sodium (approximately the amount in 1 teaspoon of salt) for many people, but they also recommend that people with high blood pressure, African Americans (because they tend to be at higher risk for sodium-sensitive hypertension), and adults of middle age or older aim even lower, for 1,500 milligrams or less per day. This is a lot less than is typical in the American diet, which has been estimated at 3,000 to 5,000 milligrams of sodium daily. A daily dietary intake of 1,500 milligrams of sodium has been shown to reduce the risk of developing high blood pressure, and for many of those who already have high blood pressure, it will significantly lower the pressure—especially when a reduced-sodium eating plan is combined with one high in potassium (from fruits and vegetables) and lower in calories. Regular physical activity also helps considerably.

If you think you can't live without salt, take heart! The less salt you use, the less you'll miss it. You can start to cut back on salt by choosing fresh over processed foods, which can be loaded with sodium, and by reading labels carefully and going for low- or lower-sodium options. For example, a look at three leading brands of jarred marinara sauce reveals big differences—respective sodium levels of 320, 440, and 590 milligrams. And the calories per serving differ widely, too.

You should also reduce your use of salty condiments like soy sauce. But perhaps the best and most rewarding way to cut back on salt is to use more herbs and spices in your cooking. Some herbs and spices—including garlic, greens like parsley, sage, and basil, and powders like curry and cinnamon—may even offer some special health benefits of their own, as well as the power to really enhance food flavors.

You'll get a great introduction to an inspiring refresher course on herbs and spices through the recipes in this book and on www.dukediet.com.

WEEK 1 EXERCISE ROUTINE

Some of our greatest fitness converts at the Duke Diet & Fitness Center tell us that what has kept them active is shifting their focus from getting results, like losing weight and dropping a size or two, to enjoying the *experience* of exercise. In fact, many even came to believe that fitness was fun. Think about the nonphysical benefits your exercise program might offer. First and foremost, when we move a little more, we start to feel better, and regular physical activity can help to reduce stress.

Beyond that, if you take a fitness class or work out at a gym or health club, you might meet new friends. If you are able to share your interests, exercise may give you quality time with a friend or a spouse. It could become an oasis of "me-time," when you can take a much needed break from life's daily challenges so that you can be refreshed and better able to meet them. Therefore, you may be more motivated to exercise if you focus on the various ways that it can satisfy your personal needs and *enhance* your day as opposed to viewing it as yet another chore.

We believe it is very important to shift your focus away from being someone who has to exercise and begin to visualize yourself as an active person. First, try to picture yourself being active and enjoying it. Imagine strong positive feelings of accomplishment, the invigoration you might feel as a result of challenging your body. By creating a clear, dynamic image of yourself in your mind—moving gracefully, being confident, and taking pleasure in exercising—you can open your mind to actually experiencing these things during a workout. Learn to enjoy the pleasure of moving and getting stronger. Attend to the feeling of satisfaction you get after an exercise session. You might be very surprised that by training your mind you can experience exercise in a whole new light. So give it a try!

The workouts you'll do each week are outlined here. The strength training and flexibility exercises correspond to the exercises and instructions in chapter 10. Do the strength training exercises in the order in which they are listed, and on nonconsecutive days, to give your muscles time to recuperate. The stretches can be done every day if you like. Be sure to follow the routine that matches the fitness level we helped you select in chapter 3 (Fitness Prep Level, Level 1, or Level 2). The program is designed to start you at the level that is right for you. Then, once you are comfortable, you can choose to challenge yourself and move to the next level. There's no hurry—for many people, staying with a level for two weeks before moving up should work well. For others, getting ready to move up may take more time. Recognize that the plan allows you to move at your own pace and invites you to increase the challenge when your body is ready.

Fitness Prep Level

If you are at the Fitness Prep Level, we want you to work gradually toward doing the more formal exercises in Level 1. Keep in mind that aiming for 10,000 steps is a solid health goal all by itself. So you will be starting your personalized fitness plan today! Use a pedometer (you can pick one up at just about any sporting goods or department store) and start adding steps to your day. Shoot for a goal of 8,000 to 10,000 steps daily. Later, when you can reach this goal consistently and comfortably—say, nearly every day for a week—you will be ready to move up to Level 1.

Level 1

In the first two weeks of the program, along with the specified strength and flexibility routine, we encourage you to continue to strive for 10,000 steps a day. Try to get at least *some* of those steps from doing more brisk walking. This is certainly a healthy level of activity. However, we feel it is useful when managing your weight to also progress gradually toward accumulating thirty minutes a day of moderate-intensity cardio exercise (for example, vig-

What Are Sets and Reps?

If you've ever been to a gym or seen an exercise video, you've heard the terms. But what do they mean? A *set* is a group of individual repetitions of an exercise—for example, twelve push-ups or twelve dumbbell curls. A *rep* is one repetition of a particular exercise—for example, one push-up or one dumbbell curl.

orous walking, swimming, or bicycling) three times a week. Remember that you don't have to do it all at one shot. You can do three 10-minute sessions if you like. Of course, on the days that you do cardio, you will not need to do 10,000 additional steps—the cardio counts! When you can comfortably achieve this amount of cardio exercise plus two sets of twelve to fifteen repetitions of the Level 1 strength training exercises, and you want more of a challenge, move to Level 2. Note that for variety, there are additional Level 1 exercises available on our website.

Level 2

If you are at Level 2, we encourage you to continue to strive for 10,000 steps a day. Try to get at least *some* of those steps from doing more brisk walking. This is certainly a healthy level of activity. However, at this level we also recommend striving for forty-five minutes a day of moderate-intensity cardio exercise (for example, vigorous walking, swimming, or bicycling) three days a week, plus two sets of twelve to fifteen reps of the Level 2 strength training exercises. To progress in this level, add five more minutes of cardio per week to each session and/or add additional sessions, until you've worked up to sixty minutes a day five days a week, plus three sets of twelve to fifteen repetitions of the exercises. Remember, on the days you are

Why Should I Warm Up before Exercising?

Warm-ups prepare your body for aerobics, strength training, and stretching by increasing your circulation and sending oxygen to your muscles. They can also help prevent injury. The best warm-ups are less intense versions of the exercise you'll be doing. For example, if you're going to do moderate-intensity walking, you should do five minutes of light walking to get ready. If you're going to do moderate-intensity swimming or cycling, do slow laps or light pedaling for five minutes to warm up.

For strength training, warm up with five minutes of light aerobics or low- or no-weight or resistance versions of your lifts and pulls.

You can also warm up with five minutes of yoga, Pilates, or tai chi. These can be good warm-ups to do before stretching.

EXERCISE AT A GLANCE, WEEKS 1 AND 2

LEVEL 1

DAY 1

Warm-up: 5 minutes
Cardio: 30 minutes

STRETCHING:
Hold each stretch for 10 to 30 seconds.
Total Body Stretch (page 365)
Lower Back and Gluteals Stretch (page 365)
Hamstrings Stretch (page 366)
Lower Back Stretch with Knees Tilted to One Side
(page 367)
Quadriceps Stretch (page 368)
Modified Hamstrings Stretch (page 369)
Triceps Stretch (page 370)

DAY 2

Warm-up: 5 minutes

STRENGTH TRAINING:
For each exercise, do 1 set of 12 to 15 reps.
Chair Squat (page 352)
Regular Push-up (alternatively, Wall Push-up)
(page 353)
Seated Leg Extension (page 355)
Straight-Leg Raise on Mat (page 356)
Hip Bridge on Mat (page 357)
Abs Curl on Mat (page 358)

STRETCHING:
Hold each stretch for 10 to 30 seconds.
Total Body Stretch (page 365)
Lower Back and Gluteals Stretch (page 365)
Hamstrings Stretch (page 366)
Lower Back Stretch with Knees Tilted to One Side
(page 367)
Quadriceps Stretch (page 368)
Modified Hamstrings Stretch (page 369)
Triceps Stretch (page 370)

DAY 3

Warm-up: 5 minutes
Cardio: 30 minutes

STRETCHING:
Hold each stretch for 10 to 30 seconds.
Total Body Stretch (page 365)
Lower Back and Gluteals Stretch (page 365)
Hamstrings Stretch (page 366)
Lower Back Stretch with Knees Tilted to One Side
(page 367)
Quadriceps Stretch (page 368)
Modified Hamstrings Stretch (page 369)
Triceps Stretch (page 370)

DAY 4

Warm-up: 5 minutes

STRENGTH TRAINING:
For each exercise, do 1 set of 12 to 15 reps.
Chair Squat (page 352)
Regular Push-up (alternatively, Wall Push-up)
(page 353)
Seated Leg Extension (page 355)
Straight-Leg Raise on Mat (page 356)
Hip Bridge on Mat (page 357)
Abs Curl on Mat (page 358)

STRETCHING:
Hold each stretch for 10 to 30 seconds.
Total Body Stretch (page 365)
Lower Back and Gluteals Stretch (page 365)
Hamstrings Stretch (page 366)
Lower Back Stretch with Knees Tilted to One Side
(page 367)
Quadriceps Stretch (page 368)
Modified Hamstrings Stretch (page 369)
Triceps Stretch (page 370)

EXERCISE AT A GLANCE, WEEKS 1 AND 2

DAY 5

Rest Day

Stretch if you wish. If you stretch, be sure to warm up for 5 minutes beforehand.

DAY 6

Warm-up: 5 minutes
Cardio: 30 minutes

STRETCHING:

Hold each stretch for 10 to 30 seconds.
Total Body Stretch (page 365)
Lower Back and Gluteals Stretch (page 365)
Hamstrings Stretch (page 366)
Lower Back Stretch with Knees Tilted to One Side (page 367)
Quadriceps Stretch (page 368)
Modified Hamstrings Stretch (page 369)
Triceps Stretch (page 370)

DAY 7

Rest Day

Stretch if you wish. If you stretch, be sure to warm up for 5 minutes beforehand.

LEVEL 2

DAY 1

Warm-up: 5 minutes
Cardio: 45 to 60 minutes

STRENGTH TRAINING:

For each exercise, do 2 sets of 12 to 15 reps.
Wall Squat with Stability Ball (page 359)
Biceps Curl and Overhead Press with Dumbbells (page 371)
Chest Press with Dumbbell Twist on Stability Ball (page 372)

Back Fly with Dumbbells on Stability Ball (page 373)
Triceps Kickback with Dumbbell (page 374)
Superman (page 375)
Hip Bridge with Stability Ball (page 376)
Abs Curl on Stability Ball (page 364)

STRETCHING:

Hold each stretch for 10 to 30 seconds.
Upper Back and Chest Stretch (page 384)
Rotary Torso Stretch (page 385)
Lat-Shoulder Stretch (page 386)
Supported Lower Back Stretch (page 387)
Seated Hamstrings Stretch (page 388)
Figure 4 Stretch (page 389)
Hip Flexor Stretch (page 390)

DAY 2

Warm-up: 5 minutes
Cardio: 45 to 60 minutes

STRETCHING:

Hold each stretch for 10 to 30 seconds.
Upper Back and Chest Stretch (page 384)
Rotary Torso Stretch (page 385)
Lat-Shoulder Stretch (page 386)
Supported Lower Back Stretch (page 387)
Seated Hamstrings Stretch (page 388)
Figure 4 Stretch (page 389)
Hip Flexor Stretch (page 390)

DAY 3

Warm-up: 5 minutes
Cardio: 45 to 60 minutes

STRENGTH TRAINING:

For each exercise, do 2 sets of 12 to 15 reps.
Wall Squat with Stability Ball (page 359)
Biceps Curl and Overhead Press with Dumbbells (page 371)

EXERCISE AT A GLANCE, WEEKS 1 AND 2

Chest Press with Dumbbell Twist on Stability Ball
  (page 372)
Back Fly with Dumbbells on Stability Ball
  (page 373)
Triceps Kickback with Dumbbell (page 374)
Superman (page 375)
Hip Bridge with Stability Ball (page 376)
Abs Curl on Stability Ball (page 364)

STRETCHING:
Hold each stretch for 10 to 30 seconds.
Upper Back and Chest Stretch (page 384)
Rotary Torso Stretch (page 385)
Lat-Shoulder Stretch (page 386)
Supported Lower Back Stretch (page 387)
Seated Hamstrings Stretch (page 388)
Figure 4 Stretch (page 389)
Hip Flexor Stretch (page 390)

DAY 4

Warm-up: 5 minutes
Cardio: 45 to 60 minutes

STRETCHING:
Hold each stretch for 10 to 30 seconds.
Upper Back and Chest Stretch (page 384)
Rotary Torso Stretch (page 385)
Lat-Shoulder Stretch (page 386)
Supported Lower Back Stretch (page 387)
Seated Hamstrings Stretch (page 388)
Figure 4 Stretch (page 389)
Hip Flexor Stretch (page 390)

DAY 5

Rest day
Stretch if you wish. If you stretch, be sure to warm
  up for five minutes beforehand.

DAY 6

Warm-up: 5 minutes
Cardio: 45 to 60 minutes

STRENGTH TRAINING:
For each exercise, do 2 sets of 12 to 15 reps.
Wall Squat with Stability Ball (page 359)
Biceps Curl and Overhead Press with Dumbbells
  (page 371)
Chest Press with Dumbbell Twist on Stability Ball
  (page 372)
Back Fly with Dumbbells on Stability Ball
  (page 373)
Triceps Kickback with Dumbbell (page 374)
Superman (page 375)
Hip Bridge with Stability Ball (page 376)
Abs Curl on Stability Ball (page 364)

STRETCHING:
Hold each stretch for 10 to 30 seconds.
Upper Back and Chest Stretch (page 384)
Rotary Torso Stretch (page 385)
Lat-Shoulder Stretch (page 386)
Supported Lower Back Stretch (page 387)
Seated Hamstrings Stretch (page 388)
Figure 4 Stretch (page 389)
Hip Flexor Stretch (page 390)

DAY 7

Rest day
Stretch if you wish. If you stretch, be sure to warm
  up for 5 minutes beforehand.

doing cardio, you do not need to do the 10,000 steps—the cardio counts! You can also log on to our website for additional customized exercise plans, and you can check out chapter 10 for what to do when you think it's time to progress from Level 2.

MAKE YOUR MARK

Research shows that people who keep daily records of how much they eat and exercise are more successful at losing weight than those who don't. At the Duke Diet & Fitness Center, we call this process *monitoring,* and we commonly see that when patients start letting it slide, the pounds start creeping back.

So we strongly urge you to monitor. To make it easy, we've developed a simple monitoring card that lets you record your food consumption and exercise routine. (You can also go to www.dukediet.com and use the interactive Food Log and the Lifestyle Journal.) The food groups on the card correspond to the groups in the Duke Diet Nutrition Plan. Note that the miscellaneous section is for foods, like Jell-O or alcohol, that do not fit into any official food group. Also, we find that if you are having trouble figuring out how to classify a particular food into the correct group, this section is a handy place to at least record the calories.

As you can see, all you have to do is note the servings you eat from each food group—it's that easy. Add up the number of servings in each group. Then multiply the number of servings by the number of calories per serving to get your subtotal for each group. Then add up the subtotals, and you'll have your daily calorie total.

On the exercise section of the card, check off your minutes of aerobic exercise and the intensity of the activity, using the RPE scale, as well as the number of sets and repetitions you completed during your strength and flexibility workout. At the Duke Diet & Fitness Center, we consider yoga part of a flexibility routine and Pilates part of a strengthening routine, so record those there. The card also has a space marked "Other" for any additional comments you want to jot down, such as how you felt during your workout or whether your levels that day fell short of or exceeded your goal (and why).

We find that people do best when they monitor daily and write down

FOOD AND CALORIE MONITORING CARD

Day of the week:

FOODS	SERVINGS PER DAY	×	CALORIES PER SERVING	=	TOTAL CALORIES	PLACE ONE CHECKMARK FOR EACH SERVING, THEN PLACE TOTAL IN "SERVINGS PER DAY" COLUMN.
Vegetable		×	25	=		
Fruit		×	60	=		
Dairy		×	90	=		
Starch		×	80	=		
Leaner protein		×	35–60	=		
Less lean protein		×	61–100	=		
Fat		×	45	=		
Miscellaneous		×		=		
Daily Calorie Total:						

DAILY EXERCISE MONITORING CARD

Aerobic	15 min ☐	30 min ☐	45 min ☐	60 min ☐	Comments
Type:			Number of steps:		
RPE:					
Strength	30 min ☐	60 min ☐	Number of exercises:		
Number of sets	1 ☐	2 ☐	3 ☐		
Number of reps		10–12 ☐	12–15 ☐		
Flexibility	15 min ☐	30 min ☐			
Other					

what they've eaten or how much they've exercised immediately, rather than trying to remember before they go to bed. We know that there will be times when you just feel too swamped to log everything, but by keeping it this simple, we hope you can keep it up. Down the road, as you get in a good rhythm with your plan, you may be fine without writing everything down. But at the first sign of trouble—if you stop making progress on your fitness routine or your food intake starts to slip off the plan—get back to monitoring. It really works. It just takes a minute if you use the card or the website, so don't think of it as a chore. It can really inspire you to see the black-and-white evidence of your daily achievements.

On the days when you veer a little off course, don't stop monitoring or view the process as a chance to beat yourself up. There's no such thing as failure! Some days you will feel that you did better than others. That's just the way it goes. We're all human. If your more challenging days start piling up, monitoring will help you recognize the pattern so you can use the behavioral tools in this book and on www.dukediet.com to break the cycle.

ASSIGNMENT FOR SUCCESS: WEEK 1

Go for Goals!

Goals can be easy to set but harder to achieve. Why? As you learned in chapter 4, goals are often abstract ("Get healthier") or unrealistic ("I want to be a size smaller by next week"). When we don't meet these vague or impossible expectations, we throw our hands up and declare that we're hopeless, doomed to failure, so we may as well not even try to change. That's why we've developed the system described in chapter 4 to help you set a range of goals and develop action plans for less-than-ideal circumstances. At first, our patients find it difficult to sit down and map out these goals and action plans, but they quickly realize how valuable the process can be. We've seen this system help so many people achieve success!

As you embark on Week 1 of the program, what are your goals? It's probably not that hard to figure out what you want to change about your eating and exercise habits. As you'll recall from chapter 4, you should set three levels of goals: your higher "next step," or optimal, goal; your current "if all goes according to plan," or desirable, goal; and your "life happens," or minimal, goal.

For example, if your next-step goal is to eat five servings of vegetables every day, consider that your optimal. If you are currently eating less than one serving of vegetables a day, your desirable goal might be to eat three servings a day. In this case, your minimal goal, which you'd aim for on a really bad day—perhaps when you're out running around doing errands or eating out where it's hard to find healthy vegetable choices—might be just one or two servings. As you get accustomed to planning and adding more vegetables into your diet, and you find yourself hitting your desirable goal more frequently, you might increase the number of servings in your desirable goal in weeks to come and work from there. If you find yourself struggling to meet this goal, an action plan might be to talk with a friend or post an online message asking for ideas on easy ways to fit vegetables in when you are out and about.

Taking a look at exercise:

• An example of an optimal goal might be: *I will work my way up to doing 30 minutes of aerobic activity three days a week, with two days of strength training per week plus stretching every day.*

• A desirable goal might be: *I think I can reasonably do 20 minutes of aerobic activity three days a week, with two days of strength training per week and stretching on at least four days.*

• A minimal goal might be: *During weeks when something comes up unexpectedly (for example, a big project is due), I can still reasonably aim for 20 minutes of aerobic activity two days a week, with one session of strength training plus three days of stretching. While this is not ideal, I would still feel successful, and I would be careful not to shoot for the minimum more often than necessary. If I am achieving the minimum two weeks in a row, then it's time for action.*

The last sentence is key. If you hit only your minimal goal for more than two weeks in a row, that is a warning flag that says it's time to launch one of your action plans to get back on track! For the preceding examples, a good action plan might be enlisting an exercise partner or working with a personal trainer to help motivate you to return to the desirable goal.

Don't be afraid to amend your goals if necessary. If the challenges you face aren't going to ease up anytime soon, maybe you need to make your minimal goal your desirable one for a while. What matters is that you don't just throw in the towel—that you keep making progress. Remember, even small changes add up to major life shifts.

Now spell out your goals for Week 1 using the following format. Be sure to apply the SMART criteria to each level of your goals: **S**pecific, **M**easurable, **A**chievable, **R**ealistic and rewarding, and **T**ime-focused.

Eating
Optimal goal:
Desirable goal:
Minimal goal:
What I will do to accomplish my goal:
How I will update my goals if I am hitting the minimal goal too often:

Exercise
Optimal goal:
Desirable goal:
Minimal goal:
What I will do to accomplish my goal:
How I will update my goals if I am hitting the minimal goal too often:

As you go through Week 1 and start meeting your goals, don't forget to pat yourself on the back and celebrate every success!

CHAPTER SIX

Week 2: Eating and Exercising with Awareness

One of the more popular classes at the Duke Diet & Fitness Center is called Mentoring Mealtime, which shows our clients how to eat with awareness, or *mindfully*. We keep the dining room silent, and everyone eats at a relaxed pace that lets them savor the aromas, flavors, and textures of the food on their plates. When people eat more slowly and fully experience their food and all its qualities, they are less likely to overeat because they experience their meal as enjoyable and fulfilling. They come away feeling much more satisfied than when they—or we—gulp down breakfast in the car on the way to work or gobble dinner in front of the TV.

So this week, we'll work on eating with full attention to the eating experience. We'll also look at how to exercise with greater self-awareness. But first, how did you do last week? Did you achieve your nutrition and exercise goals? Is your weight beginning to move in the right direction? Do you feel a little more confident or energized? It's important—and motivating—to monitor all types of progress and celebrate the steps forward you're making with each passing day.

We see so many patients who fear the scale as the ultimate goad to guilt and self-recrimination. Remember that your scale is just a tool—we want you to monitor your weight, but don't give it more importance than it deserves.

THE WAY TO WEIGH

Pounds are just one measure of the changes you're making, which include shrinking your waistline and improving your vitality, confidence, and self-esteem, as well as your health. So don't give the scale the power to intimidate you! We do believe, however, that weighing yourself regularly is important. Studies show that people who weigh themselves daily are more successful at weight loss over the long term than those who get on the scale only once a week. So we recommend that most people not only weigh themselves daily but also chart their progress. Or try the Weight Tracker on www.dukediet.com, which has a built-in graph. (Please note that it is not advisable for people with histories of eating disorders like anorexia or bulimia or for people who find the scale highly upsetting to weigh daily—in any of these cases, consult your doctor or mental health provider.)

Jane felt very strongly that daily weighing had caused her nothing but pain. I admitted that it is not for everyone, but I did ask one very specific question: Had she ever put her results on a graph? Most people who weigh daily don't. They simply weigh and carry that number—good or not so good—around in their head, and tend to remember the ones they don't like. The chart is the key because it is hard to argue with the line that is trending down.

Ultimately, charting her weight turned out to be liberating for Jane. It helped her overcome the pain she felt about the fluctuating numbers on the scale. Now she goes around handing out a graph to every new patient she sees, explaining what a powerful motivational tool it can be. So try it for yourself, and if you find it motivating, keep it up. If not, just try to weigh yourself regularly. So that you can see what we mean, here is an example of one patient's weight loss chart. Note the ups and downs!

—*Martin Binks, Ph.D.*

MY WEIGHT CHART

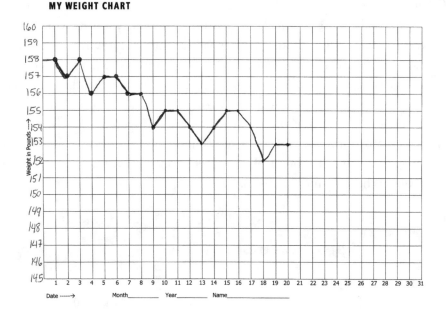

Why a chart? Because daily weighing shows you that your weight constantly fluctuates, thanks to factors like water retention. By placing the numbers where you can see them all together, you will also see that on one day weight may go up a pound or two, while on another it may drop. Once you see these shifts for yourself, you'll be less likely to despair over a single reading. If, now and then, the needle fails to budge or even moves in the "wrong" direction, the chart will help you see that the overall trend is positive, so that you focus away from the fluctuation of the day.

Charting your weight will give you the big picture, showing the trends in your progress over time. This may sound scary, especially if you have experienced a lot of anxiety around these daily ups and downs. Our experience with clients has been that, in fact, getting on the scale can reduce your anxiety about your weight.

WEEK 2 MEAL PLANS

Just as you did in Week 1, start your program by writing down your goals—optimal, desirable, and minimal—keeping the SMART principles in mind.

Visualize yourself attaining these goals and imagine how energized and successful that will make you feel. Which pillar do you want to work on this week? (To review, the Pillars of Lifestyle Change are environment [eating and exercise], stress management, body image and self-image, professional life and social life, emotional well-being, and support system.) Again, write down simple, concrete, doable actions you can take to begin shoring up the weaker areas of your program. Each positive change you make will fuel your sense of accomplishment and make new changes even easier to launch.

Here are this week's menu plans to help you stay on track, with all-new and delicious healthy meal options.

TRADITIONAL MEAL PLAN, WEEK 2
1,200–1,400 Calorie Level

DAY 1

BREAKFAST
French Toast (page 240)

LUNCH
Ham sandwich on whole-wheat bread, with 3 ounces of lean lower-sodium ham, 1 ounce of low-fat Cheddar cheese, 2 tomato slices, 1 lettuce leaf
½ medium banana with ½ cup nonfat vanilla yogurt

SNACK
Choose any from snack list (page 344)

DINNER
Pork Tenderloin with Apple Chutney (page 320)
Mediterranean Couscous (page 334)

DAY 2

BREAKFAST
2-ounce whole-grain bagel with 1 tablespoon low-fat cream cheese
4 ounces nonfat plain yogurt

LUNCH
Tuna Salad on Pita (page 290)
2 large carrots, cut into pieces, or 1 cup baby carrots

SNACK
Choose any from snack list (page 344)

DINNER
Pesto Pasta (page 335)
Broccoli with Dijon Vinaigrette (page 259)
1 medium peach

DAY 3

BREAKFAST
½ nonfat vanilla yogurt with 1 cup fresh or frozen fruit, 1½ tablespoon sliced almonds

LUNCH
Chicken Caesar Wrap (page 281)
1 small pear

SNACK
Choose any from snack list (page 344)

DINNER
Pepper-Crusted Beef Tenderloin with Horseradish Sauce (page 317)
1 cup fresh raspberries
1 cup steamed broccoli
1 medium slice sourdough bread

TRADITIONAL MEAL PLAN, WEEK 2
1,200–1,400 Calorie Level

DAY 4

BREAKFAST
Whole-Wheat Pecan Muffins (page 249)
½ cup nonfat milk

LUNCH
Tuna Salad in Tomato (page 327)
½ nonfat vanilla yogurt with 1 tablespoon chopped
    walnuts
2 slices rye bread

SNACK
Choose any from snack list (page 344)

DINNER
Pork Medallions with Orange-Rosemary Sauce
    (page 319)
Green Beans Provençal (page 267)
¼ cup couscous (measured dry; ½ cup cooked)
1 nectarine

DAY 5

BREAKFAST
Banana Bread (page 235)
½ cup nonfat milk

LUNCH
Maryland Crab Cakes (page 316)
2 slices fresh pineapple
Spinach-Pear Salad (page 279)

SNACK
Choose any from snack list (page 344)

DINNER
Grilled Shrimp (page 313)
15 spears steamed asparagus drizzled with ½
    tablespoon garlic-flavored olive oil
¼ cup sticky white rice (measured dry; ½ cup cooked)
1 cup fresh raspberries

DAY 6

BREAKFAST
Fruit smoothie with flaxseed (½ cup orange juice,
    4-ounces nonfat plain yogurt, ½ banana,
    1 tablespoon ground flaxseed, mixed in blender
    until smooth)

LUNCH
Turkey on a bagel (2-ounce whole-grain bagel,
    3 ounces lower-sodium deli turkey, 2 tomato
    slices, 1 ounce low-fat Cheddar cheese,
    1 tablespoon reduced-fat mayonnaise)
1 medium apple

SNACK
Choose any from snack list (page 344)

DINNER
Potato-Crusted Salmon (page 321)
Broccoli Salad (page 257)
1 medium apple

DAY 7

BREAKFAST
¼ cup dry oatmeal cooked with ¾ cup soy milk
¾ cup blueberries

LUNCH
Tuna Melt on English Muffin (page 289)
1 medium red bell pepper, sliced, with 2 tablespoons
    hummus

SNACK
Choose any from snack list (page 344)

DINNER
Mediterranean Wrap (page 287)
1 cup reduced-sodium minestrone soup
1 nectarine

TRADITIONAL MEAL PLAN, WEEK 2
1,400–1,600 Calorie Level

DAY 1

BREAKFAST
French Toast (page 240)
¾ cup soy milk

LUNCH
Ham sandwich on whole-wheat bread, with 3 ounces
    lean lower-sodium ham, 2 ounces low-fat
    Cheddar cheese, 2 tomato slices, 1 lettuce leaf
½ medium banana with ½ cup nonfat vanilla yogurt

SNACK
Choose any from snack list (page 344)

DINNER
Pork Tenderloin with Apple Chutney (page 320)
Mediterranean Couscous (page 334)

DAY 2

BREAKFAST
2-ounce whole-grain bagel with 2 tablespoons low-
    fat cream cheese
8 ounces plain nonfat yogurt

LUNCH
Tuna Salad on Pita (page 290)
Cucumber-Tomato Salad (page 266)
2 large carrots, cut into pieces, or 1 cup baby carrots

SNACK
Choose any from snack list (page 344)

DINNER
Pesto Pasta (page 335)
Broccoli with Dijon Vinaigrette (page 259)
3 ounces grilled chicken breast (boneless)
1 cup fresh raspberries

DAY 3

BREAKFAST
½ cup nonfat vanilla yogurt with 1 cup fresh or
    frozen pineapple, plus ½ tablespoon sliced
    almonds
½ whole-wheat English muffin, toasted
½ tablespoon trans-fat-free margarine

LUNCH
Chicken Caesar Wrap (page 281)
1 small pear
1 large carrot, sliced

SNACK
Choose any from snack list (page 344)

DINNER
Pepper-Crusted Beef Tenderloin with Horseradish
    Sauce (page 317)
1 cup fresh raspberries
1 cup steamed broccoli
2 medium slices of sourdough bread

DAY 4

BREAKFAST
Whole-Wheat Pecan Muffins (page 249)
8 ounces plain nonfat yogurt
1 cup fresh or frozen blueberries

LUNCH
Tuna Salad in Tomato (page 327)
½ cup nonfat vanilla yogurt with 1 tablespoon
    chopped walnuts
2 slices rye bread

SNACK
Choose any from snack list (page 344)

TRADITIONAL MEAL PLAN, WEEK 2
1,400–1,600 Calorie Level

DINNER
Pork Medallions with Orange-Rosemary Sauce
    (page 319)
Green Beans Provençal (page 267)
½ cup couscous (measured dry; 1 cup cooked)
1 medium apple

DAY 5

BREAKFAST
Banana Bread (page 235)
1 cup nonfat milk

LUNCH
Maryland Crab Cakes (page 316)
2 slices fresh pineapple
Spinach-Pear Salad (page 279)
1 slice oatmeal bread

SNACK
Choose any from snack list (page 344)

DINNER
Grilled Shrimp (page 313)
15 spears steamed asparagus drizzled with
    ½ tablespoon garlic-flavored olive oil
½ cup sticky white rice (measured dry; 1 cup cooked)

DAY 6

BREAKFAST
Fruit smoothie with flaxseed (½ cup orange juice,
    6 ounces low-fat plain yogurt, ½ banana,
    2 tablespoons ground flaxseed, mixed in blender
    until smooth)

LUNCH
Turkey on a bagel (3-ounce whole-grain bagel,
    3 ounces lower-sodium deli turkey, 2 tomato
    slices, 1 ounce low-fat Cheddar cheese,
    1 tablespoon reduced-fat mayonnaise)
1 medium apple

SNACK
Choose any from snack list (page 344)

DINNER
Potato-Crusted Salmon (page 321)
Broccoli Salad (page 257)
1 medium apple
1 slice flaxseed bread

DAY 7

BREAKFAST
½ cup dry oatmeal cooked with 1 cup soy milk
¾ cup blueberries

LUNCH
Tuna Melt on English Muffin (page 289)
1 medium red bell pepper sliced, with 2 tablespoons
    hummus
1 plum

SNACK
Choose any from snack list (page 344)

DINNER
Mediterranean Wrap (page 287)
1 cup reduced-sodium minestrone soup
1 nectarine

MODERATE CARBOHYDRATE MEAL PLAN, WEEK 2
1,200–1,400 Calorie Level

DAY 1

BREAKFAST
1 slice whole-wheat toast, 2 ounces lean lower-
    sodium ham, and 1 ounce low-fat cheese
½ cup fresh strawberries

LUNCH
Chicken and Wild Rice (page 300)
1 small orange
1 medium red bell pepper, sliced

SNACK
Choose any from snack list (page 344)

DINNER
Crab-Stuffed Whitefish (page 306)
Roasted Vegetables with Olive Oil and Feta Cheese
    (page 273)

DAY 2

BREAKFAST
½ small whole-grain bagel
1 tablespoon natural peanut butter
½ cup nonfat milk

LUNCH
Open-Faced Ham and Turkey Reuben
    (page 288)
Spinach–Cherry Tomato Salad (page 278)

SNACK
Choose any from snack list (page 344)

DINNER
Chicken Marsala (page 304)
⅛ cup wild rice (measured dry; ¼ cup cooked)
1 cup steamed cauliflower

DAY 3

BREAKFAST
Blueberry, Banana, and Flaxseed Smoothie
    (page 237)
Scrambled Egg Substitute with Peppers (page 245)

LUNCH
Veggie Cheeseburger (page 293)
½ cup baby carrots with 1 tablespoon hummus

SNACK
Choose any from snack list (page 344)

DINNER
Pork Chops with Bourbon Mustard Glaze
    (page 318)
Onion Ragout (page 270)
Rice Pilaf with Carrots (page 336)

DAY 4

BREAKFAST
Open-Faced Egg and Ham Sandwich (page 243)
1 small orange

LUNCH
Green Salad with Chicken, Avocado, Orange
    Segments, and Fat-Free Honey Dressing
    (page 268)

SNACK
Choose any from snack list (page 344)

DINNER
Garlic Rosemary Roasted Chicken (page 310)
Roasted Ratatouille (page 272)
1 slice cracked-wheat bread

MODERATE CARBOHYDRATE MEAL PLAN, WEEK 2
1,200–1,400 Calorie Level

DAY 5

BREAKFAST
Spinach and Cheese Omelet (page 247)
1 cup fresh raspberries

LUNCH
Turkey Roll-up with Vinaigrette (page 292)
½ cup nonfat vanilla yogurt

SNACK
Choose any from snack list (page 344)

DINNER
Fiesta Chicken Salad (page 309)
Spinach Salad with Avocado and Pear (page 276)
½ whole-wheat pita

DAY 6

BREAKFAST
Fruit salad with cottage cheese and almonds
    (¾ cup low-fat cottage cheese, ½ cup fresh or
    frozen blueberries, ½ cup fresh raspberries,
    1½ tablespoons sliced almonds)

LUNCH
Chef Salad with Turkey and Ham (page 260)
½ cup nonfat plain yogurt with 1 cup strawberry
    halves

SNACK
Choose any from snack list (page 344)

DINNER
Eggplant Parmigiana (page 307)
Grilled Flank Steak (page 311)

DAY 7

BREAKFAST
Eggs and Turkey Bacon (1 egg plus ¼ cup egg
    substitute scrambled, with 2 slices turkey bacon)
1 small orange

LUNCH
Chicken Hummus Wrap (page 283)
1 medium peach

SNACK
Choose any from snack list (page 344)

DINNER
Teriyaki Tuna Loin with Wasabi Butter and Braised
    Bok Choy (page 326)
Coconut Rice (page 333)
2 cups wilted spinach

MODERATE CARBOHYDRATE MEAL PLAN, WEEK 2
1,400–1,600 Calorie Level

DAY 1

BREAKFAST

1 slice whole-wheat toast, 2 ounces lean lower-
   sodium ham, and 1 ounce low-fat cheese

½ cup fresh strawberries

½ cup fresh raspberries

LUNCH

Chicken and Wild Rice (page 300)

1 small orange

1 medium red bell pepper, sliced, with 2 tablespoons
   hummus

SNACK

Choose any from snack list (page 344)

DINNER

Crab-Stuffed Whitefish (page 306)

Roasted Vegetables with Olive Oil and Feta Cheese
   (page 273)

Blue Cheese and Chive Potato Salad (page 332)

DAY 2

BREAKFAST

½ small whole-grain bagel

1 tablespoon natural peanut butter

½ cup nonfat milk

LUNCH

Ham and Turkey Reuben (page 286)

Spinach–Cherry Tomato Salad (page 278)

SNACK

Choose any from snack list (page 344)

DINNER

Chicken Marsala (page 304)

¼ cup wild rice (measured dry; ½ cup cooked)

1 cup steamed cauliflower

DAY 3

BREAKFAST

Blueberry, Banana, and Flaxseed Smoothie
   (page 237)

Scrambled Egg with Red Pepper (page 246)

LUNCH

Veggie Cheeseburger (page 293)

½ cup baby carrots with 1 tablespoon hummus

4 ounces nonfat vanilla yogurt

SNACK

Choose any from snack list (page 344)

DINNER

Pork Chops with Bourbon Mustard Glaze (page 318)

Onion Ragout (page 270)

Rice Pilaf with Carrots (page 336)

1 small apple

DAY 4

BREAKFAST

Open-Faced Egg, Ham, and Cheese Sandwich
   (page 243)

½ cup fresh raspberries

½ cup fresh strawberries

LUNCH

Green Salad with Chicken, Avocado, Orange
   Segments, and Fat-Free Honey Dressing
   (page 268)

½ cup raspberries and ½ cup strawberries, halved

SNACK

Choose any from snack list (page 344)

DINNER

Garlic Rosemary Roasted Chicken (page 310)

Roasted Ratatouille (page 272)

Sautéed Cabbage (page 275)

1 slice cracked-wheat bread

MODERATE CARBOHYDRATE MEAL PLAN, WEEK 2
1,400–1,600 Calorie Level

DAY 5

BREAKFAST
Spinach and Cheese Omelet (see recipe page 247, but use 2 ounces cheese)
1 cup fresh raspberries

LUNCH
Turkey Roll-up with Vinaigrette (page 292)
½ cup nonfat vanilla yogurt

SNACK
Choose any from snack list (page 344)

DINNER
Fiesta Chicken Salad (page 309)
Spinach Salad with Avocado and Pear (page 276, but use a whole pear)
½ whole-wheat pita

DAY 6

BREAKFAST
Fruit salad with cottage cheese and almonds (¾ cup low-fat cottage cheese, ½ cup fresh or frozen blueberries, ½ cup fresh raspberries, 1½ tablespoons sliced almonds)

LUNCH
Chef Salad with Turkey and Ham (page 260)
½ cup nonfat plain yogurt with 1 cup strawberry halves

SNACK
Choose any from snack list (page 344)

DINNER
Eggplant Parmigiana (page 307)
Grilled Flank Steak (page 311)

DAY 7

BREAKFAST
Eggs and Turkey Bacon (1 egg plus ¼ cup egg substitute, scrambled, with 2 slices turkey bacon)
½ cup fresh strawberries
4 ounces nonfat vanilla yogurt

LUNCH
Chicken Hummus Wrap (page 283)
½ cup baby carrots with 2 tablespoons reduced-fat dressing

SNACK
Choose any from snack list (page 344)

DINNER
Teriyaki Tuna Loin with Wasabi Butter and Braised Bok Choy (page 326)
Coconut Rice (page 333)
Asian Sesame Salad (page 256)

YOUR WEEK 2 EXERCISE ROUTINE

For Week 2, continue to follow your Week 1 regimen. We bet you're starting to get used to it, and we hope you're starting to enjoy it. It might be fun to try a new exercise, like cycling or swimming, if you've been walking so far. And, of course, don't forget to keep track of your progress on your copy of the monitoring card in chapter 5 or in your Lifestyle Journal on www.dukediet.com.

EATING WITH AWARENESS

One reason we may overeat is excessive hunger. Getting hungry is natural—it's getting *too* hungry that's a problem. The trick is to keep your appetite in balance, and eat when your hunger is in the moderate range. To help you find that range, we use a technique called the Hunger-Fullness Scale. Whenever you feel like eating, you simply pause and rate your hunger level. Then you can decide, consciously, whether it's food (and how much) or something else that you really crave.

Another reason that we tend to overeat is distraction. Have you ever bought popcorn at a movie theater and then, halfway through the film, discovered that it was all gone, though you could barely remember eating it? Most of us probably have. When we're absorbed in something else while we eat, it can be hard to keep track of what we're putting in our mouths.

So when you're watching your weight, it pays to eat with awareness, or *mindfully*. That means staying in the moment, enjoying each mouthful, and tuning in to your body's sensations of diminishing hunger, increasing satisfaction, and satiety. We see a lot of patients who struggle to lose weight because, for whatever reason (including distractions like driving, reading, and watching TV while eating), they've stopped noticing their bodies' natural cues. One of this week's Assignments for Success will be working with the Hunger-Fullness Scale to improve your ability to eat with awareness.

Here are some of the strategies that our clients find helpful for increasing

THE HUNGER-FULLNESS SCALE						
Very Hungry	Moderately Hungry	Mildly Hungry	No Feeling (Neutral)	Mildly Full	Very Full	Much Too Full
1	2	3	4	5	6	7

Desirable Zone 2.5–5.5

Interpreting the Scale

1. Very hungry: At this level, you feel ravenous, even desperate to eat. Your stomach is howling for food, and that's all you can think about. When you get food, you're at risk for overeating.

2. Moderately hungry: You're ready to eat and might even feel a bit lightheaded and irritable. Your stomach may be "talking," signaling you with hunger pangs.

3. Mildly hungry: At this level, your stomach is only whispering. You're planning to eat, perhaps within the next hour.

4. No feeling (neutral): You could eat or not—it doesn't matter. You are not really hungry.

5. Mildly full: You feel comfortable and satisfied. You've had just enough to eat, and if you had more, you'd start to feel stuffed.

6. Very full: You've had a few bites too many, and your waistband is starting to pinch.

7. Much too full: You are stuffed to the bursting point and may even be in pain.

We encourage you to try to stay within the shaded area on the scale, between 2.5 and 5.5. Try not to let your level of hunger dip as low as 1, when you're so ravenous that you could eat a horse, saddle and all. On the flip side, try never to let your level of fullness get as high as 7.

awareness of what and how much they eat, as well as for heightening enjoyment of meals.

• Eat only when you're seated at your kitchen or dining room table, with the TV off and with no reading material. Don't eat while standing over the sink, straight out of the refrigerator, on the couch in front of the TV, or in your bed.

• Make your meals pleasant occasions, with nice place mats or a tablecloth and napkins, real plates instead of take-out containers, and real, not plastic, silverware.

• Don't talk too much while eating. It's nice to have company and to enjoy the social aspects of eating, but if you get carried away with the conversation, you may eat too quickly and miss the experience completely.

• Before you start eating, take a few full, deep breaths and get ready to focus your attention on your meal. Assess where you are on the Hunger-Fullness Scale before starting to eat. Start with a moderate-sized bite, then put your knife and fork down while you chew it, fully savoring the flavors and textures. Really experience the food before you move on to the next bite.

• Pause to "check in" regularly during the meal and observe where you are on the Hunger-Fullness Scale to monitor your level of satiety.

A New Experience with Food

I came to Duke quite overweight. I'd hit my forties and thought that maybe my metabolism was slowing down, which I'd heard can happen at midlife. But the Duke program got me to focus on my behavior, not on my age. I realized that while I watched TV at night, I very often broke out the cookies and, almost without knowing it, polished off a whole box. I couldn't even remember tasting them. No wonder I'd gained weight!

So I began learning and practicing how to eat mindfully. I kept the TV off while eating and made a rule: I could eat only at my kitchen and dining room tables. I ate slowly and tried to concentrate on enjoying my food. It made a huge difference. I have truly learned to enjoy and savor my food. I get so much more pleasure out of it now!

—*Teresa, age 43*

• When you reach 5.5 on the Hunger-Fullness Scale, push away your plate and get up from the table. Remember that it can take your brain as long as fifteen to twenty minutes to register satiety. Any lingering hunger or cravings you have will quickly pass.

Keep in mind that you can have the experience of working on eating with awareness with the Duke Diet & Fitness Center behavioral health staff at home with our self-awareness CD, which can be purchased at www.dukediet.com.

KNOW YOUR EATING TRIGGERS

Ideally, we'd eat only when our appetites dipped to 2.5 on the Hunger-Fullness Scale. But hunger pangs are just one of the many factors that spur us to eat. Many of us have trigger foods—often, but not always, these are foods that are laden with fat, sugar, or salt and that we find irresistible, like dough-nuts, chocolate, pizza, and chips. They're the kind of foods that seem so dif-ficult to control once we start to eat them. We may also be triggered to eat for emotional reasons like enjoyment or gratification of unmet needs and to re-lieve stress (which we'll take up in chapter 8). Or we may just be prompted by the "eat this" messages that barrage us all day long: the muffins in the of-fice break room, the smell of a coworker's French fries, or the taco and burger chain commercials on TV.

Although urges to eat seem to strike us without warning, we see in many of our clients that these urges are actually fairly predictable, arising at certain times of day, in certain social or work situations, or in what we call "high-risk situations," including periods of stress and emotional upheaval. Becoming aware of your own patterns of urges can help you nip them in the bud. Here are some of the most common triggers we see and some examples of strate-gies to counter them.

Trigger: Unmanaged hunger, which leads to overeating.
Strategy: Avoid going longer than four or five hours between meals or snacks. It's better to eat a 100- to 200-calorie snack in the afternoon than to get so hungry that you eat 400 to 800 extra calories at dinner.

Trigger: Time of day, especially the transition from work to home.
Strategy: Plan a healthy snack right before you leave the office to take the edge off your hunger when you are most at risk of indulging.

Trigger: Unstructured time, which is filled by eating.
Strategy: Brainstorm ideas for possible activities to fill your free time. Pick things you can do in five or ten minutes—a crossword or Sudoku puzzle, a quick walk, a phone call to a friend, or the like. Write these ideas on individual strips of paper and put them into a jar

Thin Really Isn't "In"

One of my clients, Janet, a forty-two-year-old who has lost thirty-two pounds and kept them off for several years, tells me that for her, practicing trigger awareness and mindful eating was the key. She follows the guidelines from the Calories and Portions class at the Duke Diet & Fitness Center and fills half her plate with proteins and starch and the other half with nonstarchy vegetables. She focuses on the strategies for mindful eating that she learned at Duke and has significantly reduced her intake of junk food. She tells an illuminating story about how, while watching TV one night, she found herself drawn to the refrigerator and wondered what was going on—after all, she'd eaten just a short time previously.

Thinking back, she realized that she'd just watched a commercial with a stick-thin model. "I'll never look like that," she thought, "so why even bother to lose weight?" That was the trigger for what she experienced as "hunger."

Once she caught herself, she realized that she didn't even really believe that thin was so "in"—that anything but model-level skinniness was pointless. It's so easy to fall into these media-triggered traps, yet just a moment's reflection for a reality check allowed her to make the choice not to indulge in food she really didn't want or need.

—*Lucie Knapp, M.S.W., Behavioral Health Clinician
at the Duke Diet & Fitness Center*

Structure for Success

Bouts of unplanned eating strike with varying intensity, as the diagram below shows. On one end of the continuum the overeating is modest, and the feeling of being out of control is only mild. In the middle is triggered overeating, which occurs in response to an environmental cue, an emotional upset, stress, and so on. At this level, the feeling of loss of control is stronger. At the other end of the scale is what most people describe as binge eating. When binge eating, you feel very out of control. You may eat an unusually large amount of food in a short period of time, even if you're not hungry, to the point that you're uncomfortably full—and possibly experience significant guilt.

Unplanned Eating   **Triggered Overeating**   **Binge Eating**

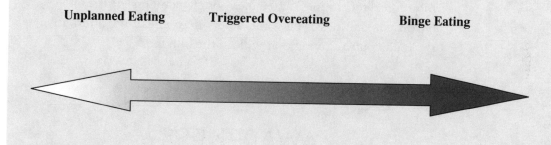

The first step in reducing unplanned eating is to structure your meal schedule, eating breakfast, lunch, dinner, and at least one snack at regularly spaced intervals and around the same time every day. If you know when you can expect to eat, you're less likely to eat off plan. Of course, if your nutritional balance is adequate and you don't let yourself get too hungry, that helps a lot, too. We will be walking you through more steps to break the unplanned eating cycle a little later.

labeled "Quick Healthy Distractions." Then make a list of activities that take a little longer—say, thirty minutes to an hour—like reading a magazine or a few chapters of a book, writing in a journal, playing computer solitaire or Scrabble, giving yourself a manicure or a home facial, working on a crafts project you enjoy like scrapbooking, surprising your spouse by vacuuming out the car, playing a board game with your kids, and so on. Put these ideas into a second "Longer Healthy Distractions" jar.

Then, when you hit a period of unstructured time, instead of reaching for the cookie jar, pull an idea out of one of these jars and act on it. One of the members of the behavioral health team at Duke, Marit Derrer, conducts a workshop in which clients actually convert a cookie jar into a "Healthy Distractions" jar. The exercise has become very popular. In fact, many participants say it has become a metaphor for reinventing themselves!

Trigger: A sense of deprivation.

Strategy: Plan in advance to include appropriate portions of the foods you love in your diet so that you avoid feeling deprived. Focus on the mouth feel (creaminess, chewiness, or crunchiness) or the taste (sweetness, saltiness) you want. There may a healthier alternative to the food you're craving that will fill the bill, too.

DEVELOP NUTRITIONAL AWARENESS

As you already know, a balanced diet is one of the keys to good health, and the Duke Diet Nutrition Plan offers you a full palette of nutrients and encourages you to enjoy a wide variety of foods. Remember that our meal plans include lots of healthy alternatives for you to choose from. We also think you might be interested to learn that there is evidence that certain "power foods" have special properties that promote health and fend off disease, so it might be worth working them into your diet on a regular basis—while staying calorie conscious, of course.

The Top Eight Power Foods

1. Blueberries: The Sweet, High-Fiber Treat. Not only are blueberries a tasty alternative to sugary desserts, they are also on the list of fruits and vegetables rich in antioxidants, which are thought to protect against cancer and heart disease. The pigment anthocyanin, found in the blueberry's skin, not only gives the berry its distinct color but also exerts an anti-inflammatory effect in blood vessels, which may be important for cardiovascular health. Fruits with similar properties are red grapes, blackberries, cherries, raspberries, boysenberries, and strawberries. Out of season, frozen are good too—just make sure there's no added sugar.

2. Broccoli: Green Power! Broccoli is a good source of nutrients such as vitamins B, C, E, and K; the minerals calcium, iron, selenium, and potassium; and fiber. All of these appear to play important roles in maintaining good health, protecting against certain cancers, heart disease, stroke, and macular degeneration; helping to build strong bones; and fortifying the immune system.

3. Dark Chocolate: The New Health Food? You might have heard in the news that this sweet treat may provide some heart-healthy benefits. Of course, chocolate should be incorporated into a meal plan in moderation because, as you are well aware, it's high in calories and fat. But certain phytochemicals found in cocoa powder, as well as stearic acid, the saturated fat in chocolate, may reduce heart disease risk by modestly increasing levels of HDL ("good") cholesterol. Chocolate's phytochemicals may also help lower blood pressure by relaxing blood vessel walls. However, these health benefits appear to be found only in dark chocolate, not in milk or white chocolate—and the darker, the better.

4. Eggs: The Tidy Protein Package. Eggs, which are an excellent source of protein, vitamins, and minerals, definitely have a place in a balanced diet. At one time we thought that the cholesterol in eggs was a major contributor to high levels of blood cholesterol, but now we know that it is saturated fat that is the more likely culprit. Meat and full-fat dairy foods are rich sources of saturated fat; eggs much less so. Still, those who have higher-than-desirable levels of cholesterol would be well advised to limit their consumption to no more than four whole eggs per week. Try stretching one whole egg with two egg whites to get many of the nutritional benefits of eggs with less cholesterol.

5. Fish: Lean Protein and Omega-3s. Fish is a great, lean protein, but it has more to offer than that. Fattier fishes contain omega-3 fatty acids, which reduce the triglycerides in the blood that have been linked to heart disease and also decrease the buildup of arterial plaque. Omega-3s can help lower blood pressure and reduce the risk of disturbances of heart rhythm. The American Heart Association recommends that people eat fatty fish (such as tuna, salmon, mackerel, or herring) twice a week to reap these benefits. Keep in mind, however, that as we said in chapter 2, certain fish are more likely to carry pollutants and should be eaten in limited quantities.

6. Low-Fat Milk: Not Just for Strong Bones. A nutrient-rich beverage, milk provides a variety of vitamins and minerals, including several B vitamins, vitamins C and D, calcium, magnesium, phosphorous, and zinc. In an effort to encourage people to consume dairy products at least three times a day, the National Dairy Council has launched a campaign highlighting calcium's positive effects on bone strength and also its "potential" to promote weight loss. The weight management claim is controversial. While some experts feel that milk may not be an appropriate beverage choice for adults, we believe that it's healthy to include moderate amounts of low-fat dairy products (including milk) as part of a balanced diet.

7. Nuts: Home to Healthy Fats. In the past, nuts were downplayed as a high-calorie, high-fat food likely to sabotage any diet. Today we know that the monounsaturated fats in nuts can help improve cholesterol levels and heart health. Also, the omega-3 fatty acids found in nuts may relax blood vessels, reduce the risk of clotting, and improve blood flow. None of these great benefits change the fact that nuts are calorie dense, so it's wise to enjoy them in moderation (a *small* cupped handful contains about 150 calories and is plenty). As always, read labels and try to enjoy nuts with minimal added salt and without the additional calories that come from treatments such as honey-roasting.

8. Oats: The Heart-Healthy Fiber Food. Oats contain soluble fiber, which binds to cholesterol and carries it from the body. In fact, one of the first health claims approved by the U.S. Food and Drug Administration for food labels holds that 3 grams of soluble fiber daily, as part of a diet low in saturated fat and cholesterol, may reduce the risk of heart disease. So oats are an excellent breakfast choice. Just be sure to check the label on the carton to see how much soluble fiber you're actually getting.

What's Not on Our Power Foods List

If you've seen articles on the top power foods, you may have noticed that we're omitting two that are often listed. One is protein-rich soy, which is lower in saturated fat than most meat and dairy sources of protein and doesn't contain cholesterol. Soy is currently being studied for its influence on bone health, the symptoms of menopause, and the development of breast cancer, and so far the results have been inconclusive.

The most controversial area of study is the potential link between soy and breast cancer. Certain phytoestrogens in soy, called isoflavones, may either block or promote breast cancer growth—and researchers are not yet sure which. For most people, it's probably fine to consume soy products such as reduced-fat soy milk, soy cheese, or meat substitutes in moderate quantities three or four times a week. But if you have a history of breast cancer or think you may be at increased risk, we suggest that you talk to your doctor about whether to incorporate soy into your diet and, if so, how much.

Our second omission from our power foods list is wine, which is often touted for its supposed health benefits as an antioxidant. Alcohol in general is thought to boost HDL, or "good," cholesterol. However, given its high calorie density, other potentially unhealthy consequences of alcohol use, and the inconclusive findings concerning its health benefits, we've chosen not to promote it as a power food. We do recognize, however, that in moderation, alcohol can be part of a healthy nutrition plan.

Which antioxidant drinks promote heart health for fewer calories? Try one to three cups of green or black tea per day.

EXERCISE WITH AWARENESS

You can enhance your workouts the same way you do your meals if you truly focus on the experience. Concentrate on what your body is doing and how it feels. While it can be helpful to fire up your iPod and listen to music while you work out, we suggest you try to avoid distraction once in a while and concentrate on the pleasurable release that comes with exercise—the ebb of stress and muscular tension and the lifting of your spirits. Mindful exercise engages the whole person—mind, body, and spirit.

Here are some ways to make your workout more mindful.

• See your workouts as a healthy escape from everyday life and worries. Work out in comfortable surroundings, wear comfortable clothes, and enjoy yourself.

• Set a performance goal (number of minutes, sets, reps, and so on) for each workout. This will help improve your focus and motivation. Ask yourself, *What do I hope this workout will help me gain? Do I want to feel more centered and calm? Less stressed out? Better able to sleep tonight?*

• Monitor your exertion using the RPE scale we described in chapter 3 to regulate the intensity of your aerobic workout. Remember that your target on the scale lies between 11 and 14, the moderate-intensity level. In chapter 3, we also described the talk test, which indicates that you should be able to carry on a conversation while exercising at moderate intensity. If you cannot only talk but sing, your intensity level is too low; if you're too winded to talk comfortably, your intensity level is too high.

If you prefer, you can use the heart rate monitor that is built into many gym exercise machines, including treadmills, stationary bikes, and elliptical trainers. Some of them are automatically programmed to compute your maximum heart rate, which is the rate your heart would be beating each minute if you were running at top speed, and target heart rate, which corresponds to moderate intensity on the RPE scale.

• Be mindful of proper form during strength training. Focus on the muscle you're working, and if it doesn't feel engaged, adjust your position or change the amount of weight or resistance. Always use slow, controlled movements instead of letting gravity pull down your weights or elasticity snap back your resistance tubes, and keep your body erect, without straining. The exercise instructions in chapter 10 and on www.dukediet.com will tell you more about proper form.

Your Target Heart Rate

At Duke we like to use either the RPE scale or the talk test to gauge the intensity of exercise because they are intuitive and simple. But like many of our clients, you may have heard that heart rate is the key. If you want to calculate your target heart rate, start by determining your resting heart rate. The first thing in the morning is the best time to do it. With your palm facing up, place two fingers lightly on the thumb side of your wrist and find your pulse. Using the second hand on your watch or a digital clock to keep time, count how many times your pulse beats in thirty seconds. Multiply by two to get your resting heart rate. The typical range is sixty to a hundred beats a minute. Just to give us an example to work with, let's say yours is 75.

Next, estimate your maximum heart rate by subtracting your age from 220. For example, if you're forty-five years old, your maximum heart rate is $220 - 45 = 175$.

Then, subtract your resting heart rate from your maximum heart rate to get what's called your *heart rate reserve*. The heart rate reserve for the preceding example numbers would be $175 - 75 = 100$.

Next, use your heart rate reserve to calculate your target heart rate range. If you're a beginning exerciser, first multiply your heart rate reserve by 40 percent, then multiply the same number by 60 percent:

$$100 \times .40 = 40$$
$$100 \times .60 = 60$$

Next, add each of these results to your resting heart rate:

$$75 + 40 = 115$$
$$75 + 60 = 135$$

Thus, the low end of your exercise range is 115 pulse beats per minute, while the higher end of the range is 135 pulse beats per minute.

If you're a more experienced exerciser, you may want to work out at a higher intensity. In this case, first multiply your heart rate reserve by 60 percent, then multiply the same number by 85 percent. Add each result to your resting heart rate to get the high and low end of your target heart rate range.

$$100 \times .60 = 60; 75 + 60 = 135$$
$$100 \times .85 = 85; 75 + 85 = 160$$

So your goal would be to stay within 135 to 160 beats per minute.

If your resting heart rate is higher or lower than the typical range, talk to your doctor about how to progress toward a moderate-intensity level of exercise. And remember that exercising regularly is more important than exercising in a precise range.

• Don't hold your breath during exercise. Breathing helps you focus on the muscle you're working, calms your mind, and helps banish stress. During strength and resistance training, *inhale* just before you begin to exert force, then *exhale* during the exertion phase of the exercise. Keep your breathing and movements synchronized and rhythmic.

• Listen to your body. Do you feel energized as certain muscles contract and expand? Do you feel pain? If the discomfort is minimal and tolerable, try adjusting your technique or posture to see if it eases up. If you are experiencing more than mild to moderate discomfort, stop immediately.

• As you exercise, try to "stay in the moment." Successful athletes often talk about being "in the zone," meaning they're so absorbed in the ex-

Should I Work through Pain While Exercising?

No one should work through pain. Exercise often causes a tolerable level of discomfort, but pain is something else!

You should also stop or ease up if your breathing gets very labored. Try the talk test. If you can't get out a sentence without gulping for air, you're working too hard.

If you get a cramp or a stitch in your side while working out, it may be caused by dehydration. Take a break, drink some water, stretch, and then resume your routine. But don't overlook any severe, persistent, or recurring pain or tightness in your chest, neck, jaw, or even shoulder or arm that occurs during or immediately after exercise. Sometimes people mistakenly blame exercise-associated chest discomfort on indigestion. These symptoms could be a sign of a serious heart problem, and they should be promptly evaluated by a physician.

Many people who are overweight have joint pain from arthritis. Though you might think that exertion would worsen the problem, lack of exercise often contributes to arthritis. The proper kinds of exercise can be powerfully beneficial for those who suffer from arthritis by strengthening the surrounding muscles that support the joint, thereby reducing impact and strain on the joint. If you have significant arthritis, consult your health care professional, who can provide you with guidance regarding the most appropriate types of exercise. Generally speaking, water exercise and other activities that are low impact are best for people with arthritis.

ercise that they seem to move through it without thinking—they are just focused on doing. The result: They push themselves harder and burn more calories.

• Stay consistent. It's natural to want to skip workouts once in a while, but if you keep to a regular exercise schedule, it will be easier to stay motivated.

ASSIGNMENTS FOR SUCCESS: WEEK 2

Eat with Awareness

You don't have to eat every meal methodically for the rest of your life, but it will help if, whenever possible, you take the time to focus on the awareness techniques we have outlined. This week, try to use the Hunger-Fullness Scale to tune in to your body's true hunger and satiety signals. Keep in mind that the scale is subjective, so one person's ravenous hunger might be more or less intense than someone else's. Experiment and learn where your own moderate-hunger (2.5 on the scale) and satisfaction (5.5 on the scale) points lie. Use these steps:

1. As mealtime approaches, listen to your body and assess your appetite level, using the Hunger-Fullness Scale.
2. Concentrate on your food as you eat. With each bite, close your eyes. Focus on the aroma, texture, and taste of your food.
3. Chew slowly, paying attention to how the food feels in your mouth.
4. Savor and completely swallow each bite before reaching out for the next.
5. Remember that it may take twenty minutes for your brain to register satiety. Slow yourself down by resting your utensils against your

plate between bites and pause midway through the meal to give your brain a chance to catch up with your stomach.

6. Throughout the meal, keep checking your hunger-fullness level using the scale.

7. When you reach 5.5 on the scale, the comfortably full level, stop eating—even if there's still food on your plate—and get up from the table.

Know Your Trigger Foods

It's common sense that the more you restrict your diet, the more deprived you'll eventually feel, and the more likely to rebel. That's why we encourage you to eat a variety of foods and, where possible, to include small amounts of even some of the higher-calorie favorites you enjoy. There are no bad or forbidden foods on the Duke Diet Nutrition Plan. As long as you count calories and follow your plan, you can have all foods in moderation. But if there are certain trigger foods—most of us have them—that are difficult to control or may prompt you to overeat, it's good to pinpoint them and rank them according to the danger they represent. Then you can approach them as you would any other challenge, by setting specific goals and learning skills to control them.

Start by listing your trigger foods on the following worksheet. It may be wise to avoid your trigger foods until you have a firm grounding in the Duke program. Then as you become more confident, you can begin to reintegrate them one at a time, starting with the least challenging foods in column 1, then moving on to column 2, and so on. When you are ready, select a food from the list and portion out just a small amount. As you eat the food, do so mindfully as we described earlier, taking small, deliberate bites and fully savoring the flavors and textures of the food. You will be encouraged each time you handle what was once a difficult food, and eventually the power that food has over you will diminish.

It's very likely that there are some foods you fear you will never be able to control. Don't worry, you don't have to tackle them right now. Don't say you'll "never" eat them again—just say "not now." For added support, we

MY TRIGGER FOODS

1. FOODS THAT ARE SLIGHT TRIGGERS:	2. FOODS THAT FEEL LESS SAFE, WHICH I FEAR MAY TRIGGER A BINGE:	3. FOODS THAT FEEL VERY UNSAFE, WHICH I AM VERY FEARFUL COULD TRIGGER A BINGE:

have included a trigger foods exercise on our awareness CD, which is available at www.dukediet.com.

Control Cravings

Cravings can strike at any time. We have seen many people learn to understand and control cravings and stop them from interfering with their weight control efforts. This week, try some or all of the following strategies to manage your own cravings.

• Make sure that your home is free of foods that might trigger a binge and that healthy alternatives are always on hand. If food commercials make you feel vulnerable, get up and walk around—it's exercise!

• If a craving strikes, try to figure out its source. Ask yourself: *Do I need food or something else?* If you recognize the source of your craving, you can fight it.

• When you're tempted to succumb to a craving, distract yourself for a few minutes by doing something relaxing and positive. Try jotting your feelings down in a journal or calling a friend for support. You will be surprised at how quickly the craving evaporates.

• Surf the urge. Cravings and urges build like waves in the ocean and then suddenly crest and fall. Cravings lessen in intensity with time— especially if you distract yourself. So when you feel a craving, try to ride it out like a surfer rides a wave. Tell yourself that you'll wait for five or ten minutes—and if necessary, add another five or ten minutes—to see if the urge passes. While you wait, do something else, like calling a friend, logging on to the message boards on www.dukediet.com, or taking a walk. Brushing your teeth is a great distraction, too—nothing tastes good after brushing your teeth.

• Plan to include a small portion of the food you crave as a substitution in your meal plan later in the week. Sometimes the promise of having the craved food is all you need to break the craving.

• Practice deep breathing. Deep breathing allows you to pause, which delays acting on your craving, but it can also help you relax and control the emotions triggering it. Just follow these instructions:

Relax by Breathing

1. Assume a relaxed posture, with your feet flat on the floor, your hands in your lap, your head facing forward, and your neck relaxed.
2. Close your eyes, or focus your gaze at a fixed point in front of you. Exhale.
3. Breathe in slowly, counting the breaths (1, 2, 3, 4 . . .).
4. Let your stomach rise as you inhale, and feel your chest fill with air.
5. Now exhale slowly, counting as you exhale (1, 2, 3, 4 . . .) and saying the word *relax*.
6. Repeat steps 3 through 6 for several minutes—and feel the relief.

• Try talking yourself through the urge. Tell yourself: *This urge won't last forever. I am in control. I am feeling uncomfortable but I can wait this out. Giving in might make me feel better for the moment, but it could leave me feeling worse in the long run. Eating for relief will not really help me solve problems.*

CHAPTER SEVEN

Week 3: Staying Motivated

Week 3—you're halfway through the core program! You've no doubt been taking lots of new, positive steps, and we hope you've seen what a difference even small changes can make. The halfway point seems like a natural time to review your big and small triumphs, and take the time to appreciate them. It is also a good time to step back and consider some of the more common obstacles that our patients tell us they find challenging to deal with. Later, in the Assignment for Success, we'll offer an exercise to help you overcome some of these.

CELEBRATING YOUR SUCCESSES

Let's start off on a positive note. Before moving on to the meal plans, we want you to pause and celebrate your success so far. What's changed since you began the program? Specifically, how have your eating and exercise habits improved? What new behavioral strategies have paid off? Are you feeling a little more confident in your workouts? Do you feel more energetic, stronger, more optimistic? Do your clothes seem to be fitting more comfortably? We tend to spend so much time solving perceived problems, planning to avoid getting off track, or looking for potential barriers that we forget to stop and smell the roses. So please pause and reflect on all the things that are getting better. Take a moment to jot them down on a piece of paper and hang on to it. Periodically, review it and add to it. Then, on a day when you are struggling, try looking it over to remind yourself of all the benefits you have experienced. It will help you stay motivated!

Now let's have a look at the Nutrition and Exercise Plans for Week 3.

WEEK 3 MEAL PLANS

Remember to start your week by setting your optimal, desirable, and minimal nutrition, exercise, and behavioral goals and establishing action plans to help achieve them. Then, enjoy this week's new, healthy meal options.

TRADITIONAL MEAL PLAN, WEEK 3
1,200–1,400 Calorie Level

DAY 1	DAY 2
BREAKFAST 2-ounce whole grain bagel with 1-ounce slice low-fat cheese	**BREAKFAST** Toasted whole-grain English muffin with 2 teaspoons natural peanut butter and 1 teaspoon all-natural fruit spread
LUNCH Mediterranean Wrap (page 287) 1 medium apple	**LUNCH** 2 ounces roasted turkey breast and 2 ounces low-fat Cheddar cheese in half a whole-wheat pita spread with 2 tablespoons hummus Broccoli Slaw (page 258) ½ cup pineapple chunks
SNACK Choose any from snack list (page 344)	**SNACK** Choose any from snack list (page 344)
DINNER Eggplant Sausage Lasagna (page 308) 1-ounce wheat roll 1 cup fresh raspberries	**DINNER** Vegetarian Chili (page 255) Roasted Pepper and Goat Cheese Polenta, 2 servings (page 337) ½ cup strawberries and 1½ tablespoons of sliced almonds mixed into ½ cup nonfat plain yogurt

TRADITIONAL MEAL PLAN, WEEK 3
1,200–1,400 Calorie Level

DAY 3

BREAKFAST
Banana Walnut Pancakes (page 236)
½ tablespoon light pancake syrup
½ cup nonfat milk

LUNCH
Grilled Cheese Sandwich (page 285)
½ cup strawberry slices in ½ cup nonfat vanilla
    yogurt

SNACK
Choose any from snack list (page 344)

DINNER
Chicken Fajitas (page 302) with 2 tablespoons
    reduced-fat sour cream
10 baked tortilla chips with 1 ounce guacamole
½ cup strawberry halves

DAY 4

BREAKFAST
Apricot-Cranberry Oatmeal (page 234)

LUNCH
Chicken Fajita Salad with Creamy Cilantro-Lime
    Sauce (page 261)
Fruit salad (1 medium orange, peeled and cubed,
    1 tablespoon orange juice, ½ cup fresh raspberries)

SNACK
Choose any from snack list (page 344)

DINNER
Eggplant Parmigiana (page 307)
1 wheat roll (1 ounce) with 1 tablespoon trans-fat-free
    margarine
Sun-Dried Tomato and Roasted Garlic Soup
    (page 253)
½ cup blueberries

DAY 5

BREAKFAST
Blueberry Bran Muffin (page 238) with
    ½ tablespoon trans-fat-free margarine
2 ounces cottage cheese (2 percent fat)

LUNCH
Vegetarian Chili (page 255)
Half a banana sliced into ½ cup low-fat cottage
    cheese mixed with 3 tablespoons sliced almonds

SNACK
Choose any from snack list (page 344)

DINNER
Fiesta Chicken Salad (page 309)
1 large whole-wheat pita
1 medium red pepper, sliced, with 1 tablespoon
    vinaigrette
½ cup blueberries

DAY 6

BREAKFAST
½ cup fiber- and protein-rich cereal (such as Kashi)
    with ¾ cup soy milk

LUNCH
2 ounces roasted chicken breast
Coconut Rice (page 333)
Asian Sesame Salad, 2 servings (page 256)
1 medium apple

SNACK
Choose any from snack list (page 344)

DINNER
Chicken Fromage with Sauce (page 303)
Rice Pilaf with Carrots (page 336)
1 cup steamed broccoli
1 cup strawberry halves

TRADITIONAL MEAL PLAN, WEEK 3
1,200–1,400 Calorie Level

DAY 7

BREAKFAST
Multigrain Pancakes (page 241)
2 tablespoons light pancake syrup
½ cup nonfat milk

LUNCH
Jerk Shrimp Skewers with Tomato-Strawberry Salsa
    (page 314)
½ cup long-grain brown rice (measured dry; 1 cup
    cooked)
1 cup cherry tomatoes with 1 tablespoon vinaigrette

SNACK
Choose any from snack list (page 344)

DINNER
Potato-Crusted Salmon (page 321)
½ cup couscous (measured dry; 1 cup cooked)
1 small pear, sliced

TRADITIONAL MEAL PLAN, WEEK 3
1,400–1,600 Calorie Level

DAY 1

BREAKFAST
2-ounce whole-grain bagel with 2 ounces low-fat
    cheese

LUNCH
Mediterranean Wrap (page 287)
1 medium apple

SNACK
Choose any from snack list (page 344)

DINNER
Eggplant Sausage Lasagna (page 308)
1-ounce wheat roll
1 cup raspberries and ½ cup blueberries

DAY 2

BREAKFAST
Toasted whole-grain English muffin with 2 teaspoons
    natural peanut butter, topped with banana slices
    (½ medium banana)
½ cup nonfat milk

LUNCH
2 ounces roasted turkey breast and 2 ounces low-fat
    Cheddar cheese in half a whole-wheat pita
    spread with 2 tablespoons hummus
Broccoli Slaw (page 258)
1 cup pineapple chunks

SNACK
Choose any from snack list (page 344)

TRADITIONAL MEAL PLAN, WEEK 3
1,400–1,600 Calorie Level

DINNER
Vegetarian Chili, 2 servings (page 255)
Roasted Pepper and Goat Cheese Polenta,
    2 servings (page 337)
½ cup strawberries mixed into ½ cup nonfat plain
    yogurt

DAY 3

BREAKFAST
Banana Walnut Pancakes (page 236)
½ tablespoon light pancake syrup
1 cup nonfat milk

LUNCH
Grilled Cheese Sandwich (page 285)
1 cup strawberry slices in ½ cup nonfat vanilla yogurt

SNACK
Choose any from snack list (page 344)

DINNER
Chicken Fajitas (page 302) with 2 tablespoons
    reduced-fat sour cream
10 baked tortilla chips with 2 ounces guacamole
1 nectarine

DAY 4

BREAKFAST
Apricot-Cranberry Oatmeal (page 234)
1 cup vanilla soy milk

LUNCH
Chicken Fajita Salad with Creamy Cilantro-Lime
    Sauce (page 261)
Fruit salad (1 medium orange, peeled and cubed,
    1 tablespoon orange juice, ½ cup fresh
    raspberries)

SNACK
Choose any from snack list (page 344)

DINNER
Eggplant Parmigiana (page 307)
1-ounce wheat roll with 1 tablespoon trans-fat-free
    margarine
Sun-Dried Tomato and Roasted Garlic Soup
    (page 253)
1 small pear

DAY 5

BREAKFAST
Blueberry Bran Muffin (page 238) with
    ½ tablespoon trans-fat-free margarine
4 ounces (2 percent fat) cottage cheese
½ medium green apple

LUNCH
Vegetarian Chili (page 255)
1 banana sliced into ½ cup low-fat cottage cheese
    mixed with 3 tablespoons sliced almonds

SNACK
Choose any from snack list (page 344)

DINNER
Fiesta Chicken Salad (page 309)
1 large whole-wheat pita
1 medium red pepper, sliced, with 1 tablespoon
    vinaigrette
1 small pear

TRADITIONAL MEAL PLAN, WEEK 3
1,400–1,600 Calorie Level

DAY 6	DAY 7
BREAKFAST 1 cup fiber- and protein-rich cereal (such as Kashi) with 1 cup soy milk	**BREAKFAST** Multigrain Pancakes (page 241) 2 tablespoons light pancake syrup 1 cup nonfat milk
LUNCH 3 ounces roasted chicken breast Coconut Rice (page 333) Asian Sesame Salad, 2 servings (page 256) 1 medium apple	**LUNCH** Jerk Shrimp Skewers with Tomato-Strawberry Salsa (page 314) ½ cup long-grain brown rice (measured dry; 1 cup cooked) 1 cup cherry tomatoes with 1 tablespoon vinaigrette 1 nectarine
SNACK Choose any from snack list (page 344)	**SNACK** Choose any from snack list (page 344)
DINNER Chicken Fromage with Sauce (page 303) Rice Pilaf with Carrots (page 336) 1 cup steamed broccoli 1 cup strawberry halves mixed with 1 cup raspberries	**DINNER** Potato-Crusted Salmon (page 321) ½ cup couscous (measured dry; 1 cup cooked) 1 small pear, sliced, dipped into ½ cup nonfat vanilla yogurt

MODERATE CARBOHYDRATE MEAL PLAN, WEEK 3
1,200–1,400 Calorie Level

DAY 1	
BREAKFAST 1 slice toasted whole-wheat bread, 1 tablespoon trans-fat-free margarine ½ cup nonfat vanilla yogurt	**SNACK** Choose any from snack list (page 344)
LUNCH Mixed Greens with Walnuts, Goat Cheese, and Pear (page 269) 3 ounces roasted chicken drizzled with 1 tablespoon vinaigrette 1 cup strawberry halves	**DINNER** Chicken Fromage with Sauce (page 303) Roasted Pepper and Goat Cheese Polenta (page 337) Cucumber–Red Onion Salad (page 265) 1 plum

MODERATE CARBOHYDRATE MEAL PLAN, WEEK 3
1,200–1,400 Calorie Level

DAY 2

BREAKFAST
Yogurt, Nut, and Fruit Parfait (page 250)

LUNCH
Chicken Salad in a Whole-Wheat Pita (page 284)
Sun-Dried Tomato and Roasted Garlic Soup
  (page 253)
¼ avocado, sliced, dusted with salt and black pepper
  to taste

SNACK
Choose any from snack list (page 344)

DINNER
Spiced Salmon (page 325)
Green Beans Provençal (page 267)
Baked potato (6 ounces) with 2 tablespoons
  reduced-fat sour cream

DAY 3

BREAKFAST
Toast with Egg Salad (page 348)
½ cup fresh raspberries

LUNCH
Turkey Roll-up with Vinaigrette (page 292)

SNACK
Choose any from snack list (page 344)

DINNER
Chicken Marsala (page 304)
Broccoli with Dijon Vinaigrette (page 259)

DAY 4

BREAKFAST
½ cup protein- and fiber-rich cold cereal (such as
  Kashi), ½ cup soy milk, topped with 1 tablespoon
  chopped walnuts

LUNCH
Peanut butter and banana sandwich (2 tablespoons
  natural peanut butter on 1 slice whole-wheat
  bread, topped with thin slices of ½ medium
  banana)
½ cup low-fat cottage cheese in a red pepper shell
  (1 medium red bell pepper, seeds removed)

SNACK
Choose any from snack list (page 344)

DINNER
Pepper-Crusted Beef Tenderloin with Horseradish
  Sauce (page 317)
Rice Pilaf with Carrots (page 336)
1 cup steamed broccoli

MODERATE CARBOHYDRATE MEAL PLAN, WEEK 3
1,200–1,400 Calorie Level

DAY 5

BREAKFAST
¼ cup dry oatmeal cooked with ½ cup nonfat milk
½ cup blueberries (fresh or frozen)
1½ tablespoons sliced almonds

LUNCH
Tuna Salad in a Tomato (page 327)
½ cup low-fat cottage cheese with 1 cup blueberries
and 2 tablespoons chopped walnuts

SNACK
Choose any from snack list (page 344)

DINNER
Pork Chops with Bourbon Mustard Glaze
(page 318)
Cucumber Leek Soup (page 252)
1 medium pear, sliced

DAY 6

BREAKFAST
Broccoli and Cheese Quiche (page 239)
¼ cup low-fat vanilla yogurt

LUNCH
Tortilla Soup (page 254)
2 ounces roasted turkey breast
½ cup fresh pineapple or canned pineapple in juice
with ½ cup low-fat cottage cheese

SNACK
Choose any from snack list (page 344)

DINNER
Chicken Breast with Ricotta and Pesto (page 301)
Sun-Dried Tomato and Roasted Garlic Soup
(page 253)
1 cup mixed berries (½ cup raspberries, ½ cup
strawberry halves) in ½ cup nonfat plain yogurt

DAY 7

BREAKFAST
Open-Faced Egg and Cheese Sandwich (page 242)

LUNCH
Chicken Salad in Whole-Wheat Pita (page 284)
1 cup cherry tomatoes with 1 tablespoon vinaigrette

SNACK
Choose any from snack list (page 344)

DINNER
MahiMahi with Pineapple Salsa, 2 servings
(page 315)
¼ cup wild rice (measured dry; ½ cup cooked)
1 cup steamed broccoli with 1 tablespoon vinaigrette

MODERATE CARBOHYDRATE MEAL PLAN, WEEK 3
1,400–1,600 Calorie Level

DAY 1

BREAKFAST

1 slice toasted whole-wheat bread, 1 tablespoon trans-fat-free margarine

1 cup nonfat vanilla yogurt

½ cup fresh raspberries

LUNCH

Mixed Greens with Walnuts, Goat Cheese, and Pear (page 269)

3 ounces roasted chicken drizzled with 1 tablespoon vinaigrette

1 medium apple, sliced

½ cup nonfat vanilla yogurt

SNACK

Choose any from snack list (page 344)

DINNER

Chicken Fromage with Sauce (page 303)

Roasted Pepper and Goat Cheese Polenta (page 337)

Cucumber–Red Onion Salad, 2 servings (page 265)

1 plum

DAY 2

BREAKFAST

Yogurt, Nut, and Fruit Parfait (page 250)

Scrambled Egg with Peppers (page 246)

LUNCH

Chicken Salad in a Whole-Wheat Pita (page 284)

Sun-Dried Tomato and Roasted Garlic Soup (page 253)

½ avocado, sliced, dusted with salt and black pepper to taste

SNACK

Choose any from snack list (page 344)

DINNER

Spiced Salmon (page 325)

Green Beans Provençal (page 267)

Baked potato (6 ounces) with 2 tablespoons reduced-fat sour cream

DAY 3

BREAKFAST

Toast with Egg Salad (page 248, but use 2 eggs)

½ cup strawberries

LUNCH

Turkey Roll-up with Vinaigrette (page 292)

½ cup nonfat vanilla yogurt

SNACK

Choose any from snack list (page 344)

DINNER

Chicken Marsala (page 304)

Broccoli with Dijon Vinaigrette (page 259)

1 cup strawberry halves

MODERATE CARBOHYDRATE MEAL PLAN, WEEK 3
1,400–1,600 Calorie Level

DAY 4

BREAKFAST

½ cup protein- and fiber-rich cold cereal (such as Kashi), 1 cup soy milk, 1 tablespoon chopped walnuts

LUNCH

Peanut butter and banana sandwich (2 tablespoons natural peanut butter on 1 slice whole-wheat bread, topped with thin slices of ½ medium banana)

½ cup low-fat cottage cheese in a red pepper shell (1 medium red bell pepper, seeds removed)

SNACK

Choose any from snack list (page 344)

DINNER

Pepper-Crusted Beef Tenderloin with Horseradish Sauce (page 317)

Rice Pilaf with Carrots (page 336)

1 cup steamed broccoli with 1 tablespoon vinaigrette

DAY 5

BREAKFAST

¼ cup dry oatmeal cooked with ½ cup nonfat milk

½ cup blueberries (fresh or frozen)

3 tablespoons sliced almonds

1 cup nonfat milk

LUNCH

Tuna Salad in a Tomato (page 327)

½ cup low-fat cottage cheese with 1 cup blueberries and 2 tablespoons chopped walnuts

SNACK

Choose any from snack list (page 344)

DINNER

Pork Chops with Bourbon Mustard Glaze (page 318)

Cucumber Leek Soup, 2 servings (page 252)

½ avocado, sliced, dusted with salt and pepper

DAY 6

BREAKFAST

Broccoli and Cheese Quiche (page 239)

1½ tablespoons sliced almonds with ½ cup fresh raspberries

½ cup nonfat plain yogurt

LUNCH

Tortilla Soup (page 254)

4 ounces roasted turkey breast

½ cup fresh pineapple or canned pineapple in juice

1 medium red bell pepper, sliced, with 2 tablespoons hummus

SNACK

Choose any from snack list (page 344)

DINNER

Chicken Breast with Ricotta and Pesto (page 301)

Sun-Dried Tomato and Roasted Garlic Soup (page 253)

1 cup mixed berries (½ cup raspberries, ½ cup strawberry halves) in 1 cup nonfat plain yogurt

DAY 7

BREAKFAST

Open-Faced Egg and Cheese Sandwich (page 242, but use 2 ounces cheese, 1 egg, and 2 egg whites)

½ cup blueberries

MODERATE CARBOHYDRATE MEAL PLAN, WEEK 3
1,400–1,600 Calorie Level

LUNCH
Chicken Salad in Whole-Wheat Pita (page 284, but use 4 ounces chicken)
1 cup cherry tomatoes with 1 tablespoon vinaigrette

SNACK
Choose any from snack list (page 344)

DINNER
MahiMahi with Pineapple Salsa, 2 servings (page 315)
$\frac{3}{8}$ cup wild rice (measured dry; $\frac{3}{4}$ cup cooked)
1 cup steamed broccoli with 1 tablespoon vinaigrette

Should I Be Taking Vitamins?

Most experts agree that consuming a balanced diet, including plenty of vegetables and fruits, whole grains, healthy fats, and lean protein, contributes to good health. However, the scientific data demonstrate inconsistent findings on the subject of vitamins, and it is not at all clear that supplementing a balanced diet with vitamins is necessary or even desirable for most people. Despite the uncertainties, we do agree with many experts that a general-purpose multivitamin is a reasonable step to help make sure you are getting all you need. But in our experience, lots of people take many more supplements (vitamins, minerals, and other add-ons) than they need, not only wasting money, but in some cases also running health risks.

Specific groups for whom supplementing a healthy diet with vitamins or minerals is widely recommended include women in their childbearing years who are encouraged to take at least 400 micrograms (mcg) of folic acid daily (and more, if they are actively seeking to become pregnant or are already pregnant). Adults can reduce their risk of fractures, and possibly other health problems, by supplementing with 400 to 800 international units (IU) of vitamin D daily (higher doses for older people). Adequate dietary calcium is important for everyone—those under age fifty are encouraged to aim for a total of 1,000 milligrams (mg) daily, from food and/or supplements; 1,200 to 1,500 mg daily is appropriate for older adults (the higher end of the range for women). Note that folic acid and vitamin D are included in multivitamins, often in adequate amounts, but read the labels to determine specific amounts. Multivitamin pills do not usually include significant amounts of calcium, so separate calcium supplements are recommended. Based on special circumstances (for instance, pregnancy and certain medical conditions where adequate nutrition has been compromised) additional supplements may be appropriate. We advise that you talk with your doctor about whether you should be augmenting your diet with any supplements beyond what you will get from a healthy diet and from the preceding recommendations.

WEEK 3 EXERCISE ROUTINE

This week, we have new strength training routines for you to try for both Level 1 and Level 2. Trying something new, although challenging, can keep your workouts interesting. If you haven't yet varied your cardio routine, this might be the week to start to diversify your exercise portfolio by trying an aerobics class, cycling, or swimming instead of just walking. The more exercises you are comfortable with, the more likely that your workout will remain interesting, challenging, and beneficial—and the better protected you will be against getting derailed if your one mode of exercise becomes unavailable (if, for instance, the swimming pool closes for renovations, or heel pain interferes with your walking). Whatever your fitness level, take a moment to pat yourself on the back for the progress you've made over the past two weeks.

Fitness Prep Level

How are you progressing toward your goal of 8,000 to 10,000 steps a day on most days?

Have you noticed how good walking can make you feel? We bet that by now you're already getting a little hooked on exercise. Many of our patients fairly quickly reach the point of missing exercise on the days when they don't work out. If you're not there yet, have faith. It can happen to you, too.

When you reach the goal of 8,000 to 10,000 steps nearly every day for a week, move ahead to Level 1.

Level 1

As you have been doing, try to get those 10,000 steps in each day, and continue to accumulate thirty minutes of moderate-intensity cardio three times a week. Add the strength training exercises listed here two times a week on nonconsecutive days and stretch on the days you exercise (or daily, if you like). When you can do thirty minutes of cardio three times a week, plus two sets of twelve to fifteen reps of the exercises, and you want more of a challenge, move to Level 2.

Level 2

If you are at Level 2, maintain those steps and keep aiming for forty-five minutes of cardio a day three days a week, plus two or three sets of twelve to fifteen reps of the Level 2 strength training exercises. Stretch on the days you exercise (or daily, if you like.) When you want to step up your workout, add five more minutes of cardio per session and, when ready, add additional sessions until you've worked up to sixty minutes five times a week, plus three sets of twelve to fifteen reps of the strength training exercises. You can find additional customized workouts at www.dukediet.com.

Where There's a Will, There's a Way

I'm often impressed by how resourceful our clients are when it comes to making time for exercise. Bob, a fifty-year-old I coached after he left the Duke Diet & Fitness Center, worked impossibly long hours every week, often with no days off. I wouldn't have been surprised if he had to struggle much of the time just to make his minimal exercise goals. But he came up with a great strategy. He worked at a large factory where the managers patrolled the grounds on golf carts. Bob gave up his golf cart and brought his bicycle to work so he could whiz from place to place. I bet that made his coworkers smile! Bob found that not only did this help him to get his aerobic workout, but the short bouts of exercise really helped him cope with stress throughout the workday as well—and it's helped him keep the weight off, too!

Another client, Debbie, discovered that she loved using a stationary bicycle. So she looked around and found a good yet affordable bike and bought two of them—one for her home and the other for her parents' house, where she spent a lot of time. Having made that investment, she wanted to keep exercising, even when her work schedule was challenging. During busy periods, she alternated evening and morning workouts—a good example of using an action plan to cope with changing circumstances. She lost twenty-six pounds and, like Bob, has maintained her weight loss.

—Marit Derrer, M.A., Behavioral Health Clinician
at the Duke Diet & Fitness Center

EXERCISE AT A GLANCE, WEEKS 3 AND 4

LEVEL 1

DAY 1

Warm-up: 5 min
Cardio: 30 min

STRETCHING:
Hold each stretch for 10 to 30 seconds.
Total Body Stretch (page 365)
Lower Back and Gluteals Stretch (page 365)
Hamstrings Stretch (page 366)
Lower Back Stretch with Knees Tilted to One Side
    (page 367)
Quadriceps Stretch (page 368)
Modified Hamstrings Stretch (page 369)
Triceps Stretch (page 370)

DAY 2

Warm-up: 5 min

STRENGTH TRAINING:
For each exercise, do 1 set of 12 to 15 reps.
Wall Squat with Stability Ball (page 359)
Standing Chest Press with Resistance Tube
    (page 360)
Back Row with Resistance Tube (page 361)
Biceps Curl with Resistance Tube (page 362)
Double Leg Heel Raise with Stability Ball Press-up
    (page 363)
Abs Curl on Stability Ball (page 364)

STRETCHING:
Hold each stretch for 10 to 30 seconds.
Total Body Stretch (page 365)
Lower Back and Gluteals Stretch (page 365)
Hamstrings Stretch (page 366)
Lower Back Stretch with Knees Tilted to One Side
    (page 367)
Quadriceps Stretch (page 368)
Modified Hamstrings Stretch (page 369)
Triceps Stretch (page 370)

DAY 3

Warm-up: 5 min
Cardio: 30 min

STRETCHING:
Hold each stretch for 10 to 30 seconds.
Total Body Stretch (page 365)
Lower Back and Gluteals Stretch (page 365)
Hamstrings Stretch (page 366)
Lower Back Stretch with Knees Tilted to One Side
    (page 367)
Quadriceps Stretch (page 368)
Modified Hamstrings Stretch (page 369)
Triceps Stretch (page 370)

DAY 4

Warm-up: 5 min

STRENGTH TRAINING:
For each exercise, do 1 set of 12 to 15 reps.
Wall Squat with Stability Ball (page 359)
Standing Chest Press with Resistance Tube
    (page 360)
Back Row with Resistance Tube (page 361)
Biceps Curl with Resistance Tube (page 362)
Double Leg Heel Raise with Stability Ball Press-up
    (page 363)
Abs Curl on Stability Ball (page 364)

STRETCHING:
Hold each stretch for 10 to 30 seconds.
Total Body Stretch (page 365)
Lower Back and Gluteals Stretch (page 365)
Hamstrings Stretch (page 366)
Lower Back Stretch with Knees Tilted to One Side
    (page 367)
Quadriceps Stretch (page 368)
Modified Hamstrings Stretch (page 369)
Triceps Stretch (page 370)

EXERCISE AT A GLANCE, WEEKS 3 AND 4

DAY 5

Rest Day
Stretch if you wish. If you stretch, be sure to warm up for 5 minutes beforehand.

DAY 6

Warm-up: 5 min
Cardio: 30 min

STRETCHING:
Hold each stretch for 10 to 30 seconds.
Total Body Stretch (page 365)
Lower Back and Gluteals Stretch (page 365)
Hamstrings Stretch (page 366)
Lower Back Stretch with Knees Tilted to One Side (page 367)
Quadriceps Stretch (page 368)
Modified Hamstrings Stretch (page 369)
Triceps Stretch (page 370)

DAY 7

Rest Day
Stretch if you wish. If you stretch, be sure to warm up for 5 minutes beforehand.

LEVEL 2

DAY 1

Warm-up: 5 min
Cardio: 45 to 60 min

STRENGTH TRAINING:
For each exercise, do 2 sets of 12 to 15 reps.
Wall Squat and Overhead Press with Medicine and Stability Balls (page 377)
Torso Twist with Resistance Tube (page 378)
Biceps Curl with Resistance Tube (page 362)
Triceps Press with Resistance Tube (page 379)

Stiff-Arm Pull-down with Resistance Tube on Stability Ball (page 380)
Leg Extension with Stability Ball (page 381)
Hamstrings Curl with Stability Ball (page 382)
Crisscross Crunch with Stability Ball (page 383)

STRETCHING:
Hold each stretch for 10 to 30 seconds.
Upper Back and Chest Stretch (page 384)
Rotary Torso Stretch (page 385)
Lat-Shoulder Stretch (page 386)
Supported Lower Back Stretch (page 387)
Seated Hamstrings Stretch (page 388)
Figure 4 Stretch (page 389)
Hip Flexor Stretch (page 390)

DAY 2

Warm-up: 5 min
Cardio: 45 to 60 min

STRETCHING:
Hold each stretch for 10 to 30 seconds.
Upper Back and Chest Stretch (page 384)
Rotary Torso Stretch (page 385)
Lat-Shoulder Stretch (page 386)
Supported Lower Back Stretch (page 387)
Seated Hamstrings Stretch (page 388)
Figure 4 Stretch (page 389)
Hip Flexor Stretch (page 390)

EXERCISE AT A GLANCE, WEEKS 3 AND 4

DAY 3

Warm-up: 5 min
Cardio: 45 to 60 min

STRENGTH TRAINING:

For each exercise, do 2 sets of 12 to 15 reps.
Wall Squat and Overhead Press with Medicine and
    Stability Balls (page 377)
Torso Twist with Resistance Tube (page 378)
Biceps Curl with Resistance Tube (page 362)
Triceps Press with Resistance Tube (page 379)
Stiff-Arm Pull-down with Resistance Tube on
    Stability Ball (page 380)
Leg Extension with Stability Ball (page 381)
Hamstrings Curl with Stability Ball (page 382)
Crisscross Crunch with Stability Ball (page 383)

STRETCHING:

Hold each stretch for 10 to 30 seconds.
Upper Back and Chest Stretch (page 384)
Rotary Torso Stretch (page 385)
Lat-Shoulder Stretch (page 386)
Supported Lower Back Stretch (page 387)
Seated Hamstrings Stretch (page 388)
Figure 4 Stretch (page 389)
Hip Flexor Stretch (page 390)

DAY 4

Warm-up: 5 min
Cardio: 45 to 60 min

STRETCHING:

Hold each stretch for 10 to 30 seconds.
Upper Back and Chest Stretch (page 384)
Rotary Torso Stretch (page 385)
Lat-Shoulder Stretch (page 386)
Supported Lower Back Stretch (page 387)
Seated Hamstrings Stretch (page 388)
Figure 4 Stretch (page 389)
Hip Flexor Stretch (page 390)

DAY 5

Rest Day
Stretch if you wish. If you stretch, be sure to warm
    up for 5 minutes beforehand.

DAY 6

Warm-up: 5 min
Cardio: 45 to 60 min

STRENGTH TRAINING:

For each exercise, do 2 sets of 12 to 15 reps.
Wall Squat and Overhead Press with Medicine and
    Stability Balls (page 377)
Torso Twist with Resistance Tube (page 378)
Biceps Curl with Resistance Tube (page 362)
Triceps Press with Resistance Tube (page 379)
Stiff-Arm Pull-down with Resistance Tube on
    Stability Ball (page 380)
Leg Extension with Stability Ball (page 381)
Hamstrings Curl with Stability Ball (page 382)
Crisscross Crunch with Stability Ball (page 383)

STRETCHING:

Hold each stretch for 10 to 30 seconds.
Upper Back and Chest Stretch (page 384)
Rotary Torso Stretch (page 385)
Lat-Shoulder Stretch (page 386)
Supported Lower Back Stretch (page 387)
Seated Hamstrings Stretch (page 388)
Figure 4 Stretch (page 389)
Hip Flexor Stretch (page 390)

DAY 7

Rest day
Stretch if you wish. If you stretch, be sure to warm
    up for 5 minutes beforehand.

STRATEGIES FOR EATING
IN RESTAURANTS

Studies have shown that frequent eating out is related to higher body fat levels. We find that clients who are able to eat at home, even just a little more often, have an easier time losing weight because they can control the ingredients, portions, and preparation methods of their meals. They also benefit by avoiding the subtle overeating triggers, such as the sights and smells of other diners' meals, the servers with dessert trays, and all those freebies like bread that we encounter in restaurants. But that doesn't mean you can't enjoy eating out. For many of us, business lunches or dinners are among our professional obligations. Even if your work doesn't require it, dining out, particularly with friends, is one of the pleasures of life. We don't want you to forgo that, so it pays to be prepared for it.

Remember that you're not "on a diet"—rather, you are changing your lifestyle and the way you eat over the long term. With a little advance planning, a few useful strategies, and some menu and nutrition know-how, you can maintain your calorie allotments and stay on track when dining in restaurants. If you eat out occasionally, then perhaps you can afford to allow yourself some of the more calorie-dense foods and even have a few extras. Relaxing your plan a little on occasion will not have a devastating impact on your weight loss. Just try to control portions and don't go overboard. If you eat out frequently, though, you will need to follow your meal plan more closely, eating fewer calorie-dense foods and consuming them in a more balanced way. We encourage you to be realistic, use common sense, and where appropriate, try some of these helpful strategies.

Strategy #1: Manage Your Mind-Set

First, realize that it is possible to eat healthfully in a restaurant without feeling that you're missing out on the overall experience. While there are no off-limits foods, some are easier to keep under control than others. Take time to consider what you will eat and what you might avoid. Develop a strategy for ordering and perhaps sharing portions. Check where your appetite is on the

Hunger-Fullness Scale at the start of your meal, and take breaks while you are eating. Remember to practice awareness. Most of all, go to the restaurant confident that you can make healthy choices.

Strategy #2: Research Your Restaurant

Often the best restaurants for people trying to control their weight are those that offer light or heart-healthy options or that are willing to accommodate special requests. How do you find that out? Look for menus online—in most major cities there are menu listing sites for restaurants, organized by cuisine and location. You can also ask friends and check the message boards at www.dukediet.com.

If possible, call ahead to see whether the restaurant will accommodate special requests like having dishes broiled or steamed rather than sautéed, and having sauces served on the side. Many will do this, especially if you go at off-peak hours when the chef isn't swamped. If you avoid the busiest times, you'll also feel more comfortable asking the server questions about the menu.

Strategy #3: Plan Ahead

Before you get to the restaurant, decide what you will order, rather than waiting to choose with the pressure of a server hovering over you. At the table, wave away the menu so you won't be tempted by the tantalizing descriptions or even the pictures of dishes, and just order what you've planned.

Consider your order in the context of everything else you have eaten or plan to eat that day. For example, you may wish to choose leaner options if you have already had a high-fat day. Try to keep your day in nutritional balance.

If you can't check the menu beforehand, go in armed with a skeleton menu that lays out the number of servings you'll eat from each food group, according to your meal plan (either the Traditional or the Moderate Carbohydrate).

Chances are, the restaurant will have chicken or fish on its menu, which might be your best options. Our nutrition manager, Elisabetta Politi, suggests that in restaurants, it can be helpful to go low carb as a strategy to con-

Skeleton Menu

Fill in the number of servings you plan to eat from each food group before you go to an unfamiliar restaurant, and do your best to stick to this plan.

	YOUR PLANNED SERVINGS	YOUR PLANNED CALORIES
Starches:		
Vegetables:		
Fruits:		
Protein:		
Fats:		
Dessert:		
Alcohol:		

trol calories. Just order the chicken or fish and a salad or a side of vegetables. Our nutrition staff members also suggest that it is a good idea to avoid combination dishes like lasagna or casseroles, which are very difficult to judge in terms of both calories and nutritional content—the more ingredients in a dish, the greater the margin for error. Simple is usually safer.

Before you order, don't be embarrassed to ask the server how dishes are prepared, so you can make informed choices. Servers are often prepared to field reasonable questions about food preparation. Request that your food arrive without salt, and ask for dressings, sauces, and toppings—where hidden calories lurk—on the side so you can decide how much to use. Here are some questions to ask:

- How is this dish prepared? Can it be modified?
- What ingredients are used?
- Do you have any low-fat or low-calorie options?

- What comes with this entrée?
- How large are the portions?
- Can I make substitutions?

Some examples of helpful (and simple) substitutions to request are a baked potato instead of fries (or even better nutritionally, a baked sweet potato), steamed vegetables instead of sautéed (over which you can lightly drizzle some olive oil and balsamic vinegar for great taste, modest calories, and a healthy helping of monounsaturated fat), or a double serving of vegetables instead of a starch. If the ingredients are already on the menu somewhere, the chef should be able to accommodate your needs. Don't be shy about asking—after all, you're paying the bill. Be "health assertive"!

At the Duke Diet & Fitness Center, we conduct a very popular role-playing class that allows clients to practice handling potentially uncomfortable situations such as ordering or dealing with others at the table in an assertive manner. This class involves applying the effective communication strategies we outlined in chapter 4.

Strategy #4: Plan Your Portions

Restaurant portions are often huge—two or three times the size you'd typically have in a meal on the Duke Diet Nutrition Plan! So, before you go out, review the "Eyeball Guide to Servings per Portion" in chapter 2, so you'll be able to gauge at a glance how much to eat. When you've decided how much of the meal you're going to eat, separate that amount and push the rest to the top of your plate. Ask to have the extra food put in a take-out bag so you can get another meal out of it, or get two plates and split your order with a dining companion.

Another good strategy is ordering from the appetizer section of the menu for your entrée. Beware of fried appetizers or those featuring cheese, cream sauces, and other high-calorie add-ons. Healthy options include steamed or raw seafood (shrimp cocktail, steamed clams, oysters on the half shell, seviche, sushi, or sashimi); hummus and raw vegetables or half a pita; and broth-based or puréed (without cream) soups like gazpacho or beef and vegetable soup. If you add a salad or soup to one or two sensible appetizers, you can create a very satisfying meal with a reasonable calorie count.

Typical Restaurant Portions and Approximate Calories

Remember that restaurants usually add a significant amount of oil, which will boost these calorie counts. Ask that your meal be prepared with minimal or no added oil.

FOOD	EDIBLE PORTION SERVED	CALORIES	CALORIE RANGE FOR PORTION
Lean meats: filet mignon, lamb chop, pork tenderloin, veal (loin cuts)	6–8 ounces*	60 per ounce	360–480
Fatty meats: rib or rack cuts (e.g., prime rib)	6–8 ounces*	100 per ounce	600–800
Skinless poultry	6–8 ounces	50 per ounce	300–400
Shellfish and fish	6–11 ounces	35 per ounce	210–385
Salmon, mackerel, trout (oily fish)	6–11 ounces	50 per ounce	300–550
Plain pasta	2–3 cups cooked	80 per ½ cup	320–480
Pasta with chicken or shrimp	1½–2 cups pasta 2–4 ounces of meat or fish	80 per ½ cup 35 to 50 per ounce	240–320 70–200
Plain tomato sauce	½ cup	50 per ½ cup	50

*These quantities may not apply at a steak house. Steak house menus usually indicate the weight of the raw steaks. Deduct one of every four ounces to calculate the edible portion. For example, an 8-ounce filet cooked medium-well will become 6 edible ounces.

Strategy #5: Skip the Extras

Many restaurants will put a basket of bread, chips (which, in most Mexican restaurants, are fried and highly caloric), or other freebies on the table as soon as you sit down. Why waste calories on these openers when you can save them for the main event? You can ask to have the breadbasket removed from the table or push it out of reach. If you really want the bread and will include it (and the butter or olive oil you put on it) in your daily calorie count, take just one serving (one slice or one small dinner roll) and send the rest back.

Strategy #6: Find the Fat and Sodium

The way your entrée is prepared makes a big difference in its calorie count. Remember, simpler is safer. For example, grilled chicken will be much lower in fat and calories than fried. When you're served chicken with skin, remove the skin to save calories. The following chart will demystify restaurant menu jargon and guide you to the better choices.

It's not easy to avoid excess fat or less-healthy fats in restaurant meals. It is important to keep in mind that most restaurants will use a significant amount of added fat in preparing many dishes, including grilled and broiled ones. Don't forget to figure the extra butter and oil into your daily calorie count. Better yet, ask the server if your entrée can be prepared without or with minimal butter or oil. Fill up on low-energy-density foods like salad and vegetables (ask that vegetables be steamed, grilled, or roasted, not sautéed). Another good way to control calories is to resist spooning sauces over your food, but instead dip your fork into the sauce dish before picking up each bite.

LOWER-FAT OPTIONS	LOWER-FAT BUT HIGH-SODIUM OPTIONS	HIGH-FAT OPTIONS	
Au jus (in its own juices)	Barbecued	Alfredo	Scalloped
Broiled	Blackened	Au gratin (with cheese)	Flaky
Flame-cooked	Creole sauce	Batter-dipped	Fried
Grilled	In broth	Béarnaise	Hollandaise
Parboiled	Marinated	Beurre blanc	Parmesan (Parmigiana)
Poached	Pickled	Breaded	Potpie
Roasted	Smoked	Creamy	Tempura
Seared		Crispy	
Steamed		En croûte	

Strategy #7: Select Salads Wisely

Not all salads are created equal. Ask the server if the one you're considering has high-fat elements like cheese, croutons, eggs, or bacon, which significantly raise the calorie count. It's usually easy for the kitchen to leave off the ingredients that you don't want, or at least to add them in smaller than usual amounts, more as a garnish, if you request that. Get your dressing on the side—low-fat vinaigrette is obviously a much better choice than high-fat blue cheese or Roquefort—and add a small amount with your teaspoon. If you've chosen a slightly thicker dressing, use the same method as for sauces: Dip your fork into the dressing before picking up each bite.

REGULAR DRESSING			FAT-FREE/LOWFAT DRESSING		
TYPE	AMOUNT	CALORIES	TYPE	AMOUNT	CALORIES
Ginger soy	2 Tbs	100	Ginger soy	2 Tbs	10
Italian	2 Tbs	100	Italian	2 Tbs	15
Thousand island	2 Tbs	110	Thousand island	2 Tbs	25
Ranch	2 Tbs	150	Ranch	2 Tbs	30
French	2 Tbs	150	French	2 Tbs	30
Raspberry vinaigrette	2 Tbs	110	Raspberry vinaigrette	2 Tbs	35
Blue cheese	2 Tbs	150	Blue cheese	2 Tbs	30

Strategy #8: Decide about Dessert

Decide ahead of time whether you're going to have dessert and, if so, what it will be. That way, you can skip the temptation of the dessert tray and the mouthwatering descriptions on the menu. If you do choose a standard dessert, ask for a half portion or share it, eat it slowly, and enjoy it!

Otherwise, consider ordering commonly available options like fruit, sorbet, and frozen yogurt, all of which contain fewer calories than rich cakes, pies, and ice cream concoctions. A coffee or cappuccino with low-fat milk and artificial sweetener can also satisfy your sweet tooth surprisingly well after a meal.

Strategy #9: Ease Up on Alcohol

Alcohol has more calories per gram than most foods and does little or nothing to fill you up. In fact, many people find it to be an appetite stimulant. Alcohol also tends to impair your sense of control (it lowers inhibitions) and lessens your resolve, leaving you more open to temptation. So it's wise to limit your intake to 150 calories' worth, or the following quantities, per day:

- 6 ounces of wine
- 1½ ounces of hard liquor
- 16 ounces of light beer
- 12 ounces of regular beer

Order wine by the glass, rather than sharing a bottle, so you can more easily monitor your intake, but be careful of the large goblets many restaurants use, which may hold ten or twelve ounces. Mixed drinks like margaritas and piña coladas can be risky choices because their ingredients vary so widely and are often high in calories. As with restaurant food, simpler is safer when it comes to cocktails; even mixers like tonic water add calories.

Decide ahead of time at which point in the meal you'll most enjoy having an alcoholic beverage—perhaps with your entrée?—and stick to calorie-free options like water, seltzer, unsweetened iced tea, or diet soda the rest of the time. The advantage of having alcohol served with your entrée is that it will have less of an impact on your inhibitions than if you drink on an empty stomach. Starting out with a cocktail might relax you so much that you'll lose sight of all your good intentions!

As you can see, although restaurant dining has its challenges, there's no reason that you can't eat out. If your companions are having steak fritas with béarnaise sauce, it doesn't have to scuttle your plan if you've prepared in advance and chosen a flavorful, satisfying alternative. Believe in yourself and your ability to choose wisely. And remember that there is a lot more to enjoy about dining out than the meal itself. There's the company of your friends, the atmosphere, the people-watching, and the celebratory feeling of being out on the town as a break from your everyday routine. Appreciate the totality of the experience and focus just as much on the fun as on the food.

FAST-FOOD FACT AND FICTION

The sheer number of fast-food outlets and their low prices make them many people's dining-out mainstay. Increasingly, fast-food restaurants are offering alternatives to the standard burger and fries, so it's getting a little easier to make better choices. Keep in mind, though, that even these "healthy" options are usually very high in sodium—meaning that fast-food restaurants may not be the best choice for people who need to limit their sodium intake.

When you make the decision to eat fast food, be sure to check the chain's website in advance for nutritional information. Once you're actually in the restaurant, it's easy to get confused by the marketing claims. For example, just because Subway promotes a "carb conscious" menu doesn't mean that these options fit into a low-calorie or low-sodium plan. Look at how the nutrients in Subway's low-carbohydrate Chicken & Bacon Ranch Wrap compare with those in its six-inch Turkey Breast Sandwich:

	CALORIES	FAT	SATURATED FAT	PROTEIN	CARBO-HYDRATE	SODIUM
Chicken & Bacon Ranch Wrap	440	27 g	10 g	41 g	18 g	1,680 mg
Six-inch Turkey Breast Sandwich	280	4.5 g	1.5 g	18 g	46 g	1,020 mg

As you can see, the Carb Conscious Chicken & Bacon Ranch Wrap contains far more saturated fat and sodium than the Turkey Breast Sandwich, as well as nearly twice the calories. So it pays to go in fully armed with information.

At most fast-food venues, the various chicken options are usually better choices than the burgers. Just know what you are eating. Here is a comparison of the nutritional values of chicken options at three major chains:

	CALORIES	FAT	SATURATED FAT	PROTEIN	CARBO- HYDRATE	SODIUM
KFC Original Recipe Chicken Breast (one piece)	380	19 g	6 g	40 g	11 g	1,150 mg
McDonald's Premium Grilled Chicken Classic Sandwich	420	10 g	2 g	32 g	51 g	1,190 mg
Subway six-inch Oven Roasted Chicken Breast Sandwich	330	5 g	2 g	24 g	47 g	1,020 mg

Take into consideration that the McDonald's and Subway sandwiches include the bun, and that the McDonald's selection includes mayonnaise. Look how many calories and how much sodium you can cut by shedding the bun and the breading:

	CALORIES	FAT	SATURATED FAT	PROTEIN	CARBO- HYDRATE	SODIUM
KFC Original Recipe Chicken **Breast without skin or breading (one piece)**	140	3 g	1 g	29 g	0 g	410 mg
McDonald's Premium Grilled **Chicken Classic Sandwich with no bun**	180	7 g	1.5 g	24 g	5 g	830 mg
Subway six-inch Oven Roasted **Chicken Breast Sandwich without bread**	130	2.5 g	1 g	16 g	7 g	660 mg

Today, most fast-food restaurants, including McDonald's, Burger King, KFC, Subway, and Wendy's, offer a variety of salads, many of which are really not healthful options. For example, Wendy's Southwest Taco Salad contains 710 calories, 41 grams of fat, and 1,620 milligrams of sodium! A better choice would be the Mandarin Chicken Salad, which contains 550 calories, 26 grams of fat, and 1,230 milligrams of sodium. If you omitted the dressing and crispy noodles that come with the salad, you could bring those numbers down to 300 calories, 13 grams of fat, and 550 milligrams of sodium.

Chains with "Healthy" Menus

Here is a comparison of "healthy" options from the menus of some popular fast-food restaurants.

• Taco Bell offers a Fresco Style menu with fifteen items containing fewer than 10 grams of fat. Several of these items are listed in the following chart. Of course, these numbers correspond to a single serving, so if you choose a double order, you have to multiply the nutrition facts accordingly.

• At Subway, an entire section of the menu, called 6 Grams of Fat or Less, is dedicated to low-fat sandwiches. Consider this combination meal: a six-inch Turkey Breast Sub, one single-serving bag of Baked Lay's Potato Chips, and one apple. You would consume about 475 calories and just 6 grams of fat. You would also take in about 85 grams of carbohydrate and 1,170 milligrams of sodium. Note that only 150 milligrams of sodium come from the potato chips—the rest are in the sandwich itself!

	CALORIES	FAT	SATURATED FAT	PROTEIN	CARBO-HYDRATE	SODIUM
Beef Soft Taco	150	8 g	2.5 g	9 g	20 g	630 mg
Ranchero Chicken Soft Taco	170	4 g	1 g	9 g	22 g	710 mg
Grilled Steak Taco	170	5 g	1.5 g	11 g	21 g	560 mg
Baja Beef Gordita	250	9 g	3 g	12 g	31 g	640 mg
Bean Burrito	350	8 g	2 g	13 g	56 g	1,220 mg
Chicken Fiesta Burrito	340	8 g	2 g	16 g	50 g	1,160 mg

• Wendy's menu doesn't have a special section for lower-fat fare, but there are a number of healthier options on the menu, such as the salads, deli-style sandwiches, grilled chicken sandwiches, baked potatoes, and chili. Try a small order of chili, a baked potato, and a side salad with reduced-fat creamy ranch dressing. The meal would total 625 calories, 14 grams of fat, and 98 grams of carbohydrate. You would also consume 1,280 milligrams of sodium.

• Even Pizza Hut now offers a Fit'N Delicious menu of lower-fat options. You could try two slices of the diced chicken, red onion, and green pepper pizza and a salad from the salad bar, with two tablespoons of low-calorie dressing. This meal provides 415 calories, 12 grams of fat, 86 grams of carbohydrate, and 1,270 mg of sodium. Many other pizzas, such as Sbarro's, would total 1,300 calories for just the two slices!

You know our philosophy: There are no forbidden foods on the Duke Diet Nutrition Plan. However, before you choose fast food, you may want to ask yourself how well it fits with your long-term health and weight loss goals. You'll find more information on fast food on www.dukediet.com.

Prediabetes, Diabetes, and a Healthy Lifestyle

Of all the health problems connected to excess weight, the link to diabetes is the most impressive. In fact, we are in the midst of a growing international epidemic of diabetes. As our weight increases beyond the healthy BMI range, the risk of developing type 2 diabetes (by far the most common kind—formerly called "adult onset" and now, sadly, often seen in overweight kids) increases very sharply. Diabetes is caused by the body's inability to produce enough of the hormone insulin—or to use it properly. The result is a condition of high blood sugar that causes many health problems, including impaired circulation, which increases our risk for heart attacks, strokes, kidney damage, nerve damage, and other problems. Diabetes is diagnosed when blood sugar, after an overnight fast, is greater than 125 milligrams per deciliter (mg/dL) on two or more occasions.

Commonly, before developing full-blown diabetes, the body goes through a stage called *prediabetes* (sometimes called *insulin resistance*) in which the fasting blood sugar is higher than normal (less than 100 mg/dL) but not yet in the diabetes range. Not everyone who has prediabetes will go on to develop full-blown diabetes, but many eventually do. The good news is that, for overweight people, even moderate, sustained weight loss (at least 5 to 10 percent of starting weight), along with regular exercise (as little as thirty minutes of moderate-intensity activity five or more days a week) is a powerful strategy for reducing the risk of progression from prediabetes to diabetes. In large clinical studies, weight loss and regular exercise were demonstrated to be more effective, in fact, than the leading oral antidiabetes medication. Not only can these measures help prevent most cases of diabetes, but they can also significantly improve control of blood glucose and reduce the occurrence of problems for overweight people who already have diabetes.

Visit www.dukediet.com or consult your doctor to learn more about prediabetes and diabetes, how they are diagnosed, and how to manage them.

If you have diabetes, you must consult your doctor before starting an exercise program. You will probably be told to check your blood sugar before, during, and after exercise—at least until you learn how your body responds. If your blood sugar is less than 100 mg/dL before you exercise, your doctor may advise you to eat a small snack, such as a box of raisins, half a bagel with cream cheese, or a few crackers with a small amount of peanut butter, so that your glucose level will not get too low (below 70 mg/dL). If your blood sugar is higher than 240 mg/dL before your workout, your doctor will probably not want you to exercise, and will make other specific recommendations.

Other precautions: Proper foot care is essential for diabetics, and polyester or polyester-cotton-blend socks without seams are recommended to help reduce dampness and friction, which can lead to blisters and skin ulcers. Also, you should drink plenty of water to prevent dehydration, which can affect blood glucose control.

ASSIGNMENT FOR SUCCESS: WEEK 3 COPE WITH HIGH-RISK SITUATIONS

Dining out can be challenging when you're trying to lose weight. It's what we call a high-risk situation. Other such situations include periods of heightened stress (which we'll cover in chapter 8) and various emotions. High-risk situations may make you vulnerable to overeating. This assignment will help you cope with high-risk situations by showing you that you have choices. You're in charge! You can take control of the situation rather than let it control you.

The following brief exercise will help you identify people, places, events, and emotions that threaten to weaken your resolve and, potentially, derail your progress; then it will help you brainstorm strategies to deal with them. Take the time to do it thoughtfully using an example you remember from the past in which you found yourself eating off plan. This is a great way to learn strategies for dealing with future situations. You may wish to repeat this exercise periodically to hone your coping skills for high-risk situations.

• Describe in detail a situation in which you were at high risk for or engaged in overeating. Be specific: Write down where you were, who you were with, what you were doing, the time of day, and so on.

• Now consider how you were feeling physically. Be specific—were you shaky, tired, sleepy, energetic? Did you have a headache or other pain?

• What thoughts were going through your mind? Again, be specific: *I'm stressed. I feel overwhelmed. I may as well eat, I'll never lose the weight anyway. I don't have time to do everything on my list.*

• What were you feeling emotionally? Again, be specific—were you sad, angry, depressed, lonely, anxious, happy, joyful, confused, frustrated, fearful, tense, or bored?

• Were you aware of any specific food or eating triggers at the time (television commercials, friends eating, difficult-to-control foods around the house)?

• Given all you have learned so far, what might be some other choices you could have made or strategies you could have used to deal with the situation? Approach this as a brainstorming exercise, which we discussed earlier in the book. Allow your mind to flow freely and be creative. See what you come up with, then evaluate to determine which options are realistic. File them away in your mind (and on a piece of paper) to pull out when you next face a high-risk situation.

CHAPTER EIGHT

Week 4: Managing Stress

Welcome to Week 4, the final week of the core Duke Plan that we hope has encouraged new and healthier nutrition, exercise, and behavior habits to take root. All you're going to need to do after this week is keep putting one foot in front of the other, using and adapting your new skills, and you'll enjoy improved weight control and better health for life.

This week's focus will be the very important subject of stress, which is an inescapable fact of life. It's our body's 911 call, the alarm that tells the brain to release hormones such as cortisol and epinephrine (also called adrenaline), chemical signals to speed up the heart, raise the blood pressure, prime the muscles, quicken the senses, and mobilize the blood sugar for action—all the metabolic requirements for responding to a perceived attack.

This primary stress response helps you deal with immediate threats to safety like the car that almost hits you as you cross the street. The stress response may also be engaged to cope with grief, trauma, and upsetting events. It may even help you make positive transitions like getting married or getting a new job. Then, too, there are the day-in, day-out demands we all face—work, family, kids, financial or health worries, noise, traffic, and so on—that can lead to a state of chronic stress, which if left unaddressed can have a detrimental impact on both our health and our overall sense of well-being.

Later in this chapter, we'll approach stress management in the two ways that we mentioned in chapter 4: by reducing or eliminating sources of stress and then by learning to unload the stress we can't escape.

But let's start out by introducing the Week 4 Nutrition and Exercise plans.

WEEK 4 MEAL PLANS

As before, start your week out right by setting your optimal, desirable, and minimal goals for nutrition, exercise, and behavioral change.

TRADITIONAL MEAL PLAN, WEEK 4
1,200–1,400 Calorie Level

DAY 1	DAY 2
BREAKFAST French Toast (page 240)	**BREAKFAST** 2-ounce whole-grain bagel with 1 tablespoon low-fat cream cheese ½ cup nonfat plain yogurt
LUNCH Chicken Caesar Wrap (page 281) 1 small pear	**LUNCH** Sloppy Turkey Joe (page 324) on whole-wheat hamburger/hot dog bun 1 medium red pepper, sliced 1 cup nonfat milk
SNACK Choose any from snack list (page 344)	**SNACK** Choose any from snack list (page 344)
DINNER Pork Tenderloin with Apple Chutney (page 320) Coleslaw (page 263) 6-ounce baked potato	**DINNER** Blackened Fish (page 299) Blue Cheese and Chive Potato Salad, 2 servings (page 332) 15 spears steamed asparagus 1 cup pineapple cubes

TRADITIONAL MEAL PLAN, WEEK 4
1,200–1,400 Calorie Level

DAY 3

BREAKFAST
½ cup nonfat vanilla yogurt with 1 cup fresh or
    frozen fruit and 1½ tablespoon sliced almonds

LUNCH
3 ounces roasted chicken breast on a whole-grain
    bun with 2 slices of tomato, ½ cup chopped
    lettuce, and 1 tablespoon hummus
Cold Dijon Carrots (page 262)
½ cup blueberries

SNACK
Choose any from snack list (page 344)

DINNER
Grilled Flank Steak (page 311)
3-ounce baked potato stuffed with 1 cup cooked
    frozen spinach
1 nectarine

DAY 4

BREAKFAST
Whole-Wheat Pecan Muffins (page 249)
½ cup nonfat milk

LUNCH
Tuna Salad in Tomato (page 327)
2 slices rye toast
½ cup nonfat vanilla yogurt with 1 tablespoon
    chopped walnuts

SNACK
Choose any from snack list (page 344)

DINNER
Teriyaki Tuna Loin with Wasabi Butter and Braised
    Bok Choy (page 326)
Coconut Rice (page 333)
½ cup blueberries

DAY 5

BREAKFAST
Banana Bread (page 235)
½ cup nonfat milk

LUNCH
Cranberry-Pecan Salad (page 264)
Top with 2 ounces roasted turkey breast and
    1 tablespoon low-calorie creamy dressing
1-ounce wheat roll
1 small pear

SNACK
Choose any from snack list (page 344)

DINNER
Thai Chicken Broccoli Salad (page 280)
½ cup strawberry halves

DAY 6

BREAKFAST
¼ cup dry oatmeal cooked with ¾ cup soy milk and
    ¾ cup blueberries

LUNCH
Ham sandwich (3 ounces lean lower-sodium ham,
    1 ounce low-fat Cheddar cheese, 2 tomato slices,
    and 1 lettuce leaf on 2 slices whole-wheat bread)
½ medium banana with ½ cup nonfat vanilla yogurt

SNACK
Choose any from snack list (page 344)

DINNER
Baked Ziti with Roasted Vegetables (page 297)
1 cup raspberries mixed with ½ cup nonfat vanilla
    yogurt and sprinkled with 1½ tablespoons sliced
    almonds

TRADITIONAL MEAL PLAN, WEEK 4
1,200–1,400 Calorie Level

DAY 7

BREAKFAST
Fruit smoothie with flaxseed (½ cup orange juice, ½ cup nonfat plain yogurt, ½ banana, and 1 tablespoon ground flaxseed, mixed in blender until smooth)

LUNCH
Maryland Crab Cakes (page 316)
Spinach-Pear Salad (page 279)
2 slices fresh pineapple

SNACK
Choose any from snack list (page 344)

DINNER
Jerk Shrimp Skewers with Tomato-Strawberry Salsa, 2 servings (page 314)
½ cup cooked long-grain brown rice (measured dry; 1 cup cooked)
1 nectarine

TRADITIONAL MEAL PLAN, WEEK 4
1,400–1,600 Calorie Level

DAY 1

BREAKFAST
French Toast (page 240)
¾ cup soy milk

LUNCH
Chicken Caesar Wrap (page 281)
1 small pear
1 large carrot, cut into pieces

SNACK
Choose any from snack list (page 344)

DINNER
Pork Tenderloin with Apple Chutney (page 320)
Coleslaw, 2 servings (page 263)
6-ounce baked potato

DAY 2

BREAKFAST
2-ounce whole-grain bagel with 2 tablespoons low-fat cream cheese
1 cup nonfat plain yogurt

LUNCH
Sloppy Turkey Joe (page 324) on whole-wheat hamburger/hot dog bun
1 medium red bell pepper, sliced
1 cup nonfat milk

SNACK
Choose any from snack list (page 344)

DINNER
Blackened Fish (page 299)
Blue Cheese and Chive Potato Salad, 2 servings (page 332)
15 spears steamed asparagus drizzled with ½ tablespoon of olive oil
1 cup pineapple cubes

TRADITIONAL MEAL PLAN, WEEK 4
1,400–1,600 Calorie Level

DAY 3

BREAKFAST
½ cup nonfat vanilla yogurt with 1 cup fresh or frozen pineapple and 1½ tablespoon sliced almonds
½ toasted whole-grain English muffin
½ tablespoon trans-fat-free margarine

LUNCH
3 ounces roasted chicken breast on a whole-grain bun with 2 slices of tomato, ½ cup chopped lettuce, and 1 tablespoon hummus
Cold Dijon Carrots (page 262)
1 cup blueberries

SNACK
Choose any from snack list (page 344)

DINNER
Grilled Flank Steak (page 311)
Roasted Ratatouille (page 272)
6-ounce baked sweet potato

DAY 4

BREAKFAST
Whole-Wheat Pecan Muffins (page 249)
1 cup nonfat plain yogurt
1 cup fresh or frozen blueberries

LUNCH
Tuna Salad in Tomato (page 327)
2 slices rye toast
½ cup nonfat vanilla yogurt with 1 tablespoon chopped walnuts

SNACK
Choose any from snack list (page 344)

DINNER
Teriyaki Tuna Loin with Wasabi Butter and Braised Bok Choy (page 326)
Coconut Rice (page 333)
1 cup blueberries

DAY 5

BREAKFAST
Banana Bread (page 235)
1 cup nonfat milk

LUNCH
Cranberry Pecan Salad (page 264)
Top with 2 ounces roasted turkey breast and 1 tablespoon low-calorie creamy dressing
1½-ounce wheat roll
1 small pear

SNACK
Choose any from snack list (page 344)

DINNER
Thai Chicken Broccoli Salad (page 280)
1 small pear, sliced

TRADITIONAL MEAL PLAN, WEEK 4
1,400–1,600 Calorie Level

DAY 6	DAY 7
BREAKFAST Fruit smoothie with flaxseed (½ cup orange juice, ¾ cup low-fat plain yogurt, ½ banana, and 1 tablespoon ground flaxseed, mixed in blender until smooth)	**BREAKFAST** ½ cup dry oatmeal cooked with 1 cup soy milk ¾ cup blueberries
LUNCH Ham sandwich (3 ounces lean lower-sodium ham, 2 ounces low-fat Cheddar cheese, 2 tomato slices, and 1 lettuce leaf on 2 slices whole-wheat bread) ½ medium banana with ½ cup nonfat vanilla yogurt	**LUNCH** Maryland Crab Cakes (page 316) 2 slices fresh pineapple Spinach-Pear Salad (page 279) 1 slice oatmeal bread
SNACK Choose any from snack list (page 344)	**SNACK** Choose any from snack list (page 344)
DINNER Baked Ziti with Roasted Vegetables (page 279) 1 cup raspberries mixed with 1 cup nonfat vanilla yogurt and sprinkled with 1½ tablespoons sliced almonds	**DINNER** Jerk Shrimp Skewers with Tomato-Strawberry Salsa, 2 servings (page 314) ¼ cup (measured dry) brown rice with 2 teaspoons trans-fat-free margarine 1 nectarine

MODERATE CARBOHYDRATE MEAL PLAN, WEEK 4
1,200–1,400 Calorie Level

DAY 1	
BREAKFAST 1 slice whole-wheat toast, 2 ounces lean lower-sodium ham, and 1 ounce low-fat cheese ½ cup strawberries	**SNACK** Choose any from snack list (page 344)
LUNCH Grilled Portobello (page 312) 2 ounces roasted chicken breast ½ cup baby carrots with 1 tablespoon hummus 1 medium apple	**DINNER** Grilled Flank Steak (page 311) Onion Ragout, 2 servings (page 270) 3-ounce baked potato

MODERATE CARBOHYDRATE MEAL PLAN, WEEK 4
1,200–1,400 Calorie Level

DAY 2

BREAKFAST
½ small whole-grain bagel
1 tablespoon natural peanut butter
½ cup nonfat milk

LUNCH
Cucumber–Red Onion Salad, 2 servings (page 265)
2 ounces roasted turkey breast on ½ whole-wheat
    English muffin, spread with 2 tablespoons
    hummus
½ cup strawberry halves

SNACK
Choose any from snack list (page 344)

DINNER
Crab-Stuffed Whitefish (page 306)
Roasted Vegetables with Olive Oil and Feta Cheese
    (page 273)
½ cup fresh raspberries

DAY 3

BREAKFAST
Blueberry, Banana, and Flaxseed Smoothie
    (page 237)
Scrambled Egg Substitute with Red Pepper
    (page 245)

LUNCH
Chicken, Cheese, and Arugula Panini (page 282)

SNACK
Choose any from snack list (page 344)

DINNER
Eggplant Sausage Lasagna (page 308)
2 cups wilted spinach tossed with 1 tablespoon
    garlic-flavored olive oil

DAY 4

BREAKFAST
Open-Faced Egg and Ham Sandwich (page 243)
1 small orange

LUNCH
Veggie Cheeseburger (page 293)
Coleslaw (page 263)

SNACK
Choose any from snack list (page 344)

DINNER
Teriyaki Tuna Loin with Wasabi Butter and Braised
    Bok Choy (page 326)
Asian Sesame Salad, 2 servings (page 256)
½ cup fresh blueberries

DAY 5

BREAKFAST
Spinach and Cheese Omelet (page 247)
1 cup fresh raspberries

LUNCH
Chicken and Wild Rice (page 300)
1 small orange
1 medium red bell pepper, sliced

SNACK
Choose any from snack list (page 344)

DINNER
Grilled Shrimp (page 313)
Mixed Greens with Walnut, Goat Cheese, and Pear
    (page 269)
2-ounce wheat roll

MODERATE CARBOHYDRATE MEAL PLAN, WEEK 4
1,200–1,400 Calorie Level

DAY 6	DAY 7
BREAKFAST Fruit salad with cottage cheese and almonds (¾ cup low-fat cottage cheese, ½ cup fresh or frozen blueberries, ½ cup fresh raspberries, and 1½ tablespoons sliced almonds)	**BREAKFAST** Eggs and Turkey Bacon (1 egg plus ¼ cup egg substitute, scrambled, with 2 slices turkey bacon) 1 small orange
LUNCH Open-faced Ham and Turkey Reuben (page 288) Spinach–Cherry Tomato Salad (page 278)	**LUNCH** Green Salad with Chicken, Avocado, Orange Segments, and Fat-Free Honey Dressing (page 268)
SNACK Choose any from snack list (page 344)	**SNACK** Choose any from snack list (page 344)
DINNER Blackberry Mustard Chicken (page 298) 2 cups fresh spinach tossed with ½ cup mandarin orange segments and 1 tablespoon vinaigrette, topped with 1½ tablespoons sliced almonds	**DINNER** Turkey, Cheese, and Kale Panini (page 291)

MODERATE CARBOHYDRATE MEAL PLAN, WEEK 4
1,400–1,600 Calorie Level

DAY 1	
BREAKFAST 1 slice whole-wheat toast, 2 ounces lean lower-sodium ham, and 1 ounce low-fat cheese ½ cup strawberries ½ cup raspberries	**SNACK** Choose any from snack list (page 344)
	DINNER Grilled Flank Steak (page 311) Onion Ragout, 2 servings (page 270) 6-ounce baked potato
LUNCH Grilled Portobello (page 312) 2 ounces roasted chicken breast 1 cup baby carrots with 2 tablespoons hummus 1 medium apple	**DAY 2** **BREAKFAST** ½ small whole-grain bagel 1 tablespoon natural peanut butter ½ cup nonfat milk

MODERATE CARBOHYDRATE MEAL PLAN, WEEK 4
1,400–1,600 Calorie Level

LUNCH

Cucumber–Red Onion Salad, 2 servings (page 265)

2 ounces roasted turkey breast on ½ whole-wheat English muffin, spread with 2 tablespoons hummus

1 cup strawberry halves

SNACK

Choose any from snack list (page 344)

DINNER

Crab-Stuffed Whitefish (page 306)

Roasted Vegetables with Olive Oil and Feta Cheese (page 273)

½ cup fresh strawberries in ½ cup nonfat plain yogurt

DAY 3

BREAKFAST

Blueberry, Banana, and Flaxseed Smoothie (page 237)

Scrambled Egg with Red Pepper (page 246)

LUNCH

Chicken, Cheese, and Arugula Panini (page 282)

SNACK

Choose any from snack list (page 344)

DINNER

Eggplant Sausage Lasagna (page 308)

2 cups wilted spinach tossed with 1 tablespoon garlic-flavored olive oil

1 plum

DAY 4

BREAKFAST

Open-Faced Egg, Ham, and Cheese Sandwich (page 244)

½ cup raspberries

½ cup strawberries

LUNCH

Veggie Cheeseburger (page 293)

Coleslaw, 2 servings (page 263)

SNACK

Choose any from snack list (page 344)

DINNER

Teriyaki Tuna Loin with Wasabi Butter and Braised Bok Choy (page 326)

Asian Sesame Salad, 2 servings (page 256)

1 cup fresh blueberries

DAY 5

BREAKFAST

Spinach and Cheese Omelet with 2 ounces cheese (page 247)

1 cup fresh raspberries

LUNCH

Chicken and Wild Rice (page 300)

1 small orange

1 medium red bell pepper, sliced, with 2 tablespoons hummus

SNACK

Choose any from snack list (page 344)

DINNER

Grilled Shrimp (page 313)

Mixed Greens with Walnut, Goat Cheese, and Pear (page 269)

2-ounce wheat roll with 1 tablespoon trans-fat-free margarine

MODERATE CARBOHYDRATE MEAL PLAN, WEEK 4
1,400–1,600 Calorie Level

DAY 6	DAY 7
BREAKFAST Fruit salad with cottage cheese and almonds (¾ cup low-fat cottage cheese, ½ cup fresh or frozen blueberries, ½ cup fresh raspberries, and 1½ tablespoons sliced almonds)	**BREAKFAST** Eggs and Turkey Bacon (1 egg plus ¼ cup egg substitute, scrambled, with 2 slices turkey bacon) ½ cup strawberries ½ cup nonfat vanilla yogurt
LUNCH Ham and Turkey Reuben (page 286) Spinach–Cherry Tomato Salad (page 278)	**LUNCH** Green Salad with Chicken, Avocado, Orange Segments, and Fat-Free Honey Dressing (page 268) ½ cup raspberries and ½ cup strawberry halves
SNACK Choose any from snack list (page 344)	**SNACK** Choose any from snack list (page 344)
DINNER Blackberry Mustard Chicken (page 298) 2 cups fresh spinach tossed with ¾ cup mandarin orange segments and 2 tablespoons vinaigrette, topped with 1½ tablespoons sliced almonds	**DINNER** Turkey, Cheese, and Kale Panini with 1 tablespoon margarine (page 291) 1 plum

WEEK 4 EXERCISE ROUTINE

This week, you will continue your cardio and stretching routines and repeat the strength training exercises from Week 3. By this point in the program, you're probably seeing definite changes. Do you have more strength? Better wind? More endurance? Keep it up. You'll make it!

STRESS MANAGEMENT, PART 1: ELIMINATING AND REDUCING STRESS

When we look back on how human beings, and the world we live in, have evolved over time, we can see that the role stress plays in our lives has changed dramatically. Historically, stress was a response to some sort of life-threatening situation that required direct, physical action—fight or flight. Our bodies were built to respond to such challenges.

But today we more commonly experience stress as an onslaught of daily mental challenges that usually cannot be resolved with quick actions. Instead, they require thought, problem solving, patience, and negotiation. As a result, many of us exist in a state of chronic stress, which can have serious physical and emotional consequences. Chronic stress suppresses the immune system and may contribute to such health problems as weight gain, cardiovascular disease, gastrointestinal distress, back pain, headaches, sleep disturbances, anxiety, and depression.

The importance of learning effective stress management skills cannot be overemphasized. Here we will review some important steps from chapter 4 and offer additional ideas on how you can disrupt the cycle of stress and reduce its impact on your healthy lifestyle.

1. Adjust your perception of stressful events. It is important to consider the way you approach stressful situations. When faced with a stressful situation, do you immediately think "I can't handle this" and panic, or are you able to focus on the elements of the situation you *can* control? As we mentioned in chapter 4, breaking down overwhelming tasks into smaller, more manageable ones is a great start—you can't beat positive action as a stress reducer. Also, simply working to stop your thoughts from spiraling out of control can interrupt the stress cycle.

2. Organize and prioritize tasks. Many of us today are just plain overcommitted and overscheduled, so, of course, we feel overwhelmed and unable to keep up with all the demands we make on ourselves. A lot of the claims on our time and attention that scream "Urgent!" aren't necessarily, and we have to be careful not to let supposedly urgent tasks trump tasks that are really more important.

That is why we advise our clients to develop skills to help them prioritize. We start by helping them distinguish between what is urgent (things that must be done in a rush) and what is important (things that really do matter). Things that are urgent aren't always important, and vice versa. An eye-opening way to establish your pri-

Hypertension

Nearly one in three American adults has high blood pressure, or *hypertension*, a leading contributor to heart attacks, strokes, kidney failure, and other problems. Because most people who have it have few, if any, symptoms, hypertension is known as the silent killer. The only way to know whether your blood pressure is elevated is to have it checked.

Blood pressure levels are considered optimal when systolic blood pressure (the top number, or the force exerted when the heart contracts and pumps blood out) is less than 120 and the diastolic (the bottom number, or the force exerted when the heart relaxes and refills with blood) is less than 80.

Prehypertension is diagnosed when the top number is between 120 and 140 and the bottom number is between 80 and 90. A person is considered to have high blood pressure when the top number is 140 or greater or the bottom is 90 or greater, and this is confirmed on several occasions.

There are many potential causes of high blood pressure, but in more than 95 percent of cases, no single one is identified. Excess weight, lack of physical activity, and a high-salt diet commonly contribute to the problem. Researchers think there may be a connection between stress and high blood pressure, but this connection is unclear. Stress hormones like cortisol and epinephrine can increase heart rate and cause blood vessels to constrict, raising blood pressure as a result—but there isn't currently enough evidence to say for sure whether the chronic stress we commonly experience in our daily lives is a cause of hypertension. However, some unhealthy reactions to stress—such as heavy alcohol consumption, and overeating that leads to weight gain—are known risk factors for hypertension. (And as you're reading in this chapter, stress reduction has so many other physical and emotional benefits that it's definitely a worthwhile pursuit.)

In the vast majority of people, it is possible to achieve good control of blood pressure via medication, with minimal, if any, side effects. However, lifestyle changes can also make a major difference. Moderate, sustained weight loss and reduced sodium intake are usually helpful. Regular, moderate aerobic exercise can also help, even if you don't lose any weight. One study found that the loss of ten pounds maintained for more than four years allowed 50 percent of patients previously on blood pressure medications to stop the drugs and stay off them.

orities is to consider what might really happen if you failed to accomplish the task. What will really happen if something isn't done a certain way? Or by a certain time? The answers may surprise you.

Start by listing the tasks that appear to be urgent but are not really that important. Put them on the back burner or take them off the stove! Then list the tasks that are both urgent *and* important. Finally, consider those that are clearly very important but do not need to be addressed immediately—in other words, they are less urgent. You'll probably also find that some things on your to-do list may be neither important nor urgent. Perhaps you can postpone doing these or, even better, take them off the list. This strategy alone will help you feel less overwhelmed by showing you where to focus your efforts and in what order to check tasks off your list. As you become more skillful at this, you will feel more in control and less stressed.

3. Problem-solve stressful situations. Stressful situations usually don't clear up on their own. It's likely that you'll have to take some kind of action. Let's say you have had some major unanticipated expenses such as car or home repairs—or perhaps the kids' college bills were higher than expected. Every problem has at least one solution, and most are likely to have several. Don't give in to the understandable urge to avoid thinking about your problem; instead, analyze it, break it down into small achievable steps, and set goals for solving it. Before you know it, you will be well on your way to reducing stress. This advice probably sounds familiar, since we've been encouraging you to apply this problem-solving method to all the lifestyle changes you're making on the Duke Plan, including your eating and exercise habits. Stress management is no different.

For the preceding example of financial stress, start by asking yourself, "What *must* be done immediately?" Do you need to get a loan or establish a realistic plan for partial payment? Once you have addressed the immediate, you should think about what got you into trouble in the first place. What are the underlying issues? Is this money crunch a recurring problem? Why? Do you need a better rainy-day plan? What steps can you take to make one? Do you need to draw up a new budget? Do you need to talk to a financial counselor? Can you ask a friend or your accountant for a referral? You know the drill. Brainstorm solutions, select the good ones, set some goals, take positive action, and evaluate the results!

This logical approach to stress, whatever the cause, will help you to feel in control. Not every problem has an easy solution, of course,

How Can I Make Healthy Choices Even When I Have No Time to Eat?

We have emphasized that when it comes to health and weight loss, it is a good strategy to sit down and eat calmly at regular intervals. However, it is important to be realistic, too, since being overscheduled has become commonplace. We all have those days when we hardly have time to catch our breath. Despite our best efforts to manage our time, many people find themselves facing the occasional "grab and go" moments.

When you're pressed for time, please don't skip a meal! What you might try is a meal replacement bar or shake as part of your meal plan. It is important to be aware that many energy bars and shakes are too high in calories to fit well into a weight control program. Look for ones that are relatively low in calories and provide a good balance of nutrients (protein, carbohydrates, healthy fat, and fiber). The brands we often recommend to patients include Slim-Fast and Glucerna.

Even beyond emergency use, you might find meal replacements helpful as a planned part of your daily routine. Some people use them regularly to replace certain meals, like breakfast, that they might otherwise be tempted to skip. Several studies have found that using meal replacements in this way can be an effective strategy for long-term weight management.

but with each small, positive action you take, you will feel less overwhelmed.

4. Practice good self-care. You will be more resistant to the negative effects of stress and better able to avoid or manage it if you eat healthfully, exercise regularly, get adequate sleep, take time to laugh and enjoy life, and stop trying to soothe yourself with food. Also be sure to try some of the stress-unloading techniques in the next section to help you.

STRESS MANAGEMENT, PART II: UNLOADING STRESS

Despite all your best efforts to limit stress, you obviously can't completely erase it from your life. That is why we recommend that you also learn skills

Stress and Transitions

Life is full of change—so much so that we often underestimate the effect that normal transitions have on us. We think that because everyone goes through certain things like job changes or retirement we shouldn't feel stress. One of our clients, Harry, recently retired. He said he couldn't figure out why, after running his own business, his retirement was stressing him out. In time, Harry came to understand that retirement meant a lessening of both the structure and the sense of purpose in life—and that this was really stressful to him. To make matters worse, there were conflicts in his family that he could no longer ignore by burying himself in his work. We worked together on identifying his thoughts about retirement and about moving on to the next stage of his life, and we examined the effectiveness of his way of communicating with his family. In time he was able to adjust to this major change and embrace his retirement.

—Kathleen Murray, M.S.W., Behavioral Health Clinician
at the Duke Diet & Fitness Center

to let go of stress. At www.dukediet.com, you can purchase a CD produced by the behavioral health staff at the Duke Diet & Fitness Center that includes several types of relaxation exercises (some of which are outlined here).

Relaxation Strategies

- Listening to soothing music
- Deep breathing, using the technique outlined in chapter 6
- Practicing visualization, which involves breathing deeply while you picture yourself in a serene environment, such as a beautiful garden, or summon to mind a soothing image, like a still pond
- Working with progressive muscle relaxation, a technique in which you alternately tense and relax one muscle group at a time as you focus on the feeling of release

- Doing mind-body exercises like Pilates, tai chi, and yoga
- Having a massage, which can help to reduce stress and relieve muscle pain and other pain associated with chronic tension
- Engaging in any kind of exercise, including walking, aerobics, and strength training

STRESS FOR ALL SEASONS

For many of us, holidays pose special weight control challenges: gifts of candy on Valentine's Day; big, traditional meals for Easter and Passover; barbecues on Memorial Day, the Fourth of July, and Labor Day; not to mention the whole party-filled holiday season that runs from Thanksgiving through New Year's. Besides the food, there are often the extra pressures of traveling to see family (perhaps with cranky kids in tow), staying in unfamiliar places where it can be hard to eat well and exercise, and other conflicts that tend to flare up at the holiday table. It's no wonder people find holidays challenging for weight control.

But you can stay in control while still enjoying these wonderful festive times. By using these season-saving holiday management strategies, you can skate through the holidays with your health and emotional well-being intact.

1. Manage your time and priorities. To avoid being hijacked by the holidays, prioritize your commitments, using the urgent/nonurgent, important/nonimportant strategy we talked about earlier in this chapter. Because holidays are about celebrating with others, decide which people mean the most to you—family, your closest friends, or out-of-town visitors. Schedule definite times to see them, rather than leaving yourself open to random drop-ins, and while you're at it, set aside some blocks of personal time for yourself, so you can catch your breath and regroup.

If year-end gift shopping and holiday card mailing seem overwhelming, tackle them in several sessions rather than in one fell swoop. You could write out a few cards every night instead of sacrificing an entire weekend to the task, create an electronic holiday

A Survival Workout
You Can Do Anywhere

There are many exercises you can perform without leaving your seat, and they're perfect for quick fitness fixes in your office, a hotel room, or even at home while you watch TV or talk on the phone. When you don't have access to dumbbells, everyday objects, such as unopened cans of food, bottles of water, or even heavy books, make excellent weights. Here is an exercise routine you can do anywhere, anytime.

- **Seated push-ups:** Sit upright, grasp the armrests of a sturdy chair, and push up until your arms are fully extended. Lower until you're almost seated, then rise back up. Repeat this process ten or twelve times. Perform two to three sets of repetitions.
- **Seated crunches:** Sit upright and press your back against the back of a sturdy chair. Your feet should be together and flat on the floor. Grasp the front edge of the seat, then slowly bring both knees as close to your chest as you can. Lower your legs, without touching the floor, and bring them back up to your chest again. Repeat ten or twelve times, and do two to three sets of repetitions.
- **Seated leg lifts:** Begin in the same position, with your back pressed against the back of a chair. Lift your right leg—keeping it straight, toes pointed up—until it's parallel with the floor. Squeeze your thigh muscles, then lower your leg slowly. Repeat ten to twelve times for each leg.
- **Arm curls:** Begin with your arms fully extended by your sides and a heavy book in each hand. Bend your elbows, lifting the books toward your shoulders while keeping your elbows tucked in by your hips, then slowly return to the starting position. Repeat ten or twelve times.
- **Stationary lunges:** Stand with your feet together and your arms down at your sides. Keep your back straight. Step forward with your right leg, bending your left knee close to, but not touching, the floor. Do not allow your right knee to travel past your toes as you step forward. Push yourself

back up to the starting position and continue lunging forward on the same leg ten to twelve times. Then switch legs.

Do these exercises at a moderate speed, maintaining control at all times and being sure to exhale when you are exerting effort and inhale when not exerting. For a quick aerobic fix, take a brisk walk outside after lunch or climb some flights of stairs. (Be sure to have a comfortable pair of flat shoes or athletic shoes on hand.)

greeting to e-mail, or make one newsletter to fill people in on your family's year, rather than composing a lot of personalized messages.

2. Safeguard your sleep. Try to get to bed on time. You may have parties to attend, but there's no rule that says you always have to be the last to leave. And try not to stay out late several nights in a row—ultimately, if you continue to shortchange your sleep, you're likely to pay a price physically and emotionally.

3. Stay active. Sticking to your regular exercise routine may help you better manage holiday stress. If you have the luxury of time off, try some new activities just for fun, like beach volleyball, ice skating, or cross-country skiing. If you'll be traveling, bring along the Survival Workout we provide in this chapter, which you can do anywhere, even in your aunt's guest room; take along easy-to-pack resistance bands; or just try to walk at least 10,000 steps every day, even in short bouts.

4. Forestall temptation. During the November-to-December holiday seasons especially, offices are overflowing with business gifts—huge drums of caramel and cheddar popcorn, cheese logs, fruitcakes, and three-pound gourmet chocolate samplers, not to mention all the homemade holiday specialties coworkers bring in to share. If you can afford to, by all means schedule a little indulgence into your meal plan. But as you know, this season goes on for weeks, and even small portions of daily treats can add up. So this might be the time to stay away from the break room. Eat at your desk, then take a walk outside during free time to avoid temptation.

Offer to bring a dish to parties and make it a healthy one so there will be something that fits in your plan. Try not to stand at or near a buffet table—before you know it, you'll be nibbling nonstop. Take a smaller plate, fill it once, and sit down across the room to eat. Instead of focusing on all the food, concentrate on the company—circulate and enjoy talking to the other guests.

Finally, try to plan holiday activities that don't involve food. Instead of going over to your in-laws' for fruitcake and homemade eggnog, invite them to join you and the kids at the holiday train show at the mall. There are lots of ways to socialize that aren't centered on food.

5. Bank your calories. Avoiding holiday treats altogether can backfire by making you feel deprived. Focus on the traditional specialties you really love, and skip the rest. Don't starve yourself, but, rather, bank some calories so you *can* enjoy your favorite foods at holiday meals and parties. Remember to eat slowly and monitor your fullness, so that you really savor the food you were anticipating and also so that you'll still have something on your plate when your host starts pressing everyone to have seconds.

6. Adopt an "everyday" attitude. Instead of viewing summer vacations and the weeks from November to January as holiday seasons, think of them as periods of ordinary life, with a few special festive events thrown in. Even on celebratory or special days you don't need to drop your healthy lifestyle plan altogether. If you are going to attend a party one night, try to stick with your meal plan for the other meals that day. Keep up at least some walking or leisure activity (enjoy the activity with visiting family or friends!), even if you take a break from the gym. This approach can help you sustain your healthy lifestyle and stay on track with your weight loss goals.

Don't be discouraged by that story news anchors trot out every year around Thanksgiving: "The average American gains five to ten pounds over the holidays." Research has shown that the average is more like one pound, and plenty of people don't gain any weight at all. You can be one of them, with careful planning and a sensible approach to holiday festivities.

7. Set realistic holiday goals. It may not be reasonable for you to expect to lose weight over the holidays. Don't set yourself up for failure and self-recrimination by vowing white-knuckled adherence to your weight loss plan. If you maintain your present weight, you're still ahead of the game.

Vacation Planning

Vacations carry their own baggage of stresses when you're trying to lose weight. You want to feel carefree, not disciplined, and you want to experience all that an exotic locale offers, including the food and drinks. Cruises or other all-inclusive vacations pose particular challenges because meals are sometimes perceived as the main events of each day, and they are often all-you-can-eat affairs. We repeatedly hear the same refrain from clients: "Every time I take a cruise, I fall off my plan and sometimes for a long time afterward find it very difficult to get back on track."

You don't have to gain weight on vacation, but you'll need to plan.

- Set a goal to maintain your weight during the vacation, rather than trying to lose.
- Shift your focus to the enjoyable aspects of the vacation that don't involve food, such as the locale, the sightseeing, and the shopping. If you're in Europe, you could determine to see all the great museums and buy gifts for your family and friends. If you're on a cruise, you can focus your days on exercise classes and luxurious spa treatments.
- Practice the dining-out strategies you now know. For example, on a cruise or at a resort, don't just stick to the buffet, but make special requests for low-fat or low-calorie options. You'll most likely be accommodated.
- If you happen to splurge a little, get right back on track—take a walk or make your next meal an on-plan, healthy one. After doing this a few times, you won't feel panicked about backsliding.

8. Go easy on alcohol. In social situations, observe the 150-calorie limit on alcoholic beverages and figure it into your daily total. If you really look forward to such special holiday treats as punch or eggnog, go ahead and enjoy them—just try to limit yourself to a single glass. If you prefer, go with lighter options like beer, wine, and spirits with no-calorie mixers. After you've had one drink, switch to juice spritzers, sparkling water, and diet sodas. If you keep a drink in your hand, you are less likely to be offered more, and your hands will be busy.

If, despite all your best intentions, you do overindulge during the holidays, don't give in to guilt. Guilt only spoils your holiday fun and undermines your resolve to maintain healthy habits. Remember, the Duke Plan is a lifestyle, and holiday celebrations are part of life. We truly believe that you should enjoy these celebrations and can do so healthfully. Go ahead and have fun.

BREAK YOUR CHAINS

Slipups, even in high-stress situations, never happen in a vacuum. They're the result of a specific chain of events and choices that you make. If you don't go grocery shopping this week, you might eat out (and, without planning, possibly go overboard). If you don't buy a warm enough coat in the fall, you probably won't walk much in the winter. By the same token, if you choose to stock up on healthy and appealing foods and have a selection of inviting recipes on hand, you will be more likely to eat at home and make wise choices. If you get the exercise gear you need, you're that much more apt to use it. Every choice has a consequence, for better or worse.

At the Duke Diet & Fitness Center, we teach clients to use *behavior chain analysis* to understand what leads them to make less-than-healthy choices and use that insight to break the chain. Behavior chains often begin with thoughts ("Ice cream will make me feel better"), which link to actions (driving to the ice cream store), which in turn link to other behaviors (buying, then eating, a whole pint of Ben & Jerry's Chunky Monkey), which may also lead to negative emotions like guilt or self-reproach, which in turn may lead to other negative thoughts, less-than-healthy behavior, and so on. Each link in the chain is a potential turning point at which the chain can be broken or at least slightly redirected. Multiple adjustments in the chain can add up to more favorable outcomes, such as weight loss and improved health.

A longer behavior chain might look like this: You have a party on Saturday, and half the dessert, a cake, is left over. You make a choice not to discard it. You come home from work on Monday, stressed and tired. You eat a large chunk of the leftover cake, and it cheers you up for a while. But then guilt kicks in, and you punish yourself by skipping dinner. The next morning you wake up starving and skip exercise so you can stop for a big breakfast on the way to work. Since your mind is telling you that you've already blown it, you continue to overeat all day. By Tuesday, you're totally demoralized about your weight loss effort and can't even make yourself go through the motions that could halt the slide for the rest of the week. All this started with a single decision that influenced each new decision made down the line. But a wonderful thing about a behavior chain is that you can always break it—no matter where you are along it—by making a different choice.

That said, the earlier in the chain you break a link, the easier it is to change the outcome. Here's an example: You bought a small cake for a dinner party but don't want to be tempted by it later. To avoid having it on hand, send the rest of the cake home with your guests. The result is that you avoid eating the leftover cake, and thus you also avoid punishing yourself by skipping dinner and waking up starving. Dr. Binks often compares working with behavioral chains to a movie in which someone goes back in time to make little changes that result in a different future. We will work on this process in this week's Assignment for Success.

Here is another example, showing a chain with big and small links: Sheila had a highly stressful day. When it was time for dinner, she decided it was too much trouble to defrost and cook something, so she ordered and ate an entire medium-sized pizza in front of the TV.

- **Link 1: Stressful day.** This chain could have been broken much earlier if Sheila had managed her stress throughout the day, possibly by taking a walk at lunchtime, pausing several times during the day for a relaxing few moments of breathing exercises, or even managing her schedule a little differently. Any of these options might have kept her stress level from reaching the boiling point.
- **Link 2: The dinnertime challenge.** The behavior chain itself may

have begun earlier in the week, when Sheila forgot to plan her meals. Or even that morning when she did not decide what she would eat that night and take it out of the freezer. By not planning, she was left with a difficult situation at dinnertime, when she was stressed, hungry, and less likely to make a healthy choice (to defrost and cook).

- **Link 3: Ordering the medium-sized pizza.** Even though the earlier links headed in a less-than-ideal direction, after she picked up the phone to call the pizzeria Sheila made a positive choice. She was on the verge of ordering a large pizza but opted for the medium one instead. Remember that even at the brink of a high-risk situation, you can still fight for control in the moment. Any small health-promoting decision is a victory, and in this case it saved quite a few calories despite not being the "perfect" decision.

- **Link 4: Eating the medium-sized pizza.** If Sheila had decided to have a healthy snack while waiting for the pizza delivery, she might not have been hungry enough to eat the whole pie when it arrived. Even with the pizza in the house, it wasn't too late for Sheila to fight the urge. She could have turned off the TV, eaten mindfully using a knife and fork to slow herself down until her brain registered fullness, and gotten away with eating only a slice or two.

As you can see, in this example, Sheila was faced with a series of difficult health choices, as many of us are every day. Most slips are the result of multiple moments of lost control, which is why Dr. Binks always tells clients to focus not on the ultimate outcomes when working with behavior chains, but rather on the little turning points. Each positive mini-decision is a battle won, which makes the next battle a little easier to face. As we've said so often throughout this book, it's the small steps that lead to serious progress.

ASSIGNMENT FOR SUCCESS: WEEK 4 PINPOINT THE LINKS

You can apply the behavior chain model to all your healthy lifestyle changes, from your eating and exercise to your behavioral health goals—for example, stress management. In this exercise, for simplicity's sake, we'll focus on unplanned eating.

1. Begin by identifying a time when you ate off plan.
2. Trace the chain of decisions back, link by link, starting with the choice you made immediately before you ate off plan. Work backward as far as necessary to reach the beginning of the chain.
3. Record the links in the chain. Don't just focus on the big ones— break them down into small ones, too.
4. Look at the whole picture. Pinpoint the links when a different decision—however small—might have turned the tide.
5. Now record the other decision(s) you could have made at each link.

This exercise is designed to help you think differently in the moment when you are faced with decisions in your daily life. Of course, you won't pull out a paper and pencil or log on to your Lifestyle Journal every time. But by doing the postgame analysis when things go wrong—and without passing judgment on yourself for every small misstep—you will begin to think automatically in terms of making different choices at every turning point.

PART THREE

The Duke Diet Recipes and Exercises

CHAPTER NINE

The Duke Diet Recipes

Healthy, low-calorie meals can be as delicious and exciting as any you might find on the menu of a fine restaurant. The team of highly skilled chefs at the Duke Diet & Fitness Center works closely with our dietitians to create portion-controlled meals that are healthy and nutritionally balanced, as well as satisfying and flavorful. One of the best perks of our jobs is that we get to sample everything on their menus. Dr. Eisenson's personal favorites include Sun-Dried Tomato and Roasted Garlic Soup, Cioppino, and for dessert, Silken Chocolate Pie. At home, his whole family enjoys Potato-Crusted Salmon, lightly marinated in honey-mustard sauce and coated with a thin crust of pan-sautéed potato flakes. Not only is it delicious, but this dish is very quick and easy to make.

Our recipes draw on a wide range of cuisines, including some that are especially popular with our clients—for example, Italian, Latin American, and Cajun. You probably didn't expect to enjoy foods like these when you're on a diet. Well, you will now. As we've been telling you all along, the Duke Plan is not about eliminating foods; it's about learning portion control, dealing more effectively with trigger, or hard-to-control, foods, and enjoying what you eat.

We love to hear clients rave about the Duke menus; and we're sure that you're going to be just as delighted as they are by the variety, sophistication, and surprising ease of preparation of our recipes. Many of our dishes can be made ahead of time and simply popped into the oven or microwave when it's time to eat. You'll find even more delicious meals—hundreds of them—on www.dukediet.com.

We encourage you not to stick solely to familiar foods and cooking methods but to approach this chapter as an adventure in good eating. Remember that our taste preferences are learned and can be broadened if we try new things. If you've been stuck on fried, salty, or sugary foods, as many of us have, you might marvel at how expert guidance in using alternative foods, seasonings, and techniques can punch up dishes and make them satisfying as well as healthy.

We will give you low-fat and low-carb cooking tips; new, healthy preparation methods; ways to cut sugar, sodium, calories, and cholesterol; and methods to boost flavor with onions, peppers, garlic, leeks, herbs, and spices. But don't worry—not all of our recipes will be exotic or require you to become an expert cook. You will also learn how to create healthier versions of your own recipes, including old favorites like crab cakes, pasta with pesto, and glazed pork chops. All the recipes come with nutritional breakdowns, so

Food Scale: The Weight Loss Warrior

Portion control is critical when you're trying to lose weight. You'll never wonder how to judge portion sizes again if you have a food scale. The best ones are digital, with an easy-to-read display. The most expensive models display not only the food's weight, but also its calories, carbohydrates, fat, cholesterol, protein, sodium, and fiber, after you input different codes. Although these extra features can be nice, a good, basic scale works just fine.

Don't worry—you won't have to weigh your food forever. Weighing will teach you what a proper portion looks like, so you will learn to eyeball food to gauge sizes. Then, periodically, you should weigh some foods again to make sure that your estimation ability hasn't drifted.

you can tell at a glance both the nutrients they contain and how many calories you're consuming.

Many of our recipes are not just easy to make but also quick. They take advantage of healthy supermarket convenience foods, such as boneless, skinless chicken breasts that are precut or prepounded for fast, even cooking. All you'll have to do is add a few finishing touches. For side dishes, you'll use quick-cooking staples like couscous, which cooks in just five minutes; prewashed greens and salad mixes; healthy, prepared low-fat salad dressings and salsas; frozen or precut vegetables; low-fat, low-sodium soups; veggie and turkey burgers; and other time-savers.

The Duke Plan recipes are designed to be prepared by anyone—in any reasonably well-equipped kitchen. You don't have to be a chef. We'll suggest a few extras you might want to invest in, apart from the standard pots, pans, and other cooking tools most people already have. If you need advice about stocking your kitchen, log on to www.dukediet.com for more helpful tips.

Helpful Kitchen Extras

These tools can help make food preparation a breeze. Try them out. You'll wonder how you ever lived without them.

- Crock-Pot or other slow cooker, for stewing
- Garlic press, for easy crushing
- Ice cube trays, to freeze broth cubes for use in sautéing
- Indoor grill, to cook foods over direct heat and drain fats
- Griddle pan
- Meat tenderizer and pounder, to flatten meats so they cook evenly and are less chewy
- Oil mister, to spray pans and cook with minimal fat
- Pastry brushes, to coat food with minimal oil

HEALTHY COOKING GUIDELINES

Low-fat and creative cooking techniques can help you significantly cut calories—as well as cholesterol, sugar, and salt—without sacrificing flavor. Here are some practical ideas to get you started. Don't hesitate to experiment. Cooking is not an exact science, and sometimes it's your own creative touches—provided, of course, that they don't add unhealthy or fattening ingredients—that make recipes even more satisfying. You might come up with some new family favorites.

Note that you won't have to make any of the suggested substitutions in the Duke recipes that we have provided you. Those recipes have been designed to incorporate healthy food prep strategies.

Proteins: Low-Fat Choices and Cooking Methods

Animal proteins from different sources vary widely in calories, from 35 to 100 per ounce. Fish and skinless white-meat poultry are on the lower end, while the dark meat from poultry and red meats tend to run higher. If you choose red meat, look for lean cuts, which often have the words *round* or *loin* in their names. For beef or veal, choose bottom round, eye of round (roast or steak), round tip (roast), flank, or top loin (New York, club, Delmonico, or strip steak). If you love lamb, opt for the leg, loin (chop or roast), or shoulder. For pork, choose the tenderloin, center loin, sirloin (boneless), or top loin chops. Whatever cut you buy, be sure to trim any visible fat before cooking to cut calories and saturated fats.

You can also cut fat by substituting Canadian bacon or turkey bacon for regular bacon. When you buy ground meat for burgers or chili, choose varieties marked "extra lean" or "lean." To reduce the amount of meat (and, hence the fat and calories) in recipes without sacrificing flavor, try replacing some of the meat by adding extra vegetables. Not only will you preserve heart health, but you will enhance the nutrients in dishes like soups, stews, casseroles, and pizza. As our executive chef, Andrew Craven, points out, substitutions include some degree of trial and error. So feel free to experiment when replacing meat with vegetables, have fun trying some things, and see how they work.

Use healthy cooking methods to prepare food. Here are some examples:

- **Baking:** Cook in the oven, using dry heat.
- **Braising:** Brown meat slowly over high heat in a pan lightly sprayed with a heart-healthy oil or cooking spray on your stove top, then add a small amount of liquid, cover, and continue cooking slowly over low heat. This is a great way to cook less-tender cuts of meat.
- **Broiling:** Cook with intense heat, under the broiler.
- **Grilling:** Cook on a rack outdoors over very hot coals, in a grill pan on the stove top, or on an indoor grill.
- **Poaching:** Immerse food in liquid that's barely simmering.
- **Roasting:** Cook uncovered in the oven using dry heat and adding very little liquid.
- **Searing:** Preheat a sauté pan, then lightly oil just before adding the meat, to seal in the juices. Quickly place the pan in a preheated oven to finish off the cooking according to the recipe.
- **Steaming:** Put food in a sieve, a woven steamer basket, or a metal steamer insert, and then suspend it over a small amount of boiling water. This is our favorite way to cook vegetables. They stay bright and fresh and keep all the nutrients that would be lost if you boiled them.
- **Stewing:** Slowly cook meats or vegetables in a covered pan in the oven, on the stove top, or in a slow cooker like a Crock-Pot. This is another great way to cook less-tender cuts.

Beyond the slow-cooking methods noted earlier, you can also tenderize meats and heighten their flavor by marinating them before cooking. You can find healthy, lower-fat, prepared marinades (or use low-fat salad dressing), but be sure to read labels—many are high in sodium. To make your own marinades, mix an acidic ingredient like lemon, lime, or orange juice, wine, vinegar, or low-fat yogurt with your favorite herbs and spices, ginger and garlic, or low-sodium chicken stock. Red meats and poultry can be marinated for one hour or, for a bigger flavor boost, overnight in the refrigerator. For more tender cuts of meat, fish, and seafood, reduce the marinating time to no more than two hours.

Meat tenderizers are another option. As with marinades, be sure to read

---

Go Low Fat with an Indoor Grill

When the weather's right and you have the time, it's great to pop virtually any food—meat, poultry, seafood, vegetables, and even fruit—onto your backyard grill. But when the weather is not great or you are in a hurry, it's even easier to use an indoor grill. You just plug it in, set the timer, put the food on the grill, close the lid—and then presto! Within minutes, it's done. No turning is needed because the grill has heating elements on both the top and the bottom. Fats drain off into a collection pan and are easily discarded. Just as for backyard barbecues, you may want to marinate or dry-rub foods before grilling for a bigger flavor wallop.

The one drawback of indoor grills is that they can fill your kitchen with cooking aromas. If you're grilling fish, especially, you'll want to use the grill near an open window or a vent. Some grills are designed to come apart easily, so the cooking plates can go right into the dishwasher, making cleanup a snap. Grills range widely in price, depending on their size and special features, so shop around to find the one that's best for you.

---

labels, because many are high in sodium or sodium preservatives like monosodium glutamate (MSG). Commercial tenderizers often contain the enzymes bromelain and papain, which come from pineapple and papaya, so they add flavor while tenderizing meat. If you use a tenderizer, don't leave it on the meat for more than two to four hours, or it will make the texture mushy.

Finally, you can tenderize meat by pounding or scoring it (making thin slashes across the surface). An added benefit of pounding is that it can flatten the meat to uniform thickness, so it cooks more evenly.

Healthy Sautéing

Sautéing usually involves cooking meat or vegetables in a skillet or wok with two tablespoons or more of butter or oil. However, it's easy to achieve the ef-

Why Press Garlic?

A garlic press crushes and shreds garlic cloves efficiently by forcing them through a grid or small holes. It will save you the trouble of mincing garlic and also spare your hands from its indelible smell. If you choose a good, heavy one with larger holes, you won't even have to peel the clove before pressing. Just pop it in, squeeze, and the garlic will pass through, leaving its papery skin behind.

Pressed garlic will have a stronger taste than chopped garlic, since pressing breaks down cell walls and releases more of the aromatic compounds, but it will be more evenly distributed in recipes. Pressed garlic can add zing to salad dressings, marinades, dips, meats, poultry, fish, vegetables, and more.

Your garlic press will also come in handy for mashing small flavor boosters like olives, capers, anchovies, and small quantities of onion or shallot.

fects of sautéing without saturating your food with unwanted fat calories. One option is to use a nonstick skillet or, if you prefer, simply coat a regular one with a light mist of vegetable oil. You can buy commercial nonstick sprays in flavors like olive oil, butter, and garlic. Here are some other strategies for sautéing with minimal fat:

- Get an oil mister at any kitchen or housewares store (Misto is one popular brand). Simply pour heart-healthy oil, such as canola or olive, into the mister, then lightly spray it over your pan or the food.
- Dip a pastry brush into a small amount of oil, then lightly brush it over foods or your skillet or griddle.
- Replace oil in sautéing with fat-free, low-sodium chicken or vegetable broth.
- Use other nonfat liquids such as a little white wine or even water in place of fats while sautéing.
- Finally, experiment with other cooking techniques. Steaming, roasting, or microwaving vegetables are good, low-calorie options. Try different methods and see which ones you like.

Super Salads

To avoid the excessive fat and sodium of many bottled dressings, make your own tasty versions. Vinaigrettes are always good choices because vinegar has very few calories and virtually no sodium or fat. You can use red or white wine vinegars, with or without added herbs like tarragon, and mix them with heart-healthy oil in a ratio of two parts vinegar to one part oil. If a dressing seems too vinegary, add a little sugar, or try balsamic or flavored vinegars, like raspberry, for calorie-free sweetness. Here's a delicious recipe for basic balsamic vinaigrette.

In a cruet or jar, mix:

1 tablespoon olive oil
2 tablespoons balsamic vinegar
1 teaspoon Dijon mustard
2 teaspoons garlic, minced
¼ cup chicken or vegetable broth

This recipe yields about ½ cup and will keep in the refrigerator for five to six days. Remember, as with many dressings and sauces, use the vinaigrette sparingly to enhance the flavor of salads, not to drown them.

For variety, try making the following substitutions:

Citrus vinaigrette: Use ¼ cup orange juice or lime juice instead of chicken broth.
Asian-style vinaigrette: Use ¼ cup rice wine vinegar instead of balsamic vinegar.

You can also customize your salad dressing with your favorite fresh herb—basil, for example. Be creative.

Nutritious Nuts

Nuts have their place in a healthy diet because they contain heart-healthy unsaturated fats. However, they're also high in calories, so use them sparingly, adding as little as a quarter to a third of the amount specified in typical recipes. You can intensify the flavor of the nuts by roasting them until brown, either in the oven at 350 degrees for ten minutes (shake the pan a few times during roasting) or on the stove top in a dry cast-iron or other heavy skillet over medium heat.

Sodium Solutions

A single teaspoon of table salt contains 2,300 milligrams of sodium—a full day's worth, according to the U.S. Department of Agriculture's Dietary Guidelines for Americans. We support the USDA recommendation of 2,300

Roasted Garlic and Peppers: Flavor Maximizers

Like nuts, which intensify in flavor when roasted, garlic and peppers transform themselves into powerful taste boosters in the oven or broiler. Here's the alchemy.

- **Garlic:** Cut the top quarter to a third from a whole, unpeeled head of garlic to expose the cloves. Lightly mist the cut surfaces of the cloves with olive oil, and if you like, top with a sprig of thyme. Wrap the head in aluminum foil and put it into a regular or toaster oven preheated to 350 degrees. At the thirty- and forty-five-minute points, squeeze the garlic gently to see if the cloves are soft (protect your hand with a dish towel). A very large head may take an hour to roast. When the cloves are soft, cool them, still in the aluminum foil, and then squeeze out the pulp. Roasted garlic pulp will keep in your refrigerator for up to a week. You can mash it into baked or boiled potatoes (no butter needed), press it to top meats and vegetables, or add it to salad dressing and sauces for a huge burst of flavor.
- **Peppers:** Cut red or yellow peppers in half, stem and seed them, and flatten the halves with your hand. Put them on a sheet of aluminum foil and place them under a preheated broiler until their skin is somewhat bubbly and charred. Remove them and transfer to a bowl just large enough to contain them, sealing it tightly with plastic wrap. Let the peppers steam until their skins soften and are cool enough to handle, about fifteen minutes. Slough off the skins and chop the roasted peppers. Add some vinegar or citrus juice to preserve them and sliced garlic or fresh herbs like basil for added flavor. Add roasted peppers to soups, sautés, sauces, and salads or just enjoy them on their own.

milligrams of sodium a day for most people. We also advise, in keeping with the same guidelines, that people who have or are at increased risk for developing high blood pressure—African Americans and adults at midlife and older, especially if they are overweight—should try to limit their intake to 1,500 milligrams a day (note that this can be difficult to do if you dine out or order take-out meals frequently—often a lot of sodium is used in their preparation).

As you reduce the salt in your diet, your taste for it will diminish. But in the meantime, here are some great ways to season with minimal salt. You won't miss the salt if your dish has full, satisfying flavors.

- If a recipe calls for salt, try using half the amount specified and keep cutting back until you find the rock-bottom minimum needed for taste.
- Replace salt with pepper (white, black, or even cayenne for a real kick); lemon or lime juice; flavored vinegars; fresh onion and garlic (or powders); cumin, curry, or chili powder; ginger; or herbs like parsley, basil, oregano, rosemary, dill, and thyme.
- Try using herbal sodium-free salt substitutes like Mrs. Dash.
- Use hot mustard sauce, Worcestershire sauce, or horseradish to boost flavor without salt. (Use sauces sparingly to keep calories in check.)

Vary the Dairy

Dairy products are rich in calcium, protein, and other nutrients, but they can also contain sodium, and some products contain a fair amount of saturated fat. One way to incorporate healthier dairy products into your cooking is by choosing low-fat cheese. In your own recipes, use nonfat, reduced-fat, or part-skim milk cheeses, decreasing the amount specified by up to one-half. Consider mixing nonfat with reduced-fat shredded cheeses to maintain flavor and heatability, since most nonfat cheeses don't melt well on their own and shredded cheese melts more quickly and evenly than sliced cheese. Many people substitute soy cheese, but check labels; some have more fat, calories, and sodium than others. And if you really want cheese flavor, remember that just a little bit of strong cheese, such as sharp Cheddar or Parmesan, can pack a powerful taste punch. You can also choose products like low-fat Swiss and part-skim mozzarella to liven things up. Remember, read the labels and pay attention to portions.

The following table shows what a difference reduced-fat cheese can make.

HIGH-FAT CHEESE	CALORIES	FAT	REDUCED-FAT CHEESE	CALORIES	FAT
Regular cottage cheese (1 cup)	240	10 g	Low-fat cottage cheese (1 cup)	160	2 g
Regular ricotta cheese (1 cup)	432	32 g	Part-skim ricotta cheese (1 cup) Nonfat ricotta cheese (1 cup)	342 200	19 g 0 g
Cream cheese, 1 ounce (2 Tbs)	100	10 g	Reduced-fat cream cheese 1 ounce (2 Tbs)	60-80	4-5 g

You'll find more information on making dairy substitutions—and for the adventurous, instructions for making yogurt cheese—at www.dukediet.com.

Better Baking

Our executive chef, Andrew Craven, has some helpful ways to cut calories that don't sacrifice flavor. To reduce saturated fats, you can try using light butter or margarine in lieu of full-fat versions. When making muffins, pancakes, and waffles, substitute canola oil in place of butter or margarine and use half the amount the recipe calls for.

To decrease the fat in baked goods, try replacing half the oil called for in the recipe with an equivalent amount of the following substitutes:

• Applesauce
• Crushed pineapple
• Grated carrots, zucchini, or apples
• Mashed bananas
• Mashed or cooked pumpkin, squash, or yams
• Prune purée or prune butter

When you decrease or replace some of the fats in a recipe, bake at a lower oven temperature (25 to 50 degrees lower) to preserve a moist consistency. After baking and cooling, refrigerate what you've made to maintain freshness.

Cholesterol and Sugar Control

You can reduce the calories, as well as the fat and cholesterol, in recipes by using egg whites or egg substitutes instead of whole eggs. In baking, use two egg whites for the first whole egg and one egg white for each additional egg. If you use an egg substitute, check the container for exact conversion. Using egg whites or egg substitutes will save you 50 calories for each egg you replace.

Every ounce of unsweetened baking chocolate you use adds 140 calories and 15 grams of fat. Try replacing it with three tablespoons of unsweetened cocoa powder and one tablespoon of heart-healthy oil (this combination has less saturated fat, but the calories and total fat are about the same). In cakes, brownies, and puddings, you can get away with using three tablespoons of unsweetened cocoa powder with two teaspoons of water in place of every ounce of unsweetened baking chocolate, which will add only 45 calories and 5 grams of fat.

Another major source of calories in baked goods is, of course, sugar. Cutting down on sugar requires some experimentation, so when you're adjusting your own recipes, expect to experiment a few times to refine them. Start by reducing the sugar by one-third to one-half. If you cut the sugar by half, decrease the liquid in the recipe by one-quarter cup. In cookie and cake recipes, you can replace the sugar that you've eliminated with nonfat dry milk powder, or try the following low-calorie sweetening tips:

- For natural sweetness, use fruits in cookies, cakes, and quick breads such as muffins, pancakes, and waffles. Good choices include raisins, dried apricots, dried cherries, dates, apples, and bananas.
- Use fruit juice instead of sugar and liquids such as milk. If the juice is acidic, add half a teaspoon of baking soda per cup of liquid.
- Enhance flavor with spices (cinnamon, allspice, nutmeg, or cloves, for example) and extracts (vanilla, lemon, almond, or chocolate).

- To reduce calories, our chefs recommend baking with one of the two sugar substitutes listed in the following chart, which indicates how to convert sugar amounts to amounts of artificial sweetener that provide a comparable amount of sweetness.

COOKING AND BAKING
WITH ARTIFICIAL SWEETENERS

SPLENDA (SUCRALOSE)		
0 (zero) calories	1 cup Splenda = 1 cup sugar	1 teaspoon Splenda = 1 teaspoon sugar
Splenda works best in foods like pie fillings, cheesecakes, sweet sauces, marinades, and glazes.		
SPLENDA BROWN SUGAR BLEND		
10 calories in 1/2 teaspoon	1/2 cup Splenda Brown Sugar Blend = 1 cup brown sugar	1/2 teaspoon Splenda Brown Sugar Blend = 1 teaspoon brown sugar
Splenda Brown Sugar Blend combines sucralose with real brown sugar, so it allows baked goods to brown and rise, with the texture, moistness, and molasses-like flavor you'd expect—but with half the calories and carbs. Use it instead of brown sugar in any recipe.		

THE DUKE DIET RECIPES

Apricot-Cranberry Oatmeal

SERVINGS: 2

*Nutritional Info
(per serving):*

Calories:	170
Carbs:	33g
Protein:	6g
Total Fat:	3g
Saturated Fat:	0.5g
Dietary Fiber:	4g
Sodium:	152mg
Cholesterol:	0mg

*Food Group
Servings:*

Starch:	0.75
Fruit:	0.5
Vegetable:	0
Protein:	0
Dairy:	0
Fat:	0

INGREDIENTS

2 cups water
½ cup steel-cut oats
1 tablespoon dried
   cranberries
1 tablespoon dried apricots
Dash salt

PREPARATION

Combine the water, oats, dried cranberries, dried apricots, and salt in a bowl. Cover and leave overnight. In the morning, transfer it to a medium saucepan and cook over medium heat for about 30 minutes.

Banana Bread

INGREDIENTS

3 cups all-purpose flour

$\frac{1}{2}$ cup plus 1 tablespoon
   packed brown sugar

2 teaspoons baking powder

$\frac{1}{2}$ teaspoon salt

$\frac{1}{4}$ teaspoon baking soda

3 tablespoons margarine,
   softened

$\frac{1}{4}$ cup reduced-fat
   buttermilk

1 teaspoon vanilla extract

2 egg whites (or $\frac{1}{4}$ cup liquid
   egg whites)

1 cup mashed banana

$\frac{1}{3}$ cup chopped walnuts

PREPARATION

Preheat the oven to 400° F. Combine the flour, $\frac{1}{2}$ cup brown sugar, baking powder, salt, and baking soda in a large mixing bowl. Using a pastry blender or fork, cut the margarine into the dry ingredients until the mixture resembles coarse meal.

Combine the buttermilk, vanilla, and egg whites in a small bowl and whisk until blended. Add the buttermilk mixture and banana to the flour mixture. Stir just until moist (dough will be wet and sticky).

Turn the dough out onto a lightly floured surface. With floured hands, knead the dough lightly four times. Coat a baking sheet with cooking spray. Put the dough on the sheet and pat it into a 9-inch circle. Sprinkle with walnuts and 1 tablespoon brown sugar. Press a knife lightly into the dough (not through the dough) to make 12 wedges. Bake for 20 minutes, or until golden.

SERVINGS: 12

*Nutritional Info
(per serving):*

Calories:	219
Carbs:	38g
Protein:	4g
Total Fat:	6g
Saturated Fat:	0.5g
Dietary Fiber:	2g
Sodium:	250mg
Cholesterol:	0mg

*Food Group
Servings:*

Starch:	2.25
Fruit:	0.25
Vegetable:	0
Protein:	0.25
Dairy:	0
Fat:	1.25

Banana Walnut Pancakes

SERVINGS: 6

Nutritional Info (per 2-pancake serving):

Calories:	197
Carbs:	32g
Protein:	7g
Total Fat:	5g
Saturated Fat:	0.5g
Dietary Fiber:	3g
Sodium:	454mg
Cholesterol:	36mg

Food Group Servings:

Starch:	1.75
Fruit:	0
Vegetable:	0
Protein:	0.25
Dairy:	0.25
Fat:	0.75

INGREDIENTS

$\frac{1}{2}$ cup all-purpose flour

$\frac{1}{2}$ cup whole-wheat flour

$\frac{1}{4}$ cup quick-cooking rolled oats

2 tablespoons yellow cornmeal

2 tablespoons packed brown sugar

$1\frac{1}{2}$ tablespoons baking powder

$\frac{1}{2}$ teaspoon salt

1 cup nonfat milk

$\frac{1}{4}$ cup nonfat plain yogurt

1 teaspoon canola oil

1 large egg

1 medium banana

$\frac{1}{4}$ cup chopped walnuts

PREPARATION

Combine the first seven ingredients in a large bowl; mix well. In a separate bowl, combine the remaining ingredients; stir well. Slowly add the wet ingredients to the dry ingredients and stir until smooth.

Heat a griddle over medium heat. When the griddle is hot, spoon about $\frac{1}{4}$ cup batter for each pancake onto the griddle. (This recipe makes about 12 pancakes.) Heat until bubbles form and each pancake is stiff enough to flip. Flip the pancakes and brown them on the other side. Remove them from the heat and serve topped with light syrup, if desired.

Blueberry, Banana, and Flaxseed Smoothie

INGREDIENTS

4 ounces low-fat plain yogurt

$\frac{1}{2}$ banana

$\frac{1}{2}$ cup blueberries

1 tablespoon flaxseeds, ground

6 ice cubes

PREPARATION

Combine all ingredients in a blender and process until smooth.

SERVING: 1

Nutritional Info (per serving):

Calories:	195
Carbs:	32g
Protein:	9g
Total Fat:	6g
Saturated Fat:	1g
Dietary Fiber:	6g
Sodium:	86mg
Cholesterol:	7mg

Food Group Servings:

Starch:	0
Fruit:	2
Vegetable:	0
Protein:	0.25
Dairy:	0.5
Fat:	0

Blueberry Bran Muffins

SERVINGS: 12

*Nutritional Info
(per 1-muffin
serving):*

Calories:	122
Carbs:	27g
Protein:	4g
Total Fat:	1g
Saturated Fat:	1g
Dietary Fiber:	4g
Sodium:	264mg
Cholesterol:	18mg

*Food Group
Servings:*

Starch:	1.50
Fruit:	0.25
Vegetable:	0
Protein:	0
Dairy:	0
Fat:	0

INGREDIENTS

1½ cups wheat bran

1 cup nonfat milk

½ cup unsweetened
   applesauce

1 large egg

⅔ cup packed brown sugar

½ teaspoon vanilla extract

½ cup all-purpose flour

½ cup whole-wheat flour

1 teaspoon baking soda

1 teaspoon baking powder

½ teaspoon salt

1 cup blueberries

PREPARATION

Preheat the oven to 375° F. Grease muffin cups or use paper liners. Mix together the wheat bran and milk, and let stand for 10 minutes.

In a large bowl, combine the applesauce, egg, brown sugar, and vanilla. Add the bran mixture and beat. Sift together the all-purpose flour, whole-wheat flour, baking soda, baking powder, and salt. Stir this into the bran mixture until just blended. Fold in the blueberries.

Scoop the batter into the muffin cups. Bake for 15 to 20 minutes, until the tops spring back when lightly tapped.

Broccoli and Cheese Quiche

INGREDIENTS

2 tablespoons fine, dry bread
    crumbs

2 large eggs

$\frac{1}{2}$ cup egg substitute

$1\frac{1}{4}$ cups low-fat milk

$\frac{1}{2}$ teaspoon Tabasco sauce

Salt to taste

Pepper to taste

2 slices light whole-wheat
    bread, toasted and diced

2 cups broccoli florets

2 teaspoons olive oil (may
    substitute salad or
    cooking oil)

1 cup chopped white onion

$\frac{1}{2}$ cup shredded Cheddar
    cheese

SERVINGS: 6

*Nutritional Info
(per serving):*

Calories:	155
Carbs:	12g
Protein:	11g
Total Fat:	8g
Saturated Fat:	3g
Dietary Fiber:	2g
Sodium:	207mg
Cholesterol:	83mg

*Food Group
Servings:*

Starch:	0.25
Fruit:	0
Vegetable:	0.25
Protein:	1.25
Dairy:	0.25
Fat:	0.25

PREPARATION

Preheat the oven to 350° F. Coat a 9-inch pie pan with cooking spray. Add the bread crumbs, tilting to coat the bottom and sides. Whisk the eggs, egg substitute, milk, Tabasco, salt, and pepper in a large bowl. Add the bread to the egg mixture and stir to coat. Refrigerate until ready to use.

Steam the broccoli until just tender, 3 or 4 minutes. Rinse under cold water and drain well. Chop coarsely.

Heat the oil in a medium nonstick skillet over medium-high heat. Add the onion, stirring often, until soft and light golden, 3 to 5 minutes. Remove the bowl of wet ingredients from the refrigerator and stir in the onion, broccoli, and cheese. Spread evenly into the prepared pan. Bake the quiche 45 to 50 minutes, until light golden and set. Let it cool slightly, cut into wedges, and serve.

French Toast

SERVING: 1

Nutritional Info (per 2-slice serving):

Calories:	235
Carbs:	43g
Protein:	8g
Total Fat:	3g
Saturated Fat:	2g
Dietary Fiber:	2g
Sodium:	470mg
Cholesterol:	0mg

Food Group Servings:

Starch:	3
Fruit:	0
Vegetable:	0
Protein:	0
Dairy:	0.5
Fat:	0

INGREDIENTS

4¾ teaspoons egg substitute

⅛ teaspoon vanilla extract

¼ teaspoon heat-stable sugar substitute (such as Splenda)

⅛ teaspoon ground cinnamon

2 slices Texas toast (or white bread)

PREPARATION

Beat together the egg substitute, vanilla, sugar substitute, and cinnamon. Heat a griddle over medium heat. Dip the bread into the batter and cook on the hot griddle until the underside is brown. Flip the bread and brown it on the other side.

Multigrain Pancakes

INGREDIENTS

1 tablespoon sunflower seeds

1 tablespoon dry millet

2 tablespoons dry pearl barley

$\frac{1}{2}$ cup wheat-bran cereal

$\frac{1}{4}$ cup whole-wheat flour

$\frac{1}{4}$ cup all-purpose flour

$\frac{3}{4}$ teaspoon baking soda

$\frac{1}{2}$ teaspoon baking powder

$\frac{1}{4}$ teaspoon salt

$\frac{1}{4}$ teaspoon ground cinnamon

$\frac{1}{8}$ teaspoon ground nutmeg

1 large egg

1 tablespoon canola oil

1 tablespoon unsweetened apple juice

$\frac{2}{3}$ cup reduced-fat buttermilk

PREPARATION

Combine the dry ingredients in a large mixing bowl. In a separate bowl, whisk together the egg, oil, and apple juice. Stir in the buttermilk. Add the egg mixture to the dry ingredients, stirring just until combined (do not overmix).

Lightly grease a griddle (or coat it with cooking spray) and heat it over medium heat until the griddle is hot (325° F to 350° F on an electric skillet). Pour $\frac{1}{4}$ cup batter for each pancake onto the hot griddle. (This recipe makes about 12 pancakes.) Cook the pancakes until bubbles form on the surface, and then turn the pancakes and cook until golden brown.

SERVINGS: 6

Nutritional Info (per 2-pancake serving):

Calories:	122
Carbs:	16g
Protein:	5g
Total Fat:	5g
Saturated Fat:	1g
Dietary Fiber:	2g
Sodium:	356mg
Cholesterol:	37mg

Food Group Servings:

Starch:	1
Fruit:	0
Vegetable:	0
Protein:	0
Dairy:	0
Fat:	0.25

Open-Faced Egg and Cheese Sandwich

SERVING: 1

*Nutritional Info
(per serving):*

Calories: 194
Carbs: 16g
Protein: 16g
Total Fat: 7g
Saturated Fat: 3g
Dietary Fiber: 2g
Sodium: 446mg
Cholesterol: 218mg

*Food Group
Servings:*

Starch: 1
Fruit: 0
Vegetable: 0
Protein: 2
Dairy: 0
Fat: 0

INGREDIENTS

1 large egg
1 ounce low-fat cheese
   (Cheddar or flavor of your
   choice)

½ whole-wheat English
   muffin

PREPARATION

Coat a skillet with cooking spray and heat it over medium heat. Crack the egg into the skillet and cook until the egg is set; flip carefully. When the egg is almost done, top it with cheese. Cover the skillet and heat until the cheese is slightly melted (watch carefully!).

Toast the English muffin half as desired. Top with the cooked egg and cheese.

Variation: For the 1,400–1,600-calorie Moderate Carbohydrate plan, add another ounce of low-fat Cheddar cheese and 2 egg whites.

Open-Faced Egg and Ham Sandwich

INGREDIENTS

1 large egg

½ whole-wheat English
   muffin

1 ounce cooked low-sodium
   ham

PREPARATION

Coat a skillet with cooking spray and heat it over medium heat. Crack the egg into the skillet and cook until the egg is set; flip carefully. Toast the English muffin half as desired. Top it with the cooked egg and ham.

SERVING: 1

*Nutritional Info
(per serving):*

Calories:	174
Carbs:	15g
Protein:	14g
Total Fat:	7g
Saturated Fat:	2g
Dietary Fiber:	2g
Sodium:	508mg
Cholesterol:	224mg

*Food Group
Servings:*

Starch:	1
Fruit:	1
Vegetable:	0
Protein:	2
Dairy:	0
Fat:	0.5

Open-Faced Egg, Ham, and Cheese Sandwich

Nutritional Info (per serving):

Calories:	253
Carbs:	17g
Protein:	27g
Total Fat:	9g
Saturated Fat:	3g
Dietary Fiber:	2g
Sodium:	797mg
Cholesterol:	230mg

Food Group Servings:

Starch:	1
Fruit:	0
Vegetable:	0
Protein:	2
Dairy:	0
Fat:	0

INGREDIENTS

1 large egg

¼ cup egg substitute

1 ounce reduced-fat cheese (Cheddar or flavor of your choice)

½ whole-wheat English muffin

1 ounce cooked low-sodium ham

PREPARATION

Coat a skillet with cooking spray and heat it over medium heat. Add the egg and egg substitute to the pan. Cook until the egg is set; flip. When the egg is almost done, top it with cheese. Cover the skillet and heat until the cheese is slightly melted (watch carefully!).

Toast the English muffin half as desired. Top with the cooked egg-cheese mixture and ham.

Scrambled Egg Substitute with Peppers

INGREDIENTS

¼ cup egg substitute

¼ cup diced red or green bell
   pepper

PREPARATION

Coat a skillet with cooking spray and heat it over medium heat.
Pour the egg substitute into the skillet, scrambling with a fork
until the egg begins to cook. Add the diced red or green pepper
and cook until softened.

SERVING: 1

*Nutritional Info
(per serving):*

Calories:	40
Carbs:	3g
Protein:	6g
Total Fat:	0g
Saturated Fat:	0g
Dietary Fiber:	1g
Sodium:	116mg
Cholesterol:	0mg

*Food Group
Servings:*

Starch:	0
Fruit:	0
Vegetable:	0.25
Protein:	1
Dairy:	0
Fat:	0

Scrambled Egg with Peppers

SERVING: 1

Nutritional Info (per serving):

Calories:	118
Carbs:	4g
Protein:	12g
Total Fat:	5g
Saturated Fat:	2g
Dietary Fiber:	1g
Sodium:	178mg
Cholesterol:	212mg

Food Group Servings:

Starch:	0
Fruit:	0
Vegetable:	0.25
Protein:	1
Dairy:	0
Fat:	0

INGREDIENTS

1 large egg

$1/4$ cup egg substitute

$1/4$ cup diced red or green bell pepper

PREPARATION

Coat a skillet with cooking spray and heat it over medium heat. Pour the egg and egg substitute into the pan, scrambling the egg mixture with a fork until it begins to cook. Add the diced red or green pepper and cook until softened.

Spinach and Cheese Omelet

INGREDIENTS

1 large egg

¼ cup egg substitute

1 ounce reduced-fat cheese
(Swiss or flavor of your
choice)

2 cups spinach, finely
chopped

PREPARATION

Whisk together the egg, egg substitute, and cheese in a medium bowl. Coat a medium frying pan with cooking spray and place it over medium-high heat. Add the spinach to the pan and sauté for 2 to 3 minutes. Add the egg mixture. As the eggs begin to set, lift the edges with a spatula so the uncooked eggs will flow to the bottom of the pan and cook. When the eggs are set and fully cooked, fold in half and serve.

Variation: For 1,400–1,600-calorie Moderate Carbohydrate plan, add an additional 1 ounce reduced-fat cheese to the omelet.

SERVING: 1

*Nutritional Info
(per serving):*

Calories:	171
Carbs:	5g
Protein:	21g
Total Fat:	7g
Saturated Fat:	3g
Dietary Fiber:	2g
Sodium:	399mg
Cholesterol:	218mg

*Food Group
Servings:*

Starch:	0
Fruit:	0
Vegetable:	0
Protein:	4
Dairy:	0
Fat:	0

Toast with Egg Salad

SERVING: 1

Nutritional Info (per serving):

Calories:	162
Carbs:	16g
Protein:	9g
Total Fat:	8g
Saturated Fat:	2g
Dietary Fiber:	2g
Sodium:	333mg
Cholesterol:	187mg

Food Group Servings:

Starch:	1
Fruit:	0
Vegetable:	0
Protein:	2
Dairy:	0
Fat:	1

INGREDIENTS

1 large egg

1 tablespoon light mayonnaise

Ground pepper to taste

1 slice whole-wheat bread

PREPARATION

Place the egg in a medium saucepan and fill it with water until the egg is completely covered. Cook over medium heat until the water boils. Turn the heat down to low and simmer about 15 minutes. Remove the egg from the pan and run it under cold water to cool. Peel and chop the egg and mix it with the mayonnaise; add ground pepper to taste. Toast the bread if desired and top it with the egg salad.

NOTE: You can hard-boil many eggs at one time for later use. Hard-boiled eggs last for up to a week in the refrigerator.

Whole-Wheat Pecan Muffins

INGREDIENTS

1/3 cup whole-wheat flour

2 tablespoons all-purpose flour

1/2 teaspoon baking powder

Dash baking soda

Dash salt

2 tablespoons cornmeal

1/3 cup low-fat buttermilk

2 tablespoons packed brown sugar

2/3 tablespoon margarine, melted

1/3 teaspoon almond extract

1 large egg white

2 tablespoons chopped pecans

PREPARATION

Preheat oven to 375° F.

To measure the flours, lightly spoon them into dry measuring cups and level with a knife. Combine the flours, baking powder, baking soda, salt, and cornmeal in a medium bowl. Make a well in the center of the mixture.

In a small bowl, whisk together the buttermilk, brown sugar, margarine, almond extract, and egg white. Add to the flour mixture, stirring just until moist.

Spoon the batter into four muffin cups coated with cooking spray; sprinkle with nuts. Bake for 20 minutes, or until the muffins spring back when touched lightly in the center. Remove them from the pans immediately.

SERVINGS: 4

Nutritional Info (per serving):

Calories:	149
Carbs:	22g
Protein:	4g
Total Fat:	5g
Saturated Fat:	1g
Dietary Fiber:	2g
Sodium:	179mg
Cholesterol:	1mg

Food Group Servings:

Starch:	1.75
Fruit:	0
Vegetable:	0
Protein:	0.25
Dairy:	0
Fat:	1

Yogurt, Nut, and Fruit Parfait

SERVING: 1

Nutritional Info (per serving):

Calories:	221
Carbs:	27g
Protein:	15g
Total Fat:	11g
Saturated Fat:	0g
Dietary Fiber:	4g
Sodium:	136mg
Cholesterol:	5mg

Food Group Servings:

Starch:	0
Fruit:	0.5
Vegetable:	0
Protein:	0.5
Dairy:	1
Fat:	2

INGREDIENTS

1 cup nonfat plain yogurt

$\frac{1}{2}$ cup strawberries, halved

2 tablespoons chopped walnuts

PREPARATION

Mix the strawberries into the yogurt. Top with the chopped walnuts.

SOUPS AND STEWS

Butternut Squash Soup

INGREDIENTS

Soup:

1¼ cups cubed butternut
   squash

1 cup chicken broth, divided

¼ teaspoon ground nutmeg

¼ teaspoon white pepper

¼ teaspoon salt

Roasted onion crème fraîche topping:

⅓ cup chopped white onion

2 tablespoons nonfat plain
   yogurt

2 tablespoons reduced-fat
   sour cream

PREPARATION

For soup: Preheat the oven to 375° F. Lay the cubed squash on a lightly oiled baking sheet. Roast the squash until soft (about 25 minutes). Let it cool. In a blender or food processor, purée the squash with ¾ cup chicken broth. Transfer to a large saucepan, season with nutmeg, white pepper, and salt and simmer for 15 minutes. Add the remaining broth until desired consistency is reached.

For topping: In a small frying pan coated with cooking spray, heat the onion until caramelized. Place the onions in a food processor and add the yogurt and sour cream. Pulse until smooth. Strain the yogurt mixture and then put it in a squirt bottle. Use it to decorate the surface of the soup.

SERVINGS: 2

Nutritional Info (per serving):

Calories:	144
Carbs:	22g
Protein:	6g
Total Fat:	4g
Saturated Fat:	2g
Dietary Fiber:	4g
Sodium:	484mg
Cholesterol:	14mg

Food Group Servings:

Starch:	0
Fruit:	0
Vegetable:	1
Protein:	0
Dairy:	0
Fat:	0

Cucumber Leek Soup

SERVINGS: 2

Nutritional Info (per serving):

Calories:	97
Carbs:	16g
Protein:	5g
Total Fat:	2g
Saturated Fat:	1g
Dietary Fiber:	2g
Sodium:	220mg
Cholesterol:	4mg

Food Group Servings:

Starch:	0.5
Fruit:	0
Vegetable:	0.5
Protein:	0
Dairy:	0
Fat:	0

INGREDIENTS

3/4 teaspoon butter

1 cup chopped cucumber, divided

1/3 cup chopped leeks

1/4 cup chopped celery

2/3 cup peeled and cubed potatoes

1/2 cup water

3/4 cup reduced-sodium chicken broth

1/8 teaspoon salt

1/8 teaspoon ground black pepper

1/4 cup nonfat plain yogurt

PREPARATION

Combine the butter, 3/4 cup cucumber, leeks, celery, potatoes, water, chicken broth, salt, and pepper in a large pot. Cook over medium-high heat until boiling. Reduce to medium-low heat, cover, and cook until the vegetables are tender (about 45 minutes). Let cool.

Pour into a blender or food processor and purée until smooth. Strain to remove any lumps. Top the soup with the remaining diced cucumber and the yogurt.

Sun-Dried Tomato and Roasted Garlic Soup

INGREDIENTS

2 teaspoons olive oil

2/3 cup chopped red onion

1/3 cup diced celery

1/3 cup diced carrots

1 teaspoon fennel seed

1 teaspoon thyme

1 teaspoon ground coriander

1/2 teaspoon white pepper

1/2 bay leaf

1 ounce reduced-sodium tomato paste

7 cups reduced-sodium chicken broth

3 ounces sun-dried tomatoes

1 tablespoon garlic, roasted and minced

2 teaspoons honey

PREPARATION

Heat the oil in a Dutch oven or stockpot over medium-high heat. Add the onion and sauté for 2 minutes. Add the celery and carrot and continue to sauté. Stir in the seasonings and tomato paste, and continue cooking, stirring mixture constantly. Pour in the broth and bring to a boil. Add the sun-dried tomatoes, roasted garlic, and honey. Simmer for 1 hour.

SERVINGS: 5

Nutritional Info (per serving):

Calories:	60
Carbs:	10g
Protein:	2g
Total Fat:	2g
Saturated Fat:	0g
Dietary Fiber:	3g
Sodium:	380mg
Cholesterol:	0mg

Food Group Servings:

Starch:	0
Fruit:	0
Vegetable:	2
Protein:	0
Dairy:	0
Fat:	0

Tortilla Soup

SERVINGS: 8

Nutritional Info (per serving):

Calories:	144
Carbs:	15g
Protein:	8g
Total Fat:	6g
Saturated Fat:	1g
Dietary Fiber:	2g
Sodium:	108mg
Cholesterol:	12mg

Food Group Servings:

Starch:	1
Fruit:	0
Vegetable:	0
Protein:	0
Dairy:	0
Fat:	0

INGREDIENTS

1 12-inch flour tortilla

2 tablespoons extra-virgin olive oil

$1/3$ cup chopped white onion

1 raw jalapeño pepper

1 clove garlic

$1/3$ cup chopped red bell pepper

$2/3$ cup garbanzo beans (chickpeas)

$2/3$ cup diced zucchini

$1\frac{1}{8}$ cup no-salt-added canned diced tomatoes

$1\frac{1}{3}$ cups reduced-sodium chicken broth

4 ounces chicken breast, cubed

$1\frac{1}{2}$ teaspoons lemon juice

$1/3$ cup chopped cilantro leaves

PREPARATION

Preheat the oven to 375° F. Lightly brush the tortilla with olive oil and slice it into thin strips. Place it on a cookie sheet and bake until slightly browned and crispy; cool and set aside.

In a Dutch oven or stockpot, sauté the onion, jalapeño, and garlic with the remaining oil. When the onions are soft, add the red bell pepper, garbanzo beans, and zucchini. Add the tomatoes, chicken broth, and chicken breast.

Simmer on medium-low heat for 30 minutes. Finish with the lemon juice and cilantro.

To serve, divide tortilla strips among bowls and pour the soup over them.

Vegetarian Chili

INGREDIENTS

2 cups fresh whole
  mushrooms

1 cup chopped white onion

$\frac{1}{2}$ cup chopped green bell
  pepper

8 teaspoons diced green chile
  pepper

1 teaspoon minced garlic

2 cups whole no-salt-added
  canned tomatoes

1 teaspoon reduced-sodium
  vegetable broth (no MSG)

$\frac{1}{2}$ cup water

2 teaspoons chili powder

$\frac{1}{8}$ teaspoon dried, ground
  cayenne pepper

$\frac{1}{2}$ teaspoon ground cumin

$\frac{1}{3}$ cup canned chili-style
  beans, drained and rinsed

$\frac{2}{3}$ cup canned black beans,
  drained and rinsed

$5\frac{1}{4}$ ounces vegetarian
  crumbles (soy burger
  substitute)

PREPARATION

Spray a skillet with cooking spray and heat it over medium heat. Slice the mushrooms and sauté them in the skillet until browned. Remove from the pan.

Spray a Dutch oven or stockpot with cooking spray and heat it over medium heat. Add the onions and peppers to the kettle and sauté until the vegetables are soft. Add the garlic, tomatoes, broth, water, chili powder, cayenne pepper, cumin, beans, and soy crumbles, and simmer gently for about 20 minutes. Add the mushrooms and simmer another 15 minutes. Serve hot.

SERVINGS: 4

*Nutritional Info
(per serving):*

Calories:	170
Carbs:	27g
Protein:	14g
Total Fat:	3g
Saturated Fat:	0g
Dietary Fiber:	8g
Sodium:	492mg
Cholesterol:	0mg

*Food Group
Servings:*

Starch:	1
Fruit:	0
Vegetable:	2
Protein:	2
Dairy:	0
Fat:	0

Asian Sesame Salad

SERVINGS: 4

Nutritional Info (per serving):

Calories:	49
Carbs:	4g
Protein:	1g
Total Fat:	4g
Saturated Fat:	1g
Dietary Fiber:	1g
Sodium:	11mg
Cholesterol:	0mg

Food Group Servings:

Starch:	0
Fruit:	0
Vegetable:	0.5
Protein:	0
Dairy:	0
Fat:	0.5

INGREDIENTS

$\frac{1}{4}$ cup carrot strips or slices

$\frac{1}{4}$ cup sliced asparagus, cut into 2-inch lengths

2 jalapeño peppers

1 tablespoon sesame seeds

2 cloves garlic, minced

2 teaspoons grated ginger root

1 teaspoon sesame oil, divided

1 tablespoon lemongrass

1 teaspoon extra-virgin olive oil

1 teaspoon lime juice

$\frac{1}{2}$ teaspoon honey

$\frac{1}{2}$ teaspoon white pepper

$\frac{1}{2}$ cup fresh arugula, chopped

PREPARATION

Preheat the oven to 375° F. Steam the carrots and asparagus until crisp; transfer them quickly to an ice bath to seal in the flavor.

Place the jalapeños on a baking sheet and roast in the preheated oven until their skins are brown. Remove the peppers and place them in a covered bowl for 10 minutes.

Heat a sauté pan over medium heat. Rapidly toast the sesame seeds, garlic, and ginger with half a teaspoon of the sesame oil. Remove from the heat when the sesame seeds turn golden brown.

Trim off the outer leaves of the lemongrass, remove the base of the stem, and slice the stalk into thin rounds. Remove the skin and seeds from the jalapeños and dice small. In a large bowl, combine the lemongrass, jalapeño, asparagus, carrot, sesame-garlic mixture, remaining sesame oil, olive oil, lime juice, honey, and pepper. Place the marinated salad over a bed of the arugula, adding a little low-sodium soy sauce if desired.

Broccoli Salad

INGREDIENTS

$\frac{1}{3}$ cup nonfat sour cream

8 teaspoons light mayonnaise

8 teaspoons cider vinegar

2 teaspoons granulated sugar

$3\frac{1}{4}$ cups broccoli florets

$\frac{2}{3}$ cup chopped red onion

$3\frac{1}{4}$ teaspoons raisins

$3\frac{1}{4}$ teaspoons sunflower seeds

PREPARATION

Mix the sour cream, mayonnaise, vinegar, and sugar to make a dressing. In a large bowl, toss the broccoli, onion, raisins, and sunflower seeds to combine. Mix with the dressing.

SERVINGS: 6

Nutritional Info (per serving):

Calories:	111
Carbs:	15g
Protein:	4g
Total Fat:	5g
Saturated Fat:	1g
Dietary Fiber:	3g
Sodium:	114mg
Cholesterol:	5mg

Food Group Servings:

Starch:	0
Fruit:	0
Vegetable:	0.5
Protein:	0
Dairy:	0
Fat:	0.5

Broccoli Slaw

SERVINGS: 2

Nutritional Info (per serving):

Calories:	63
Carbs:	9g
Protein:	3g
Total Fat:	2g
Saturated Fat:	0g
Dietary Fiber:	3g
Sodium:	238mg
Cholesterol:	2mg

Food Group Servings:

Starch:	0
Fruit:	0
Vegetable:	2
Protein:	0
Dairy:	0
Fat:	0.5

INGREDIENTS

$\frac{3}{4}$ slice vegetarian bacon

2 teaspoons low-fat yogurt

2 teaspoons light mayonnaise

$1\frac{1}{2}$ teaspoons cider vinegar

$\frac{1}{2}$ teaspoon granulated sugar

$\frac{1}{8}$ teaspoon salt

$\frac{1}{8}$ teaspoon ground black pepper

4 ounces broccoli florets

4 teaspoons chopped red onion

$1\frac{1}{2}$ ounces water chestnuts, chopped

PREPARATION

Cook the vegetarian bacon in a large skillet over medium heat, turning frequently until crisp. Chop coarsely.

Whisk the yogurt, mayonnaise, vinegar, sugar, salt, and pepper in a large bowl. Add the broccoli, red onion, water chestnuts, and bacon; toss to coat.

Broccoli with Dijon Vinaigrette

INGREDIENTS

1 pound broccoli florets

2 teaspoons extra-virgin olive oil

2 tablespoons chopped green onion

1/4 teaspoon dried tarragon

1/4 teaspoon dry mustard

1 1/2 cloves garlic, minced

1 tablespoon red wine vinegar

1 tablespoon water

1 1/2 teaspoons Dijon mustard

1/8 teaspoon ground black pepper

PREPARATION

Steam the broccoli, covered, for 6 minutes, or until tender-crisp. Drain; place in a serving bowl.

Heat the olive oil in a small saucepan over medium heat. Add the green onion, tarragon, mustard, and garlic, and sauté for 3 minutes. Remove from the heat. Add the vinegar and remaining ingredients, stirring with a whisk until blended. Drizzle over the broccoli, tossing gently to coat.

SERVINGS: 4

Nutritional Info (per serving):

Calories:	57
Carbs:	7g
Protein:	4g
Total Fat:	3g
Saturated Fat:	0g
Dietary Fiber:	4g
Sodium:	56mg
Cholesterol:	0mg

Food Group Servings:

Starch:	0
Fruit:	0
Vegetable:	1.25
Protein:	0
Dairy:	0
Fat:	0.5

Chef Salad with Turkey and Ham

SERVING: 1

Nutritional Info (per serving):

Calories:	339
Carbs:	5g
Protein:	35g
Total Fat:	20g
Saturated Fat:	4g
Dietary Fiber:	1g
Sodium:	636mg
Cholesterol:	247mg

Food Group Servings:

Starch:	0
Fruit:	0
Vegetable:	2
Protein:	5
Dairy:	0
Fat:	1

INGREDIENTS

1 medium egg

2 cups romaine lettuce

1 ounce lean low-sodium ham

2 ounces roasted turkey breast

1 ounce sliced low-fat Cheddar cheese

1 tablespoon low-fat balsamic vinaigrette

PREPARATION

Place the egg in a saucepan. Fill the pan with water until the egg is completely submerged. Heat to boiling over medium heat, then reduce the heat and simmer about 15 minutes. Remove the egg from the pan and run it under cold water to cool. Peel the egg and slice it.

In a large bowl, combine the lettuce, ham, turkey, cheese, and egg slices. Add the vinaigrette and toss to coat.

Chicken Fajita Salad with Creamy Cilantro-Lime Sauce

INGREDIENTS

Salad:

1 tablespoon olive oil

1 teaspoon ground cumin

1 teaspoon paprika

1 teaspoon chili powder

1/4 teaspoon ground black pepper

1 pound chicken breast, skinned, boned, and cut into thin strips

6 cups shredded romaine lettuce

1 1/3 cups thinly sliced green bell pepper rings

1 cup sliced red onion, separated into rings

1/2 cup grated Cheddar cheese

1 cup cooked black beans

1 medium tomato, cut into wedges

Sauce:

1/2 cup nonfat sour cream

1/2 cup light mayonnaise

1/3 cup nonfat milk

3 tablespoons lime juice

3 tablespoons cilantro leaves, chopped

1 tablespoon balsamic vinegar

2 cloves garlic, minced

SERVINGS: 4

Nutritional Info (per serving):

Calories:	355
Carbs:	26g
Protein:	36g
Total Fat:	13g
Saturated Fat:	4g
Dietary Fiber:	6g
Sodium:	581mg
Cholesterol:	87mg

Food Group Servings:

Starch:	0.75
Fruit:	0
Vegetable:	1.5
Protein:	3.5
Dairy:	0
Fat:	0.75

PREPARATION

For salad: In a medium bowl, combine the olive oil, cumin, paprika, chili powder, and black pepper. Add the chicken; toss to coat. Coat a large nonstick skillet with cooking spray and place it over medium heat until hot. Add the chicken mixture; sauté 8 minutes, or until the chicken is done. Set aside.

Divide the lettuce, bell pepper rings, red onion, cheese, beans, and tomato evenly among four bowls; top with the chicken mixture. Serve with Creamy Cilantro-Lime Sauce (recipe below).

For sauce: In a medium bowl, whisk together the sour cream, mayonnaise, milk, lime juice, cilantro, vinegar, and garlic. Cover the sauce and chill until ready for use.

Cold Dijon Carrots

SERVINGS: 4

*Nutritional Info
(per serving):*

Calories:	86
Carbs:	12g
Protein:	2g
Total Fat:	4g
Saturated Fat:	0g
Dietary Fiber:	2g
Sodium:	206mg
Cholesterol:	0mg

*Food Group
Servings:*

Starch:	0
Fruit:	0
Vegetable:	1
Protein:	0
Dairy:	0
Fat:	0.5

INGREDIENTS

4 cups baby carrots

1 clove garlic, minced

1 tablespoon water

1 tablespoon extra-virgin
    olive oil

2 tablespoons Dijon mustard

1 tablespoon whole-grain
    mustard (may substitute
    Dijon mustard)

PREPARATION

Cook the carrots in boiling water 5 to 10 minutes, or until the carrots are tender. Drain the carrots and run them under cold water to stop the cooking process. Allow to cool completely. In a small bowl, whisk together the garlic, water, olive oil, and mustards. Pour over the cooled carrots and toss to coat.

Coleslaw

INGREDIENTS

8 ounces cabbage, shredded

$\frac{1}{2}$ cup grated carrots

8 teaspoons light mayonnaise

$\frac{1}{2}$ teaspoon celery seed

$\frac{1}{2}$ teaspoon cider vinegar

$\frac{1}{2}$ teaspoon Dijon mustard

$\frac{3}{4}$ teaspoon heat-stable sugar substitute (such as Splenda)

PREPARATION

In a large bowl, combine all ingredients. Chill for at least one hour. Serve cold.

SERVINGS: 4

Nutritional Info (per serving):

Calories:	55
Carbs:	6g
Protein:	1g
Total Fat:	4g
Saturated Fat:	1g
Dietary Fiber:	2g
Sodium:	116mg
Cholesterol:	4mg

Food Group Servings:

Starch:	0
Fruit:	0
Vegetable:	2
Protein:	0
Dairy:	0
Fat:	1

Cranberry Pecan Salad

SERVING: 1

*Nutritional Info
(per serving):*

Calories:	133
Carbs:	10g
Protein:	5g
Total Fat:	9g
Saturated Fat:	3g
Dietary Fiber:	3g
Sodium:	230mg
Cholesterol:	17mg

*Food Group
Servings:*

Starch:	0
Fruit:	0
Vegetable:	0
Protein:	1.25
Dairy:	0
Fat:	1.5

INGREDIENTS

1½ cups mixed greens

1 tablespoon pecan halves

2 tablespoons crumbled feta
    cheese

1 tablespoon dried
    cranberries

PREPARATION

Place the greens in a salad bowl. Top with the pecans, feta, and
dried cranberries.

Cucumber–Red Onion Salad

INGREDIENTS

2 cups sliced cucumber

¼ cup chopped red onion

¼ cup light mayonnaise

¼ cup reduced-fat sour
   cream

2 tablespoons white vinegar

¼ teaspoon ground black
   pepper

⅛ teaspoon onion powder

PREPARATION

Combine the cucumbers and red onion in a medium bowl.

Combine the mayonnaise, sour cream, vinegar, pepper, and onion powder; mix well. Fold into the cucumbers and onions until coated. Add cherry tomatoes, if desired.

SERVINGS: 4

Nutritional Info (per serving):

Calories:	86
Carbs:	5g
Protein:	1g
Total Fat:	7g
Saturated Fat:	1g
Dietary Fiber:	1g
Sodium:	136mg
Cholesterol:	13mg

Food Group Servings:

Starch:	0
Fruit:	0
Vegetable:	0.5
Protein:	0
Dairy:	0
Fat:	1

Cucumber-Tomato Salad

SERVING: 1

Nutritional Info (per serving):

Calories: 73
Carbs: 7g
Protein: 1g
Total Fat: 5g
Saturated Fat: 1g
Dietary Fiber: 1g
Sodium: 8mg
Cholesterol: 0mg

Food Group Servings:

Starch: 0
Fruit: 0
Vegetable: 0.75
Protein: 0
Dairy: 0
Fat: 1

INGREDIENTS

4 slices tomato
½ cup sliced cucumber
1 tablespoon balsamic vinegar

1 teaspoon extra-virgin
    olive oil
Salt and pepper to taste

PREPARATION

Arrange the cucumber and tomato slices on a plate. Drizzle with the balsamic vinegar and olive oil. Add salt and pepper to taste.

Green Beans Provençal

INGREDIENTS

2 teaspoons extra-virgin
olive oil

8 cherry tomatoes, halved

3 tablespoons chopped red
onion

1 clove garlic, minced

4 teaspoons white wine
vinegar

2¾ cups green beans, ends
trimmed and cut to
desired length

⅛ teaspoon dried thyme

⅛ teaspoon ground black
pepper

3½ tablespoons chopped
parsley

4 teaspoons water

2 teaspoons grated Parmesan
cheese

PREPARATION

Heat the oil in a nonstick pan over medium heat. Add the tomatoes, onion, and garlic. Cook for 2 minutes.

In a saucepan, combine the white wine vinegar, green beans, thyme, black pepper, parsley, and water. Cover and simmer for 10 minutes, or until the beans are tender. Drain the beans and sprinkle with the Parmesan cheese.

SERVINGS: 4

*Nutritional Info
(per serving):*

Calories:	63
Carbs:	8g
Protein:	2g
Total Fat:	3g
Saturated Fat:	1g
Dietary Fiber:	3g
Sodium:	30mg
Cholesterol:	1mg

*Food Group
Servings:*

Starch:	0
Fruit:	0
Vegetable:	1
Protein:	0
Dairy:	0
Fat:	0.5

Green Salad with Chicken, Avocado, Orange Segments, and Fat-Free Honey Dressing

SERVINGS: 2

Nutritional Info (per serving):

Calories:	381
Carbs:	33g
Protein:	41g
Total Fat:	11g
Saturated Fat:	2g
Dietary Fiber:	6g
Sodium:	100mg
Cholesterol:	96mg

Food Group Servings:

Starch:	1
Fruit:	0.5
Vegetable:	2
Protein:	4
Dairy:	0
Fat:	1

INGREDIENTS

¼ cup water

¼ cup white wine vinegar

2 tablespoons honey

2 heads butter lettuce, washed, dried, and torn into bite-size pieces

1 head radicchio, washed, dried, and torn into bite-size pieces

8 ounces precooked chicken breast, sliced into strips

⅛ avocado, sliced

1 orange, peeled and separated into segments, with seeds removed

3 tablespoons sliced almonds

PREPARATION

To make the dressing, mix the water, vinegar, and honey until thoroughly combined.

In a large bowl, combine the lettuce and radicchio leaves. Add the sliced chicken, sliced avocado, and orange segments. Add the dressing to the salad and toss; sprinkle with almonds.

Mixed Greens with Walnut, Goat Cheese, and Pear

INGREDIENTS

1 tablespoon extra-virgin
   olive oil

2 teaspoons balsamic vinegar

½ teaspoon ground black
   pepper

2 teaspoons Dijon mustard

4 cups chopped romaine
   lettuce

2 ounces goat cheese,
   crumbled

4 tablespoons chopped
   walnuts

¼ cup sliced pears

PREPARATION

To make the dressing, whisk together the oil, vinegar, pepper, and mustard in a small bowl. Place the lettuce in large bowl, add the dressing, and toss. Top with the goat cheese, walnuts, and pears.

SERVINGS: 4

Nutritional Info (per serving):

Calories:	137
Carbs:	5g
Protein:	5g
Total Fat:	12g
Saturated Fat:	3g
Dietary Fiber:	2g
Sodium:	90mg
Cholesterol:	7mg

Food Group Servings:

Starch:	0
Fruit:	0
Vegetable:	1
Protein:	1.5
Dairy:	0
Fat:	1

Onion Ragout

SERVINGS: 4

Nutritional Info (per serving):

Calories: 87
Carbs: 10g
Protein: 2g
Total Fat: 5g
Saturated Fat: 1g
Dietary Fiber: 3g
Sodium: 10mg
Cholesterol: 0mg

Food Group Servings:

Starch: 0
Fruit: 0
Vegetable: 0.5
Protein: 0
Dairy: 0
Fat: 1

INGREDIENTS

4 teaspoons extra-virgin olive oil

$\frac{1}{2}$ teaspoon minced garlic

$\frac{3}{4}$ cup plus 1 tablespoon chopped tomatoes

$\frac{1}{8}$ teaspoon ground black pepper

$2\frac{1}{2}$ medium onions, peeled and thinly sliced

$\frac{1}{2}$ teaspoon ground coriander

$\frac{1}{8}$ teaspoon ground cinnamon

$\frac{1}{3}$ cup fat-free, sodium-free chicken broth

$1\frac{1}{4}$ teaspoons dried thyme

$\frac{1}{2}$ bay leaf

$\frac{1}{2}$ teaspoon orange peel

2 teaspoons orange juice

2 teaspoons fresh cilantro

$\frac{1}{2}$ teaspoon packed brown sugar

PREPARATION

Heat the oil in a large nonstick skillet over medium heat. Add all the remaining ingredients, reduce the heat to low, cover, and simmer for 10 minutes, stirring occasionally.

Pomegranate, Steak, and Spinach Salad

INGREDIENTS

4½ teaspoons pomegranate
    juice

1½ teaspoons white wine
    vinegar

1 teaspoon Dijon mustard

1 teaspoon extra-virgin
    olive oil

¼ teaspoon honey

3 cups baby spinach

¼ cup mandarin oranges,
    drained

1 ounce pomegranate
    seeds

1 tablespoon dry-roasted,
    unsalted almonds

Salt and pepper to taste

4 ounces lean beef flank steak
    (London broil)

PREPARATION

For dressing, in a small bowl, whisk together the pomegranate juice, vinegar, mustard, oil, and honey.

In a large bowl, combine the spinach, oranges, pomegranate seeds, and almonds. Toss, adding all but 2 teaspoons of the dressing. Season with salt and pepper to taste.

Heat a small skillet over medium-high heat. Lightly spray the steak with cooking spray and sauté in a hot skillet 3 minutes per side for medium-rare. Remove from the heat and let the meat rest for 3 minutes before slicing thinly. Top the salad with the steak slices and drizzle it with the remaining dressing.

SERVING: 1

*Nutritional Info
(per serving):*

Calories:	387
Carbs:	35g
Protein:	28g
Total Fat:	17g
Saturated Fat:	4g
Dietary Fiber:	5g
Sodium:	232mg
Cholesterol:	47mg

*Food Group
Servings:*

Starch:	0
Fruit:	0.25
Vegetable:	2.25
Protein:	3
Dairy:	0
Fat:	2

Roasted Ratatouille

SERVINGS: 4

Nutritional Info (per serving):

Calories:	104
Carbs:	7g
Protein:	2g
Total Fat:	8g
Saturated Fat:	1g
Dietary Fiber:	1g
Sodium:	84mg
Cholesterol:	0mg

Food Group Servings:

Starch:	0
Fruit:	0
Vegetable:	0.5
Protein:	0
Dairy:	0
Fat:	2

INGREDIENTS

$\frac{1}{3}$ cup peeled eggplant, cut into cubes

2 tablespoons olive oil

$\frac{1}{3}$ cup diced zucchini

$\frac{1}{3}$ cup diced yellow summer squash

$\frac{1}{3}$ cup julienned red bell pepper

$\frac{1}{3}$ cup chopped tomato

$\frac{1}{3}$ cup chopped red onion

4 teaspoons minced garlic

$\frac{3}{4}$ teaspoon dried thyme

$\frac{1}{8}$ teaspoon salt

$\frac{1}{2}$ teaspoon ground black pepper

2 tablespoons red wine vinegar

7 tablespoons fat-free, sodium-free chicken broth

PREPARATION

Preheat the broiler. Place the cubed eggplant in a single layer in a pan or broiler rack sprayed with cooking spray. Broil 5 minutes, or until browned.

Heat the oil in a large saucepan over medium heat. Add the rest of the vegetables, garlic, and seasonings. Sauté until softened and slightly browned. Remove the vegetables and deglaze the pan with the red wine vinegar. Return the vegetables to the pan, add the cooked eggplant and chicken stock, and simmer for 30 minutes.

Roasted Vegetables with Olive Oil and Feta Cheese

INGREDIENTS

²⁄₃ cup baby carrots

²⁄₃ cup cauliflower florets

²⁄₃ cup chopped zucchini

²⁄₃ cup chopped yellow
   squash

¹⁄₃ cup chopped red bell
   pepper

¹⁄₃ cup chopped green bell
   pepper

1¹⁄₃ cups chopped tomato

4 teaspoons extra-virgin
   olive oil

¹⁄₂ teaspoon dried basil

¹⁄₂ teaspoon dried oregano

¹⁄₂ teaspoon garlic powder

¹⁄₂ teaspoon ground black
   pepper

¹⁄₂ teaspoon paprika

2 ounces feta cheese,
   crumbled

PREPARATION

Preheat the oven to 350° F. Mix the vegetables, oil, and spices in large bowl until the vegetables are well coated. Spread the vegetables out evenly in a single layer on a sheet pan well coated with cooking spray. Roast for 15 to 20 minutes, until done (the vegetables should be softened and browned). Serve the vegetables topped with the feta cheese.

SERVINGS: 4

Nutritional Info (per serving):

Calories:	123
Carbs:	10g
Protein:	4g
Total Fat:	8g
Saturated Fat:	3g
Dietary Fiber:	3g
Sodium:	182mg
Cholesterol:	13mg

Food Group Servings:

Starch:	0
Fruit:	0
Vegetable:	1
Protein:	0.25
Dairy:	0
Fat:	1

Roasted Winter Vegetables

SERVINGS: 4

Nutritional Info (per serving):

Calories:	164
Carbs:	36g
Protein:	4g
Total Fat:	2g
Saturated Fat:	0.5g
Dietary Fiber:	7g
Sodium:	252mg
Cholesterol:	0mg

Food Group Servings:

Starch:	0
Fruit:	0
Vegetable:	1.5
Protein:	0
Dairy:	0
Fat:	0.25

INGREDIENTS

8 ounces roughly chopped beets

$2\frac{1}{4}$ cups roughly chopped butternut squash

$1\frac{1}{2}$ cups roughly chopped turnips

1 cup roughly chopped white onion

1 cup roughly chopped carrots

$\frac{1}{2}$ cup unpeeled, roughly chopped potatoes

4 cloves garlic, roughly chopped

$1\frac{1}{2}$ teaspoons extra-virgin olive oil

$\frac{1}{4}$ teaspoon salt

$\frac{1}{4}$ teaspoon ground black pepper

PREPARATION

Preheat the oven to 450° F. Place the beets, squash, turnips, onion, carrots, potatoes, and garlic in a 9×13-inch baking dish coated with cooking spray. Drizzle with the oil. Sprinkle with the salt and pepper. Bake for 45 minutes, stirring occasionally, until the vegetables are softened and browned.

Sautéed Cabbage

INGREDIENTS

1½ tablespoons extra-virgin
olive oil

4 cups shredded red cabbage

PREPARATION

Heat the oil in a 10-inch skillet over medium heat. Add the cabbage and reduce the heat to low. Cover and simmer, stirring occasionally, until the cabbage is tender-crisp.

SERVINGS: 4

*Nutritional Info
(per serving):*

Calories:	64
Carbs:	4g
Protein:	1g
Total Fat:	5g
Saturated Fat:	1g
Dietary Fiber:	1g
Sodium:	13mg
Cholesterol:	0mg

*Food Group
Servings:*

Starch:	0
Fruit:	0
Vegetable:	1
Protein:	0
Dairy:	0
Fat:	1

Spinach Salad with Avocado and Pear

SERVING: 1

Nutritional Info (per serving):

Calories:	254
Carbs:	21g
Protein:	5g
Total Fat:	18g
Saturated Fat:	3g
Dietary Fiber:	8g
Sodium:	176mg
Cholesterol:	0mg

Food Group Servings:

Starch:	0
Fruit:	0.5
Vegetable:	2
Protein:	0.25
Dairy:	0
Fat:	3

INGREDIENTS

2 cups fresh spinach
1/2 medium pear, sliced
1 1/2 ounces avocado, sliced
1 tablespoon low-fat balsamic vinaigrette
1 1/2 tablespoons sliced almonds

PREPARATION

In a large bowl, combine the spinach and the pear and avocado slices. Pour the vinaigrette over the salad and toss to combine. Sprinkle with the almonds before serving.

Variation: For the 1,400–1,600-calorie Moderate Carbohydrate plan, use a whole pear in the salad.

Spinach Soy Nut Salad

INGREDIENTS

2 cups fresh spinach

1 medium nectarine, sliced

3/4 ounce soy nuts, roasted
   and salted

2 tablespoons reduced-fat
   dressing

Vinegar to taste

PREPARATION

In a medium bowl, combine the spinach, nectarine slices, and soy nuts; toss with the dressing. If desired, add vinegar to taste.

Variation: For the 1,400–1,600-calorie Moderate Carbohydrate plan, add another 3/4 ounce soy nuts.

SERVING: 1

*Nutritional Info
(per serving):*

Calories:	222
Carbs:	28g
Protein:	11g
Total Fat:	7g
Saturated Fat:	2g
Dietary Fiber:	6g
Sodium:	404mg
Cholesterol:	5mg

*Food Group
Servings:*

Starch:	0
Fruit:	1
Vegetable:	2
Protein:	1
Dairy:	0
Fat:	2

Spinach-Cherry Tomato Salad

SERVING: 1

Nutritional Info (per serving):

Calories:	157
Carbs:	17g
Protein:	5g
Total Fat:	8g
Saturated Fat:	2g
Dietary Fiber:	6g
Sodium:	368mg
Cholesterol:	5mg

Food Group Servings:

Starch:	0
Fruit:	0
Vegetable:	3
Protein:	0
Dairy:	0
Fat:	2

INGREDIENTS

1 cup cherry tomatoes

¼ avocado

2 cups fresh spinach

2 tablespoons reduced-fat dressing

Vinegar to taste

PREPARATION

Slice the cherry tomatoes in half and dice the avocado. Combine the tomatoes, avocado, and spinach in a medium bowl. Pour the dressing over the salad and toss to coat. If desired, add vinegar to taste.

Spinach-Pear Salad

INGREDIENTS

1½ cups chopped fresh
   spinach

½ cup chopped raw carrots

½ medium pear, thinly sliced

5 cherry tomatoes

1 tablespoon low-calorie
   creamy dressing

PREPARATION

Place the spinach in a bowl. Top with the carrots, pear slices, cherry tomatoes, and dressing. Toss to coat.

SERVING: 1

*Nutritional Info
(per serving):*

Calories:	134
Carbs:	26g
Protein:	3g
Total Fat:	3g
Saturated Fat:	0g
Dietary Fiber:	6g
Sodium:	181mg
Cholesterol:	0mg

*Food Group
Servings:*

Starch:	0
Fruit:	0.5
Vegetable:	2
Protein:	0
Dairy:	0
Fat:	1

Thai Chicken Broccoli Salad

SERVINGS: 2

*Nutritional Info
(per serving):*

Calories:	446
Carbs:	43.5g
Protein:	37.5g
Total Fat:	13.5g
Saturated Fat:	3g
Dietary Fiber:	4.5g
Sodium:	348mg
Cholesterol:	72mg

*Food Group
Servings:*

Starch:	2
Fruit:	0
Vegetable:	0.5
Protein:	4
Dairy:	0
Fat:	1

INGREDIENTS

3 ounces dry linguine

9 ounces skinless chicken breast, cubed

$3/4$ cup raw broccoli florets

$4^{1}/_{2}$ teaspoons water

4 tablespoons chopped red bell pepper

2 scallions (green onions), chopped

$1^{1}/_{2}$ tablespoons peanut butter

$2^{1}/_{4}$ teaspoons reduced-sodium soy sauce

$3/4$ teaspoon sesame oil

$1/8$ teaspoon crushed red pepper

$1/8$ teaspoon garlic powder

$1^{1}/_{2}$ tablespoons dry-roasted, unsalted peanuts

PREPARATION

Cook the pasta according to the package directions, omitting salt. Drain; set aside.

Spray a large nonstick skillet with cooking spray; heat it over medium-high heat. Add the chicken; stir-fry 5 minutes or until the chicken is no longer pink. Remove the chicken from the skillet.

Add the broccoli and $2^{1}/_{2}$ teaspoons cold water to the skillet. Cook, covered, 2 minutes. Uncover; cook and stir 2 minutes or until the broccoli is tender-crisp. Remove the broccoli from the skillet.

Combine the pasta, chicken, broccoli, bell pepper, and scallions in a large bowl. In a small bowl, mix the peanut butter, $2^{1}/_{2}$ teaspoons hot water, soy sauce, oil, red pepper, and garlic powder until well blended. Drizzle over the pasta mixture; toss to coat. Top with the peanuts before serving.

SANDWICHES

Chicken Caesar Wrap

INGREDIENTS

1 medium whole-wheat flour
    tortilla

2 cups fresh spinach

3 ounces grilled chicken

2 tablespoons low-calorie
    Caesar dressing

PREPARATION

Place the tortilla on a plate. Top with the spinach, chicken, and dressing. Tightly roll up the tortilla and cut it in half diagonally.

SERVING: 1

*Nutritional Info
(per serving):*

Calories:	336
Carbs:	29g
Protein:	34g
Total Fat:	8g
Saturated Fat:	2g
Dietary Fiber:	4g
Sodium:	592mg
Cholesterol:	78mg

*Food Group
Servings:*

Starch:	1.5
Fruit:	0
Vegetable:	0
Protein:	3
Dairy:	0
Fat:	1

Chicken, Cheese, and Arugula Panini

SERVING: 1

*Nutritional Info
(per serving):*

Calories:	421
Carbs:	33g
Protein:	41g
Total Fat:	13g
Saturated Fat:	5g
Dietary Fiber:	5g
Sodium:	750mg
Cholesterol:	69mg

*Food Group
Servings:*

Starch:	2
Fruit:	0
Vegetable:	1
Protein:	3
Dairy:	0
Fat:	0

INGREDIENTS

½ cup fresh arugula

2 slices whole-wheat bread

1 ounce low-fat Cheddar
   cheese

1 ounce reduced-fat
   provolone cheese

3 slices tomato

2 ounces roasted chicken
   breast

Dash salt

Dash ground black pepper

PREPARATION

Wash the arugula leaves, remove the stems if necessary, and pat the leaves dry with a paper towel. On one slice of bread, layer the cheese, tomato, arugula, and chicken; season with salt and pepper and top with the second slice of bread. Coat a medium frying pan with cooking spray and heat it over medium-high heat. Cook the sandwich, flipping it when the underside is golden brown, until the cheese is melted and both sides are browned.

Chicken Hummus Wrap

INGREDIENTS

1 medium whole-wheat flour
    tortilla

2 tablespoons hummus (store-
    bought)

3 ounces chicken breast

1 ounce low-fat Cheddar
    cheese, sliced

2 slices tomato

PREPARATION

Lay the tortilla on a plate. Spread the hummus over the tortilla to
within 1 inch of the edge. Place the chicken, cheese, and tomato
slices in the center third. Tightly roll up the tortilla and cut it in
half diagonally.

SERVING: 1

*Nutritional Info
(per serving):*

Calories:	376
Carbs:	27g
Protein:	30g
Total Fat:	11g
Saturated Fat:	3g
Dietary Fiber:	4g
Sodium:	513mg
Cholesterol:	78mg

*Food Group
Servings:*

Starch:	2
Fruit:	0
Vegetable:	0.25
Protein:	4
Dairy:	0
Fat:	1

Chicken Salad in a Whole-Wheat Pita

SERVING: 1

Nutritional Info (per serving):

Calories:	284
Carbs:	24g
Protein:	30g
Total Fat:	8g
Saturated Fat:	4g
Dietary Fiber:	3g
Sodium:	518mg
Cholesterol:	72mg

Food Group Servings:

Starch:	1
Fruit:	0
Vegetable:	0
Protein:	3
Dairy:	0
Fat:	2

INGREDIENTS

3 ounces roasted chicken breast

2 tablespoons diced celery

2 tablespoons diced onion

2 tablespoons reduced-fat mayonnaise

½ whole-wheat pita

PREPARATION

Dice the chicken and combine it with the celery, onion, and mayonnaise in a small bowl. Mix well. Stuff the chicken salad into the pita and serve.

Variation: For the 1,400–1,600-calorie Moderate Carbohydrate plan, add one more ounce of roasted chicken breast.

Grilled Cheese Sandwich

INGREDIENTS

2 slices 100%-whole-wheat
   bread

1 ounce low-fat Cheddar
   cheese, sliced

1 ounce reduced-fat
   provolone cheese

3 slices tomato

PREPARATION

Heat a frying pan over medium-high heat. Coat the pan with cooking spray. Layer one slice of bread with the cheeses and tomato, and cover with the other slice of bread. Cook until the underside is golden brown. Flip the sandwich and cook until the cheese is melted and both sides are brown.

SERVING: 1

*Nutritional Info
(per serving):*

Calories:	324
Carbs:	33g
Protein:	23g
Total Fat:	11g
Saturated Fat:	4g
Dietary Fiber:	5g
Sodium:	705mg
Cholesterol:	21mg

*Food Group
Servings:*

Starch:	2
Fruit:	0
Vegetable:	0.5
Protein:	2
Dairy:	0
Fat:	0

Ham and Turkey Reuben

SERVING: 1

*Nutritional Info
(per serving):*

Calories: 310
Carbs: 35g
Protein: 32g
Total Fat: 8g
Saturated Fat: 2g
Dietary Fiber: 4g
Sodium: 1,015mg
Cholesterol: 66mg

*Food Group
Servings:*

Starch: 2
Fruit: 0
Vegetable: 1
Protein: 4
Dairy: 0
Fat: 0.5

INGREDIENTS

2 slices rye bread

5 squirts spray margarine
   (such as I Can't Believe
   It's Not Butter! spray)

2 ounces lower-sodium ham

2 ounces roasted turkey
   breast

½ cup low-sodium sauerkraut

PREPARATION

Spray one side of one slice of bread with spray margarine. Turn the slice over (margarine side down) and top it with the ham, turkey, and sauerkraut. Top this with the second slice of bread and spray the top with margarine. Heat a frying pan over medium-high heat. Cook the sandwich until the underside is golden brown. Flip it and cook until both sides are brown.

Mediterranean Wrap

INGREDIENTS

1 whole-wheat flour tortilla

2 tablespoons hummus (store-bought)

¼ cup chopped red bell pepper

3 ounces cooked turkey breast

2 ounces low-fat Cheddar cheese

2 tablespoons fresh mint, chopped

¼ cup romaine lettuce, chopped

PREPARATION

Lay the tortilla on a large cutting board. Spread the hummus evenly over the tortilla to within ½ inch of the edge. Lay the peppers evenly over the hummus. Layer slices of the turkey and cheese, sprinkle with the mint, and then top with the lettuce leaves. Tightly roll up the tortilla and cut it in half diagonally.

SERVING: 1

Nutritional Info (per serving):

Calories:	333
Carbs:	37g
Protein:	34g
Total Fat:	10g
Saturated Fat:	4g
Dietary Fiber:	4g
Sodium:	1,328mg
Cholesterol:	58mg

Food Group Servings:

Starch:	2
Fruit:	0
Vegetable:	0.25
Protein:	4
Dairy:	0
Fat:	0

Open-Faced Ham and Turkey Reuben

SERVING: 1

Nutritional Info (per serving):

Calories:	247
Carbs:	20g
Protein:	29g
Total Fat:	7g
Saturated Fat:	2g
Dietary Fiber:	3g
Sodium:	878mg
Cholesterol:	66mg

Food Group Servings:

Starch:	1
Fruit:	0
Vegetable:	1
Protein:	4
Dairy:	0
Fat:	0.5

INGREDIENTS

1 slice rye bread

5 squirts spray margarine (such as I Can't Believe It's Not Butter! spray)

2 ounces lower-sodium ham

2 ounces roasted turkey breast

½ cup low-sodium sauerkraut

PREPARATION

Spray one side of the slice of bread with the spray margarine. Turn the bread over (margarine side down) and top it with the ham, turkey, and sauerkraut. In a frying pan over medium-high heat, cook the sandwich, bread side down, until the bread is golden brown and the meat and sauerkraut are warm.

Tuna Melt on English Muffin

INGREDIENTS

3 ounces albacore tuna,
  packed in water

1 tablespoon light mayonnaise

2 tablespoons diced celery

2 tablespoons chopped white
  onion

1 whole-wheat English
  muffin

2 slices tomato

1 ounce low-fat Cheddar
  cheese

PREPARATION

Combine the tuna, mayonnaise, celery, and onion in a medium bowl; mix well. Scoop onto the English muffin and top with the sliced tomato and Cheddar cheese. Heat in a broiler or toaster oven until the cheese is melted.

SERVING: 1

Nutritional Info (per serving):

Calories:	320
Carbs:	33g
Protein:	33g
Total Fat:	6g
Saturated Fat:	2g
Dietary Fiber:	5g
Sodium:	769mg
Cholesterol:	43mg

Food Group Servings:

Starch:	2
Fruit:	0
Vegetable:	0.25
Protein:	4
Dairy:	0
Fat:	0.5

Tuna Salad on Pita

SERVING: 1

*Nutritional Info
(per serving):*

Calories:	331
Carbs:	41g
Protein:	29g
Total Fat:	8g
Saturated Fat:	2g
Dietary Fiber:	6g
Sodium:	830mg
Cholesterol:	37mg

*Food Group
Servings:*

Starch:	2
Fruit:	0
Vegetable:	0
Protein:	3
Dairy:	0
Fat:	1

INGREDIENTS

3 ounces tuna, packed in water

2 tablespoons light
   mayonnaise

1 stalk celery, diced

1 whole-wheat pita

PREPARATION

In a medium bowl, combine the tuna with the mayonnaise. Add the diced celery and mix well. Stuff the pita with the tuna salad.

Turkey, Cheese, and Kale Panini

INGREDIENTS

1 cup fresh kale

Salt and pepper to taste

2 slices 100%-whole-wheat
   bread

1 ounce low-fat Cheddar
   cheese, sliced

1 ounce reduced-fat
   provolone cheese

3 slices tomato

2 ounces roasted turkey
   breast

PREPARATION

Thoroughly wash the kale leaves and remove the stems. Bring 1 cup water to a boil. Add the kale to the pot and cook until tender. Drain the kale, pressing out the water if necessary, and season with salt and pepper. On one slice of bread, layer the cheeses, tomato, kale, and turkey; top with the second slice of bread. Spray a medium frying pan with cooking spray and heat it over medium-high heat. Cook the sandwich until the underside is golden brown. Flip the sandwich and continue cooking until both sides are golden brown and the cheese is melted.

Variation: For 1,400–1,600-calorie Moderate Carbohydrate plan, spread ½ tablespoon of trans-fat-free margarine on the bread before assembling the sandwich.

SERVING: 1

Nutritional Info (per serving):

Calories:	465
Carbs:	40g
Protein:	39g
Total Fat:	15g
Saturated Fat:	5g
Dietary Fiber:	6g
Sodium:	770mg
Cholesterol:	63mg

Food Group Servings:

Starch:	2
Fruit:	0
Vegetable:	1.5
Protein:	4
Dairy:	0
Fat:	0

Turkey Roll-up with Vinaigrette

SERVING: 1

*Nutritional Info
(per serving):*

Calories:	403
Carbs:	30g
Protein:	29g
Total Fat:	17g
Saturated Fat:	3g
Dietary Fiber:	6g
Sodium:	576mg
Cholesterol:	48mg

*Food Group
Servings:*

Starch:	2
Fruit:	0
Vegetable:	2.5
Protein:	3
Dairy:	0
Fat:	1

INGREDIENTS

1 tablespoon low-fat balsamic
  vinaigrette
1 medium whole-wheat flour
  tortilla
2 cups fresh spinach

½ cup shredded carrots
2 ounces cooked turkey
  breast
1 ounce low-fat Cheddar
  cheese

PREPARATION

Spread the vinaigrette over the tortilla. Top with the spinach, carrots, turkey, and cheese. Tightly roll up the tortilla and cut it in
half diagonally.

Veggie Cheeseburger

INGREDIENTS

1 veggie burger (such as Boca
  Meatless Burgers)

2 slices tomato

½ cup shredded lettuce

¼ avocado, sliced

½ whole-grain hamburger bun

2 ounces low-fat Cheddar
  cheese

PREPARATION

Prepare the veggie burger according to the package directions.
Place the tomato slices, lettuce, avocado, and burger on the bun.
Top with the cheese and heat until melted.

SERVING: 1

*Nutritional Info
(per serving):*

Calories:	316
Carbs:	26g
Protein:	27g
Total Fat:	13g
Saturated Fat:	4g
Dietary Fiber:	7g
Sodium:	811mg
Cholesterol:	12mg

*Food Group
Servings:*

Starch:	1
Fruit:	0
Vegetable:	1
Protein:	4
Dairy:	0
Fat:	1.5

Almond-Crusted Salmon

SERVINGS: 4

*Nutritional Info
(per serving):*

Calories:	308
Carbs:	3g
Protein:	34g
Total Fat:	17g
Saturated Fat:	2g
Dietary Fiber:	0.5g
Sodium:	119mg
Cholesterol:	81mg

*Food Group
Servings:*

Starch:	0.25
Fruit:	0
Vegetable:	0
Protein:	4
Dairy:	0
Fat:	0.25

INGREDIENTS

1 tablespoon canola oil

$\frac{1}{2}$ cup egg substitute

4 tablespoons sliced almonds

4 teaspoons all-purpose flour

21 ounces salmon fillet, cut
  into four equal portions

PREPARATION

Preheat the oven to 350° F. Heat the oil in a medium sauté pan over high heat. Pour the egg substitute into a small bowl. Place the almonds and flour on separate plates. Dip one side of a salmon fillet in the flour, then dip it into the egg substitute, and then into the almonds. Place the salmon, almond side down, in the hot pan and cook until the nuts are brown. Flip the fillet and cook 1 minute. Remove from the pan, and place on a baking sheet, almond side up. Repeat for the remaining fillets. Bake the fillets until the fish is flaky.

Asian Duck Salad

INGREDIENTS

6 ounces precooked duck

$\frac{1}{2}$ tablespoon reduced-
sodium teriyaki sauce

$\frac{1}{2}$ teaspoon honey

$\frac{1}{2}$ teaspoon reduced-sodium
soy sauce

$\frac{1}{2}$ head red cabbage,
chopped

2 ounces roasted red bell
pepper (jarred or canned)

$1\frac{1}{2}$ teaspoons dry-roasted
peanuts, chopped

PREPARATION

Thinly slice the duck. Combine the teriyaki sauce, honey, and soy sauce in a medium bowl and mix well. Add the duck and toss to coat. Place the chopped cabbage in the center of a plate and top with the duck. Add the red pepper to the salad. Top with the chopped peanuts.

SERVINGS: 2

Nutritional Info
(per serving):

Calories:	144
Carbs:	6g
Protein:	14g
Total Fat:	7g
Saturated Fat:	2g
Dietary Fiber:	0.5g
Sodium:	253mg
Cholesterol:	47mg

Food Group
Servings:

Starch:	0
Fruit:	0
Vegetable:	0
Protein:	3
Dairy:	0
Fat:	0

Baked Salmon with Citrus Salsa

SERVINGS: 4

*Nutritional Info
(per serving):*

Calories:	243
Carbs:	9g
Protein:	29g
Total Fat:	9g
Saturated Fat:	1g
Dietary Fiber:	1g
Sodium:	81mg
Cholesterol:	65mg

*Food Group
Servings:*

Starch:	0
Fruit:	1
Vegetable:	0
Protein:	2
Dairy:	0
Fat:	0

INGREDIENTS

3 tablespoons chopped red bell pepper

3 tablespoons chopped red onion

7 teaspoons cilantro leaves

1⅔ cups diced fresh pineapple

1 pound wild Atlantic salmon fillet, cut into four equal portions

PREPARATION

To make the salsa, combine the red pepper, onion, cilantro, and pineapple in a small bowl and mix well. Cover and refrigerate for at least 8 hours.

Preheat the oven to 350° F. Spray a baking sheet with cooking spray and place the salmon fillets on it. Bake for 10 to 15 minutes, until the fish is flaky. Top each serving with ½ cup of the salsa.

Baked Ziti with Roasted Vegetables

INGREDIENTS

4 ounces ziti pasta

2 cups zucchini

2 cups chopped red bell
    peppers

2 cups chopped white onions

1 cup chopped asparagus

1 cup chopped carrots

1 cup 1% fat cottage cheese

3 cups low-sodium tomato
    sauce

½ cup part-skim mozzarella
    cheese

¼ cup grated Parmesan
    cheese

PREPARATION

Cook the ziti according to the directions on the package. Preheat the oven to 400° F. Spray two baking sheets with cooking spray and spread the vegetables in a single layer on them. Roast the vegetables for 15 to 20 minutes, stirring once. When the vegetables are soft and slightly browned, fill four individual casserole dishes with equal amounts of the cooked ziti.

Reduce the oven temperature to 350° F. Divide the vegetables evenly on top of the casseroles. Layer each alternately with ¼ cup of cottage cheese and ¾ cup tomato sauce. Sprinkle with mozzarella and Parmesan cheese. Bake for 20 to 30 minutes, until the casseroles are heated through and the cheese is melted.

SERVINGS: 4

*Nutritional Info
(per serving):*

Calories:	329
Carbs:	49g
Protein:	22g
Total Fat:	8g
Saturated Fat:	4g
Dietary Fiber:	8g
Sodium:	658mg
Cholesterol:	17mg

*Food Group
Servings:*

Starch:	2
Fruit:	0
Vegetable:	2
Protein:	1.5
Dairy:	0
Fat:	0

Blackberry Mustard Chicken

SERVINGS: 2

*Nutritional Info
(per serving):*

Calories:	240
Carbs:	12g
Protein:	36g
Total Fat:	6g
Saturated Fat:	1g
Dietary Fiber:	1g
Sodium:	388mg
Cholesterol:	94mg

*Food Group
Servings:*

Starch:	0
Fruit:	0
Vegetable:	0
Protein:	6
Dairy:	0
Fat:	0

INGREDIENTS

3 tablespoons blackberries

4 teaspoons Dijon mustard

2½ teaspoons honey mustard

2 teaspoons honey

½ teaspoon balsamic vinegar

¼ teaspoon dry mustard

2 chicken breasts, approximately 6 ounces each

PREPARATION

Add the blackberries to the work bowl of a food processor. Process for about 1 minute, until smooth; strain and discard the seeds. Combine the blackberry purée, Dijon mustard, honey mustard, honey, balsamic vinegar, and dry mustard in a small bowl and stir well.

Preheat the oven to 350° F. Baste each chicken breast with the blackberry-mustard mixture and marinate for at least 30 minutes. Bake for 20 to 30 minutes or grill until done.

Blackened Fish

INGREDIENTS

Seasoning:

⅛ teaspoon white pepper

½ teaspoon ground red chile pepper

½ teaspoon ground black pepper

½ teaspoon onion powder

½ teaspoon salt substitute

⅛ teaspoon dried ground sage

½ teaspoon paprika

2 teaspoons dried oregano

4 teaspoons dried thyme

1 teaspoon ground saffron

4 teaspoons Cajun seasoning

Fish:

4 teaspoons extra-virgin olive oil

1¾ pounds red snapper

PREPARATION

For the blackened fish seasoning, combine all the spices and flavorings in a small bowl.

Preheat the oven to 350° F. Add the olive oil to a nonstick skillet and heat it over medium-high heat. Wash the fish, pat it dry, and sprinkle one side lightly with the seasoning. Put the fish in the hot skillet, spice side down. Sprinkle the top with the seasoning. Turn the fish over after 1 minute. Cook 1 minute longer. Place the fish on a baking sheet and bake until flaky, approximately 10 minutes per inch of thickness. Cut into four equal portions to serve.

SERVINGS: 4

Nutritional Info (per serving):

Calories:	218
Carbs:	3g
Protein:	35g
Total Fat:	8g
Saturated Fat:	2g
Dietary Fiber:	2g
Sodium:	682mg
Cholesterol:	60mg

Food Group Servings:

Starch:	0
Fruit:	0
Vegetable:	0
Protein:	4.75
Dairy:	0
Fat:	0

Chicken and Wild Rice

SERVING: 1

*Nutritional Info
(per serving):*

Calories:	326
Carbs:	18g
Protein:	31g
Total Fat:	15g
Saturated Fat:	4g
Dietary Fiber:	2g
Sodium:	219mg
Cholesterol:	72mg

*Food Group
Servings:*

Starch:	1
Fruit:	0
Vegetable:	0
Protein:	3
Dairy:	0
Fat:	3

INGREDIENTS

$\frac{1}{8}$ cup dry wild rice

3 ounces roasted chicken
breast

1 tablespoon trans-fat-free
margarine

Salt-free garlic and herb
seasoning blend or
other salt-free seasoning
blend

PREPARATION

Cook the rice according to the package directions. Dice the chicken
and add it to the rice with the margarine; toss to combine. Sprinkle
with the seasoning.

Chicken Breast with Ricotta and Pesto

INGREDIENTS

6 basil leaves

¼ teaspoon minced garlic

1¼ teaspoons pine nuts

⅛ teaspoon diced jalapeño pepper

⅛ teaspoon white pepper

¼ teaspoon lemon juice

6½ tablespoons chopped parsley

1¼ teaspoons grated Parmesan cheese

3½ teaspoons olive oil

¼ cup low-fat ricotta cheese

4 broiler-fryer chicken breasts (just under 7 ounces each), skinless

3¼ tablespoons egg whites

¼ cup fine, dry bread crumbs

PREPARATION

Preheat the oven to 400° F.

In a food processor, combine the basil leaves, garlic, pine nuts, jalapeño pepper, white pepper, lemon juice, parsley, Parmesan cheese, and oil. Pulse until a smooth paste forms. Transfer the pesto to a mixing bowl and stir in the ricotta cheese.

Pound out the chicken breasts by placing them, one at a time, between two sheets of wax paper and pounding with a wooden mallet or rolling pin. Place ¼ of the ricotta-pesto mixture in the center of each breast, and fold in the sides. Place the stuffed breasts on a baking sheet, seam side down. Brush the top and sides with egg white, then cover the top of each breast with ¼ of the bread crumbs. Bake until the internal temperature reaches 160° F.

SERVINGS: 4

Nutritional Info (per serving):

Calories:	343
Carbs:	6g
Protein:	51g
Total Fat:	12g
Saturated Fat:	3g
Dietary Fiber:	0.5g
Sodium:	222mg
Cholesterol:	134mg

Food Group Servings:

Starch:	0
Fruit:	0
Vegetable:	0
Protein:	4.75
Dairy:	0
Fat:	1.25

Chicken Fajitas

SERVINGS: 4

*Nutritional Info
(per serving):*

Calories:	319
Carbs:	35g
Protein:	23g
Total Fat:	10g
Saturated Fat:	2g
Dietary Fiber:	5g
Sodium:	720mg
Cholesterol:	28mg

*Food Group
Servings:*

Starch:	1
Fruit:	0
Vegetable:	1.5
Protein:	3
Dairy:	0
Fat:	0

INGREDIENTS

- 4 flour tortillas
- 12 ounces chicken breast, cubed
- 1 teaspoon chili powder
- ½ teaspoon ground cumin
- ½ teaspoon ground black pepper
- ¼ teaspoon salt
- 1 tablespoon lime juice
- ⅔ cup sliced scallions (green onions)
- ⅓ cup cilantro leaves
- ½ cup nonfat plain yogurt
- 4 green lettuce leaves
- 1 medium tomato, quartered

PREPARATION

Preheat the oven to 350° F. Wrap the tortillas in damp paper towels and then in aluminum foil. Bake for 7 minutes, or until softened; set aside.

Coat a large nonstick skillet with cooking spray; place it over medium-high heat until hot. Add the chicken, chili powder, and cumin; sauté 5 minutes, or until chicken is heated. Remove the chicken to a large bowl. Add the pepper, salt, and lime juice; toss well. Add the scallions, cilantro, and yogurt and toss well. Place a lettuce leaf on each tortilla; place an equal amount of chicken mixture over each lettuce leaf. Top each with tomato pieces and roll up.

Chicken Fromage with Sauce

INGREDIENTS

1 large egg

4 teaspoons shredded part-
   skim mozzarella cheese

2 teaspoons grated Parmesan
   cheese

$2/3$ cup nonfat ricotta cheese

$1/4$ cup baby spinach

1 red sweet pepper, roasted
   and diced

$1/2$ teaspoon dried basil

$1/8$ teaspoon dried oregano

$1/8$ teaspoon white pepper

$1/2$ teaspoon garlic powder

4 skinless broiler-fryer
   chicken breasts (about
   $5 1/2$ ounces each)

Paprika

Sauce:

$3/4$ cup plus 4 teaspoons
   reduced-sodium chicken
   broth

2 teaspoons dry sherry

1 tablespoon cornstarch

Fresh herbs (chives or
   parsley), if desired

SERVINGS: 4

*Nutritional Info
(per serving):*

Calories:	267
Carbs:	8g
Protein:	40g
Total Fat:	6g
Saturated Fat:	2g
Dietary Fiber:	0.5g
Sodium:	265mg
Cholesterol:	152mg

*Food Group
Servings:*

Starch:	0
Fruit:	0
Vegetable:	0
Protein:	4.25
Dairy:	0
Fat:	0

PREPARATION

Preheat the oven to 350° F. Combine the egg, cheeses, spinach, red pepper, basil, oregano, white pepper, and garlic powder; mix well. Make a slit in each chicken breast with a small, sharp knife, starting at the thick end of the breast, to make a pocket. Put the filling in a pastry bag with a round tip. Pipe $1/4$ of the mixture into each breast.

Coat a baking sheet with cooking spray. Place the filled breasts on the baking sheet, sprinkle each breast lightly with paprika, and bake for about 25 minutes, until done.

To make the sauce, bring $3/4$ cup chicken broth to a boil, add the sherry, reduce the heat, and simmer for 10 minutes. Combine the cornstarch with 4 teaspoons cold broth to make a smooth paste. Whisk the cornstarch into the broth mixture, stirring constantly. Cook until thickened to desired sauce consistency. Simmer for 5 minutes.

To serve, pour the sauce over the chicken breasts and garnish with the fresh chopped herbs.

Chicken Marsala

SERVINGS: 4

*Nutritional Info
(per serving):*

Calories:	476
Carbs:	23g
Protein:	37g
Total Fat:	18g
Saturated Fat:	3g
Dietary Fiber:	1g
Sodium:	117mg
Cholesterol:	96mg

*Food Group
Servings:*

Starch:	1
Fruit:	0
Vegetable:	1
Protein:	4
Dairy:	0
Fat:	3.5

INGREDIENTS

$\frac{1}{4}$ cup all-purpose flour

$\frac{1}{4}$ teaspoon ground black
pepper

4 broiler-fryer chicken
breasts, (approximately
5 ounces each) skinless

$\frac{1}{4}$ cup extra-virgin olive oil,
divided

2 cups chopped mushrooms

$\frac{1}{4}$ teaspoon chicken bouillon
powder

$\frac{1}{2}$ cup water, divided

1 cup dry Marsala wine

$\frac{1}{4}$ cup cornstarch

$\frac{1}{4}$ cup chopped parsley

PREPARATION

Preheat the oven to 300° F.

Blend the flour and pepper in a small bowl. Dredge each chicken breast in the flour mixture and shake off the excess. Heat half the olive oil in a nonstick skillet over medium-high heat. Brown the chicken breasts on both sides until the flesh is firm. Do not crowd the breasts in the skillet; brown them in batches if necessary, wiping the skillet occasionally to remove the burned flour residue. Remove the cooked breasts from the skillet and place them on a baking sheet.

Heat the remaining olive oil in a clean skillet over medium-high heat. Sauté the mushrooms in the skillet until browned.

Dissolve the chicken bouillon powder in $\frac{1}{4}$ cup hot water. Combine the bouillon with the Marsala in a medium stainless-steel saucepan. Stir the remaining $\frac{1}{4}$ cup water into the cornstarch, forming a smooth paste. Heat the Marsala-bouillon mixture to a simmer over medium heat and gradually whisk in the cornstarch mixture, gently whisking until all of the cornstarch has been added and the sauce reaches the consistency of pancake syrup. Add the sautéed mushrooms along with their juices to the Marsala sauce. Ladle the Marsala-mushroom sauce evenly over the four chicken breasts. Cook 15 to 20 minutes, until the chicken is done (160° F on an instant-read thermometer). Sprinkle with the fresh parsley before serving.

Cioppino

INGREDIENTS

8 teaspoons extra-virgin
  olive oil

$2\frac{1}{2}$ cloves garlic, minced

$1\frac{1}{2}$ medium onions, diced

$\frac{1}{2}$ bay leaf

$\frac{1}{2}$ teaspoon dried oregano

$\frac{1}{2}$ teaspoon crushed red
  pepper flakes

$\frac{1}{2}$ teaspoon ground black
  pepper

$\frac{1}{2}$ green bell pepper, chopped

4 teaspoons tomato paste

1 cup red table wine

$18\frac{1}{2}$ ounces whole canned
  tomatoes

$\frac{2}{3}$ cup clam juice

$\frac{2}{3}$ cup reduced-sodium
  chicken broth

$10\frac{1}{2}$ ounces Dungeness
  crabmeat

9 large clams, rinsed
  thoroughly

$10\frac{1}{2}$ ounces large shrimp

8 teaspoons chopped
  parsley

Basil

PREPARATION

Pour the oil into a large kettle or Dutch oven and tilt to coat the bottom. Place the kettle over medium heat until hot. Add the garlic, onions, bay leaf, oregano, red pepper flakes, and black pepper, and sauté until the onions are softened. Stir in the bell pepper and tomato paste and cook about 1 minute. Add the wine and bring to a boil. Continue cooking until the liquid is reduced by half, 5 to 6 minutes. Add the tomatoes with their juice, the clam juice, and the broth; simmer, covered, 30 minutes. Add the crabmeat and clams and continue simmering, covered, until the clams just open, about 10 minutes. Remove the clams from the pot; discard any that didn't open during the 10 minutes of simmering. Lightly season the shrimp with pepper; add to the stew and simmer about 5 minutes. Discard the bay leaf. Return the cooked clams to the pot, stirring gently. Serve with the chopped parsley and basil.

SERVINGS: 4

Nutritional Info (per serving):

Calories:	413
Carbs:	17g
Protein:	41g
Total Fat:	16g
Saturated Fat:	2g
Dietary Fiber:	3g
Sodium:	766mg
Cholesterol:	191mg

Food Group Servings:

Starch:	0
Fruit:	0
Vegetable:	2
Protein:	5.5
Dairy:	0
Fat:	2

Crab-Stuffed Whitefish

SERVINGS: 4

Nutritional Info (per serving):

Calories:	366
Carbs:	9g
Protein:	50g
Total Fat:	14g
Saturated Fat:	3g
Dietary Fiber:	0.5g
Sodium:	623mg
Cholesterol:	204mg

Food Group Servings:

Starch:	0.5
Fruit:	0
Vegetable:	0
Protein:	6.75
Dairy:	0
Fat:	0

INGREDIENTS

$1\frac{1}{2}$ teaspoons light mayonnaise

$1\frac{1}{2}$ teaspoons Worcestershire sauce

1 large egg

$\frac{1}{2}$ teaspoon parsley

$1\frac{1}{2}$ teaspoons baking powder

8 ounces Dungeness crabmeat

6 tablespoons fine, dry bread crumbs

$1\frac{1}{2}$ pounds whitefish fillet, divided into 8 equal portions of approximately 3 ounces each

$\frac{1}{2}$ teaspoon seafood seasoning

PREPARATION

Combine the mayonnaise, Worcestershire sauce, and egg in a medium bowl; stir well. Add the parsley, baking powder, and crabmeat; mix well. Divide the mixture into four equal portions, shaping each into a $\frac{1}{2}$-inch-thick patty. Place the bread crumbs in a shallow dish; dredge the patties in the bread crumbs. Lightly coat a large nonstick skillet with cooking spray and heat the skillet over medium heat.

Add 2 patties to the skillet and cook until the undersides are golden brown, approximately 3 minutes. Carefully turn over the patties and cook for 3 minutes, or until both sides are golden brown. Remove the patties from the skillet; set them aside and keep them warm. Wipe any burned crumbs from the skillet and cook the remaining two patties as described above.

Preheat the oven to 325° F. Spray a shallow baking dish lightly with cooking spray. Arrange 4 of the fillets in the baking dish. Place 1 patty over each fillet and top each with the remaining fillets. Sprinkle the fillets with the seafood seasoning. Cover the baking dish and bake for 15 minutes. Remove the cover and bake an additional 10 minutes, or until the fish flakes easily when tested with a fork.

Eggplant Parmigiana

INGREDIENTS

1 pound eggplant, peeled

1 medium egg

¼ cup nonfat milk

1 tablespoon plus 4½ tea-
spoons grated Parmesan
cheese

¼ cup all-purpose flour

½ cup fine, dry bread crumbs

2¼ cups low-sodium
marinara sauce

4 ounces part-skim moz-
zarella cheese, shredded

PREPARATION

Preheat the oven to 325° F. Slice the peeled eggplant crossways into quarter-inch-thick rounds. Whisk together the egg, milk, and 1 tablespoon of the Parmesan cheese, to form a batter. Dredge each eggplant slice in the flour, shaking off the excess. Dip each eggplant slice in the batter and then coat with the bread crumbs. Spray a baking pan or cookie sheet with cooking spray, or line with parchment paper. Place the eggplant on the sheet and bake 15 to 20 minutes, until the eggplant is golden brown and a little crisp.

Lightly cover the bottom of a small baking pan with marinara sauce. Add a layer of the baked eggplant slices and cover with half of the remaining sauce. Sprinkle lightly with half of the remaining grated Parmesan cheese (2¼ teaspoons) and half the mozzarella cheese. Make a second layer of eggplant, top with the remaining marinara sauce, remaining 2¼ teaspoons Parmesan cheese, and remaining mozzarella cheese. Bake for 15 to 20 minutes, until cheese is golden and bubbly.

SERVINGS: 4

*Nutritional Info
(per serving):*

Calories:	261
Carbs:	32g
Protein:	15g
Total Fat:	9g
Saturated Fat:	4g
Dietary Fiber:	2g
Sodium:	461mg
Cholesterol:	68mg

*Food Group
Servings:*

Starch:	1
Fruit:	0
Vegetable:	1
Protein:	1.25
Dairy:	0
Fat:	0

Eggplant Sausage Lasagna

SERVINGS: 4

Nutritional Info (per serving):

Calories:	383
Carbs:	40g
Protein:	30g
Total Fat:	12g
Saturated Fat:	5g
Dietary Fiber:	3g
Sodium:	1,170mg
Cholesterol:	115mg

Food Group Servings:

Starch:	1.5
Fruit:	0
Vegetable:	1.5
Protein:	3.25
Dairy:	0
Fat:	0

INGREDIENTS

$1\frac{1}{2}$ cups sliced mushrooms

1 cup peeled, cubed eggplant

8 ounces turkey sausage or links, sliced

$\frac{3}{4}$ cup nonfat ricotta cheese

1 large egg

$\frac{3}{4}$ teaspoon dried basil leaves

$\frac{1}{2}$ teaspoon dried oregano

$\frac{1}{8}$ teaspoon ground nutmeg

2 cups tomato sauce

$4\frac{1}{2}$ ounces lasagna noodles

2 tablespoons grated Parmesan cheese

$\frac{3}{4}$ cup shredded part-skim mozzarella cheese

PREPARATION

Preheat the oven to 350° F. Spray a large frying pan with cooking spray and heat it over medium-high heat. Add the mushrooms and eggplant and sauté until softened and slightly browned. Remove from the pan and set aside. Add the sausage to the pan and sauté until browned and heated through. In a small bowl, mix the ricotta, egg, basil, oregano, and nutmeg. Assemble the lasagna in a 9 × 13-inch baking pan, distributing the layers as follows:

$\frac{1}{3}$ of the tomato sauce

$\frac{1}{3}$ of the lasagna noodles

All of the ricotta mixture

$\frac{1}{3}$ of the lasagna noodles

All of the mushroom-sausage mixture

Remaining sauce

All of the eggplant

Remaining lasagna noodles

Parmesan and Mozzarella cheese

Cover and bake for 45 minutes. Uncover and bake an additional 5 minutes, or until the cheese is browned.

Fiesta Chicken Salad

INGREDIENTS

1½ teaspoons lemon juice

¼ teaspoon caraway seeds

⅛ teaspoon ground cumin

⅛ teaspoon ground coriander

⅛ teaspoon salt

⅛ teaspoon ground black pepper

¼ cup nonfat plain yogurt

½ cup chopped or sliced tomatoes

5 ounces cooked, skinless broiler-fryer chicken breast, cut into pieces

2 tablespoons chopped red bell pepper

2 tablespoons chopped green bell pepper

2 tablespoons chopped red onion

1 tablespoon chopped parsley

1 cup shredded lettuce

PREPARATION

In a small bowl, combine the lemon juice, caraway seeds, cumin, coriander, salt, pepper, and yogurt; mix well. In a medium bowl, combine the tomatoes, chicken, red and green peppers, onion, parsley, and lettuce. Toss until thoroughly combined. Top with the yogurt mixture. Chill thoroughly.

SERVINGS: 2

Nutritional Info (per serving):

Calories:	155
Carbs:	8g
Protein:	24g
Total Fat:	3g
Saturated Fat:	0.5g
Dietary Fiber:	2g
Sodium:	229mg
Cholesterol:	61mg

Food Group Servings:

Starch:	0
Fruit:	0
Vegetable:	1
Protein:	2.5
Dairy:	0
Fat:	0

Garlic Rosemary Roasted Chicken

SERVINGS: 4

Nutritional Info (per serving):

Calories:	325
Carbs:	8g
Protein:	54g
Total Fat:	7g
Saturated Fat:	2g
Dietary Fiber:	0.5g
Sodium:	129mg
Cholesterol:	145mg

Food Group Servings:

Starch:	0
Fruit:	0
Vegetable:	0.25
Protein:	5
Dairy:	0
Fat:	0.25

INGREDIENTS

$1\frac{1}{2}$-pound broiler-fryer chicken

$1\frac{1}{2}$ teaspoons fresh rosemary

10 cloves garlic, crushed

$1\frac{1}{4}$ red onions, diced into 1-inch pieces

12 cloves garlic, peeled

1 teaspoon olive oil

PREPARATION

Preheat the oven to 400° F. Rinse the chicken under cold water; pat it dry. Smear the rosemary and crushed garlic on the top skin of the breast and drumsticks.

Place the onions and whole, peeled garlic cloves in a layer in a roasting pan. Coat the garlic and onions with olive oil, and roast in the oven for 10 minutes. Cover the onions and garlic loosely with foil; let stand 10 minutes. Remove foil, then add the chicken to the roasting pan, skin side down, on the layer of onion and garlic. Bake for 45 minutes.

Grilled Flank Steak

INGREDIENTS

4 ounces lean beef chuck
  steak

Dash salt and black pepper

PREPARATION

Heat the grill to medium. Remove the excess fat from the steak.
Season with salt and pepper. Place the steak on the grill, flipping
it a little before the halfway point, and cook to desired doneness.
Cooking time will depend on the thickness of the steak, the heat
of the grill, and the distance from the heat source. Allow 8 to
10 minutes to cook a 1-inch-thick steak medium rare.

SERVING: 1

*Nutritional Info
(per serving):*

Calories:	270
Carbs:	0g
Protein:	32g
Total Fat:	15g
Saturated Fat:	6g
Dietary Fiber:	0g
Sodium:	237mg
Cholesterol:	80mg

*Food Group
Servings:*

Starch:	0
Fruit:	0
Vegetable:	0
Protein:	3
Dairy:	0
Fat:	0

Grilled Portobello

SERVINGS: 4

*Nutritional Info
(per serving):*

Calories:	139
Carbs:	8g
Protein:	9g
Total Fat:	8g
Saturated Fat:	5g
Dietary Fiber:	3g
Sodium:	419mg
Cholesterol:	25mg

*Food Group
Servings:*

Starch:	0
Fruit:	0
Vegetable:	1.5
Protein:	1
Dairy:	0
Fat:	0

INGREDIENTS

4 portobello mushrooms
Olive-oil flavored cooking
   spray
1 red bell pepper, chopped
½ cup chopped spinach
4 ounces blue cheese,
   crumbled

PREPARATION

Wash the mushrooms, remove the stems and gills, and coat lightly with cooking spray. Broil or grill the mushrooms 4 inches from the flame for 2 to 3 minutes. Coat a medium frying pan with the cooking spray and heat over medium heat. Add the peppers and spinach, and sauté until the peppers soften and the spinach wilts. Top the mushrooms with the spinach-pepper mixture. Sprinkle the crumbled blue cheese over each mushroom.

Grilled Shrimp

INGREDIENTS

1 pound raw, peeled shrimp

1 cup mushrooms, halved

½ cup red bell pepper, cut into 2-inch pieces

½ cup coarsely chopped red onion

½ cup low-sodium barbecue sauce

PREPARATION

Thread the shrimp onto wooden skewers, alternating shrimp with the mushroom halves, red pepper pieces, and onion pieces. Place the skewers in a glass dish and cover with the barbecue sauce, reserving about 2 tablespoons for basting during cooking. Cover and refrigerate for 1 hour.

Clean the grill surface and coat it with oil. The grill is ready when the coals are covered with gray ash and no longer flaming. Place the skewers on the grill about 6 inches from the coals. Grill the shrimp for 3 to 4 minutes on each side, basting with the reserved sauce before turning.

SERVINGS: 4

Nutritional Info (per serving):

Calories:	184
Carbs:	16g
Protein:	24g
Total Fat:	2g
Saturated Fat:	0.5g
Dietary Fiber:	1g
Sodium:	212mg
Cholesterol:	173mg

Food Group Servings:

Starch:	0
Fruit:	0
Vegetable:	0.5
Protein:	3
Dairy:	0
Fat:	0

Jerk Shrimp Skewers with Tomato-Strawberry Salsa

SERVINGS: 4

*Nutritional Info
(per serving):*

Calories:	136
Carbs:	11g
Protein:	20g
Total Fat:	1g
Saturated Fat:	0.5g
Dietary Fiber:	3g
Sodium:	248mg
Cholesterol:	166mg

*Food Group
Servings:*

Starch:	0
Fruit:	0.25
Vegetable:	1.75
Protein:	3
Dairy:	0
Fat:	0

INGREDIENTS

½ cup chopped scallion (green onion), tops and bulb

2 jalapeño peppers, or 2 serrano chiles chopped with seeds, or ½ Scotch bonnet chile chopped without seeds

½ tablespoon reduced-sodium soy sauce

1 tablespoon fresh lime juice

2 teaspoons ground allspice

1 clove garlic, chopped

¼ teaspoon sugar

½ teaspoon ground black pepper

½ teaspoon dried thyme

¼ teaspoon ground cinnamon

¼ teaspoon ground ginger

⅛ teaspoon fresh-grated nutmeg

1 pound shrimp, peeled and deveined

1 red onion, peeled and quartered

Salsa:

1 pound Roma tomatoes, seeded and diced

1 serrano chile pepper, seeded and minced

½ cup fresh minced cilantro leaves

1 teaspoon minced garlic

¼ pound strawberries, diced

1½ tablespoons fresh lime juice

PREPARATION

In a blender or in the work bowl of a food processor, combine the scallion, jalapeño, soy sauce, lime juice, allspice, garlic, sugar, black pepper, thyme, cinnamon, ground ginger, and nutmeg. Pulse until a thick paste forms. Transfer to a resealable plastic bag. Add the shrimp and ¾ of the quartered red onion to the bag and marinate in the refrigerator for at least 30 minutes.

To make the salsa, dice the remaining ¼ red onion. Combine

with the tomatoes, serrano pepper, cilantro, garlic, strawberries, and lime juice.

Preheat the grill. Thread the shrimp and the quartered onions onto skewers. Grill the skewers 2 to 3 minutes on each side, until the shrimp become just firm to the touch. Serve with the salsa.

MahiMahi with Pineapple Salsa

INGREDIENTS

Salsa:

1½ cups fresh diced pineapple

¼ cup chopped red bell pepper

¼ cup chopped green bell pepper

2 tablespoons cilantro leaves

½ teaspoon lime zest

2 tablespoons lime juice

Fish:

12 ounces mahimahi

1 tablespoon extra-virgin olive oil

½ teaspoon white pepper

PREPARATION

For salsa: Combine the pineapple, red and green peppers, cilantro, lime zest, and 1 tablespoon of the lime juice in a medium bowl. Set aside.

For fish: Preheat the broiler. Spray the rack of the broiler pan with cooking spray. Rinse the mahimahi and pat it dry with paper towels. Place the mahimahi on the rack. Combine the remaining lime juice and the olive oil; brush on the mahimahi. Broil for 2 minutes, 4 inches from the heat. Turn and brush the second side with the olive oil mixture; sprinkle with the white pepper. Continue to broil 2 minutes, or until the mahimahi flakes when tested with a fork. Divide into 4 equal portions and serve with the pineapple salsa.

SERVINGS: 4

Nutritional Info (per serving):

Calories:	162
Carbs:	9g
Protein:	21g
Total Fat:	5g
Saturated Fat:	0.5g
Dietary Fiber:	1g
Sodium:	98mg
Cholesterol:	80mg

Food Group Servings:

Starch:	0
Fruit:	0.5
Vegetable:	0
Protein:	3
Dairy:	0
Fat:	0.75

Maryland Crab Cakes

SERVINGS: 4

Nutritional Info (per serving):

Calories:	163
Carbs:	5g
Protein:	25g
Total Fat:	4g
Saturated Fat:	0.5g
Dietary Fiber:	0.5g
Sodium:	1,010mg
Cholesterol:	155mg

Food Group Servings:

Starch:	0
Fruit:	0
Vegetable:	0
Protein:	3.25
Dairy:	0
Fat:	0

INGREDIENTS

1 tablespoon light mayonnaise

$\frac{1}{4}$ teaspoon salt

1 tablespoon Worcestershire sauce

1 large egg

1 tablespoon chopped parsley

1 tablespoon baking powder

1 pound canned blue crabmeat

2 tablespoons fine, dry bread crumbs

PREPARATION

Combine the mayonnaise, salt, Worcestershire sauce, and egg in a medium bowl; stir well. Add the parsley, baking powder, and crabmeat; stir well. Divide the mixture into 4 equal portions, shaping each into a $\frac{1}{2}$-inch-thick patty. Place the bread crumbs in a shallow dish; dredge the patties in the bread crumbs.

Lightly coat a large nonstick skillet with cooking spray and heat it over medium heat. Add 2 patties to the skillet and cook until the undersides are golden brown, approximately 3 minutes. Carefully turn over the patties and cook for 3 minutes, or until both sides are golden brown. Remove the patties from the skillet; set aside and keep warm. Wipe any burned crumbs from the skillet and cook the remaining two patties as described above.

Pepper-Crusted Beef Tenderloin with Horseradish Sauce

INGREDIENTS

21 ounces beef tenderloin roast, cleaned and trimmed

$\frac{1}{2}$ teaspoon olive oil

2$\frac{1}{4}$ teaspoons fine, dry bread crumbs

1$\frac{1}{2}$ teaspoons chopped parsley

$\frac{1}{4}$ teaspoon ground black pepper

$\frac{1}{4}$ teaspoon salt

$\frac{1}{4}$ cup nonfat sour cream

1$\frac{1}{2}$ teaspoons horseradish

$\frac{3}{4}$ teaspoon grated lemon peel

$\frac{1}{8}$ teaspoon Worcestershire sauce

$\frac{1}{8}$ teaspoon hot sauce

PREPARATION

Preheat the oven to 425° F. Clean the tenderloin and rub it with the olive oil. Mix the bread crumbs, parsley, pepper, and salt together thoroughly. Rub the crumb mixture over the tenderloin until coated. Bake until the internal temperature reaches 140° F (about 30 minutes).

While the tenderloin is cooking, combine the sour cream, horseradish, lemon peel, Worcestershire sauce, and hot sauce in a mixing bowl.

Once the tenderloin is cooked, remove it from the oven and let it stand for 10 minutes before cutting it into 4 portions. Top each portion with 1 ounce (2 tablespoons) of the sauce.

SERVINGS: 4

Nutritional Info (per serving):

Calories:	259
Carbs:	4g
Protein:	34g
Total Fat:	11g
Saturated Fat:	5g
Dietary Fiber:	0g
Sodium:	239mg
Cholesterol:	106mg

Food Group Servings:

Starch:	0.25
Fruit:	0
Vegetable:	0
Protein:	4
Dairy:	0
Fat:	0

Pork Chops with Bourbon Mustard Glaze

SERVINGS: 4

Nutritional Info (per serving):

Calories:	251
Carbs:	2g
Protein:	36g
Total Fat:	9g
Saturated Fat:	3g
Dietary Fiber:	0.5g
Sodium:	397mg
Cholesterol:	93mg

Food Group Servings:

Starch:	0
Fruit:	0
Vegetable:	0
Protein:	4
Dairy:	0
Fat:	0

INGREDIENTS

4 lean boneless center pork
    loin chops, approximately
    5 ounces each
4 teaspoons bourbon

8 teaspoons Dijon mustard
2 teaspoons reduced-sodium
    soy sauce
2 teaspoons water

PREPARATION

Preheat the grill. Grill the pork chops on both sides until grill marks form; set aside. Combine the bourbon, mustard, soy sauce, and water in a medium-heavy saucepan. Simmer over medium heat, whisking occasionally, until the sauce is reduced enough to coat a spoon (about 4 minutes). Brush 1 side of the chops generously with the sauce.

    Preheat the oven to 350° F. Place the chops, sauce side down, on a sheet pan. Brush the chops generously with the remaining sauce. Put the chops in the oven and cook until they reach an internal temperature of 155° F.

Pork Medallions with Orange-Rosemary Sauce

INGREDIENTS

21 ounces lean pork tenderloin

$\frac{1}{8}$ teaspoon salt

$\frac{1}{4}$ teaspoon ground black pepper

4 teaspoons olive oil

$1\frac{1}{2}$ teaspoons minced garlic

$\frac{1}{4}$ cup red table wine

$\frac{1}{4}$ teaspoon dried rosemary

1 tablespoon reduced-sodium tomato paste

1 tablespoon paprika

$1\frac{1}{2}$ teaspoons chopped fresh oregano

6 tablespoons fat-free chicken broth

2 tablespoons orange juice

PREPARATION

Trim the fat from the pork, and cut it crosswise into 1-inch-thick rounds. Place each piece between 2 sheets of heavy-duty plastic wrap; flatten to $\frac{1}{2}$-inch thickness using a meat mallet or rolling pin. Remove the plastic wrap. Sprinkle both sides of the pork with salt and pepper.

Heat the oil in a 9-inch cast-iron skillet over medium-high heat. Add the pork; cook 3 minutes on each side, or until done. Remove the pork from the pan; set aside.

Add the garlic to the pan and spray the pan with cooking spray; sauté 45 seconds. Stir in the wine and rosemary, scraping the pan to loosen the browned bits. Add the tomato paste; cook 2 minutes. Add the paprika and oregano. Stir in the broth and orange juice; cook until thick. Add the pork to the sauce; coat well. Divide into four equal portions to serve.

SERVINGS: 4

Nutritional Info (per serving):

Calories:	284
Carbs:	3g
Protein:	36g
Total Fat:	12g
Saturated Fat:	4g
Dietary Fiber:	0g
Sodium:	188mg
Cholesterol:	114mg

Food Group Servings:

Starch:	0
Fruit:	0
Vegetable:	0
Protein:	4
Dairy:	0
Fat:	1

Pork Tenderloin with Apple Chutney

SERVINGS: 4

*Nutritional Info
(per serving):*

Calories:	258
Carbs:	21g
Protein:	30g
Total Fat:	5g
Saturated Fat:	2g
Dietary Fiber:	1g
Sodium:	88mg
Cholesterol:	84mg

*Food Group
Servings:*

Starch:	1
Fruit:	0
Vegetable:	0
Protein:	4
Dairy:	0
Fat:	0

INGREDIENTS

$\frac{1}{2}$ large apple

3 tablespoons chopped green bell pepper

3 tablespoons chopped white onion

$\frac{1}{3}$ cup diced green chili peppers

$\frac{1}{2}$ teaspoon minced garlic

$\frac{1}{2}$ teaspoon ginger root, peeled and grated

4 teaspoons brown sugar

3 tablespoons granulated sugar

3 tablespoons cider vinegar

2 teaspoons raisins

$3\frac{1}{2}$ tablespoons water

$\frac{1}{8}$ teaspoon ground cayenne pepper

$\frac{1}{8}$ teaspoon curry powder

21 ounces lean pork tenderloin

PREPARATION

Peel and core the apple, and cut it into small pieces. In a large saucepan, combine the apple and all the other ingredients except the pork. Mix thoroughly. Heat the apple mixture over low heat until simmering, stirring frequently. Cover and continue to heat until the apple pieces turn translucent but still retain their shape.

Cool completely; add the pork and marinate in the refrigerator for at least 1 hour. Preheat the oven to 375° F. Spray a baking sheet with cooking spray. Remove the pork from the marinade, place it on the baking sheet, and bake for approximately 20 minutes, until thoroughly cooked (pork should register between 150 and 155° F on a meat thermometer).

Potato-Crusted Salmon

INGREDIENTS

21 ounces salmon fillet

4 teaspoons honey

4 teaspoons Dijon mustard

½ cup instant mashed potato flakes

4 teaspoons olive oil

PREPARATION

Pat the salmon fillet with a paper towel to remove excess moisture. Combine the honey and mustard to form a paste. Smear the paste on top of the salmon. Place the potato flakes on a plate. Press the top of the salmon into the flakes to form a crust.

Preheat the oven to 350° F. Heat the olive oil in a nonstick skillet over medium heat. Lay the fillet in the skillet, crust side down, and sauté until the crust is golden brown. Place the salmon in a baking dish lined with aluminum foil and bake for approximately 15 minutes or until thoroughly cooked (the fish will flake with a fork when done). Divide into 4 equal portions and serve.

SERVINGS: 4

Nutritional Info (per serving):

Calories:	304
Carbs:	13g
Protein:	30g
Total Fat:	14g
Saturated Fat:	2g
Dietary Fiber:	0.5g
Sodium:	207mg
Cholesterol:	81mg

Food Group Servings:

Starch:	0.75
Fruit:	0
Vegetable:	0
Protein:	4
Dairy:	0
Fat:	1

Salmon with Peanut Sauce

SERVINGS: 4

Nutritional Info (per serving):

Calories:	252
Carbs:	2g
Protein:	30g
Total Fat:	13g
Saturated Fat:	2g
Dietary Fiber:	0.5g
Sodium:	188mg
Cholesterol:	83mg

Food Group Servings:

Starch:	0
Fruit:	0
Vegetable:	0
Protein:	4.25
Dairy:	0
Fat:	0.5

INGREDIENTS

4 teaspoons peanut butter

4 teaspoons reduced-sodium chicken broth

2 teaspoons light mayonnaise

1/2 teaspoon reduced-sodium soy sauce

1 teaspoon dry sherry

1 teaspoon chili paste

1/4 teaspoon ginger root

1/2 teaspoon minced garlic

1/2 teaspoon water

1 pound salmon fillet

PREPARATION

Preheat the oven to 350° F. Add the peanut butter and all the other ingredients except the salmon to a blender or the work bowl of a food processor. Purée until smooth and thoroughly combined. Place the salmon on a cookie sheet and bake approximately 15 minutes (the fish will flake with a fork when done). Evenly distribute the sauce over the fillet and divide it into four equal servings.

Shrimp Jambalaya

INGREDIENTS

2 teaspoons extra-virgin olive oil

4 ounces turkey kielbasa, halved lengthwise and sliced

1 cup minced white onion

1 cup diced green bell pepper

1 cup long-grain rice

$\frac{1}{4}$ teaspoon salt

$\frac{1}{4}$ teaspoon dried thyme

$\frac{1}{4}$ teaspoon ground black pepper

$\frac{1}{4}$ teaspoon ground red pepper

2 cups water

2 teaspoons chicken broth

1 pound canned diced tomatoes, no salt added

$\frac{3}{4}$ pound medium shrimp, peeled and deveined

$\frac{1}{4}$ teaspoon hot sauce

2 tablespoons chopped parsley

PREPARATION

Heat the oil in a medium saucepan over medium heat. Add the kielbasa, onion, and bell pepper. Sauté 5 minutes, or until the vegetables are tender. Add the rice and sauté 2 more minutes. Add the salt, thyme, black pepper, and red pepper. Sauté 1 minute.

Add the water, chicken broth, and tomatoes and bring to a boil. Cover, reduce the heat, and simmer 15 minutes or until the rice is tender.

Stir in the shrimp and hot sauce; cover and cook 5 minutes, or until the shrimp are done. Remove from the heat. Stir in the parsley.

SERVINGS: 4

Nutritional Info (per serving):

Calories:	353
Carbs:	48g
Protein:	27g
Total Fat:	6g
Saturated Fat:	1g
Dietary Fiber:	3g
Sodium:	1,117mg
Cholesterol:	185mg

Food Group Servings:

Starch:	2.5
Fruit:	0
Vegetable:	1.5
Protein:	3
Dairy:	0
Fat:	0.5

Sloppy Turkey Joes

SERVINGS: 8

*Nutritional Info
(per serving):*

Calories:	301
Carbs:	41g
Protein:	16g
Total Fat:	9g
Saturated Fat:	3g
Dietary Fiber:	3g
Sodium:	433mg
Cholesterol:	43mg

*Food Group
Servings:*

Starch:	3
Fruit:	0
Vegetable:	0.25
Protein:	1.5
Dairy:	0
Fat:	0

INGREDIENTS

1 tablespoon molasses

2 teaspoons chili powder

1 cup canned diced tomatoes,
    no salt added

$1/3$ cup white wine vinegar

$1/2$ cup low-sodium ketchup

$1/3$ cup dark corn syrup

$1/2$ cup water

$1/2$ cup orange juice

1 pound ground turkey
    breast

$1/2$ cup chopped white onion

$1/2$ cup chopped green bell
    pepper

$1/2$ teaspoon salt

$1/2$ teaspoon ground black
    pepper

PREPARATION

In a heavy saucepan, stir together the molasses and chili powder. Whisk in the tomatoes, vinegar, ketchup, corn syrup, water, and orange juice. Bring to a boil, reduce the heat, and simmer uncovered for 30 minutes, stirring occasionally.

In a separate pan, sauté the ground turkey until it is no longer pink. Add the onions, bell pepper, salt, and black pepper. Continue cooking until the vegetables soften slightly.

Add the sauce to the meat mixture, reduce the heat to low, and simmer until thick. Serve on whole-wheat buns.

Spiced Salmon

INGREDIENTS

4 salmon fillets, approx-
   imately 4.5 ounces each

4 teaspoons honey

4 teaspoons chili-garlic sauce

PREPARATION

Preheat the oven to 400° F. Place the salmon fillets on a baking sheet and brush the fillets with honey and chili-garlic sauce. Cook for 8 to 10 minutes.

SERVINGS: 4

*Nutritional Info
(per serving):*

Calories:	267
Carbs:	6g
Protein:	25g
Total Fat:	14g
Saturated Fat:	3g
Dietary Fiber:	0.5g
Sodium:	288mg
Cholesterol:	76mg

*Food Group
Servings:*

Starch:	0
Fruit:	0
Vegetable:	0
Protein:	4
Dairy:	0
Fat:	0

Teriyaki Tuna Loin with Wasabi Butter and Braised Bok Choy

SERVINGS: 4

Nutritional Info (per serving):

Calories:	349
Carbs:	18g
Protein:	40g
Total Fat:	14g
Saturated Fat:	7g
Dietary Fiber:	6g
Sodium:	803mg
Cholesterol:	84mg

Food Group Servings:

Starch:	0
Fruit:	0
Vegetable:	2
Protein:	4
Dairy:	0
Fat:	3

INGREDIENTS

4 tuna steaks, approximately 5 ounces each

¼ cup teriyaki marinade

1 tablespoon extra-virgin olive oil, divided

3 tablespoons butter

2 tablespoons wasabi powder

2 tablespoons minced chives

2 heads bok choy, halved

Salt and pepper to taste

PREPARATION

Place the tuna in a 9 × 9-inch baking dish. Pour the teriyaki marinade over the tuna and turn to coat. Let the tuna stand 10 minutes at room temperature, or cover and refrigerate 1 hour.

Preheat the grill (medium heat). Remove the tuna from the marinade; use 1 teaspoon of the oil to brush both sides. Sprinkle with pepper. Grill the fish, brushing it occasionally with the remaining marinade, about 2 minutes per side for medium-rare. Transfer the tuna to a platter.

Mix the butter, wasabi powder, and chives in a small bowl. Top the tuna with the wasabi butter and serve.

For bok choy: Season the bok choy with salt and pepper. Then brush it with 2 teaspoons olive oil, and cook in 400° F oven for 20 minutes, or until the bok choy is soft, or grill until the bok choy is slightly charred.

Tuna Salad in Tomato

INGREDIENTS

3 ounces white albacore tuna, packed in water, drained

1 tablespoon light mayonnaise

2 tablespoons diced celery

2 tablespoons chopped white onion

½ large tomato

PREPARATION

Combine the tuna, mayonnaise, celery, and onion; mix well. Scoop the seeds and pulp out of the tomato half and fill with the tuna mixture.

SERVING: 1

Nutritional Info (per serving):

Calories:	150
Carbs:	8g
Protein:	21g
Total Fat:	3g
Saturated Fat:	1g
Dietary Fiber:	2g
Sodium:	183mg
Cholesterol:	37mg

Food Group Servings:

Starch:	0
Fruit:	0
Vegetable:	0.5
Protein:	3
Dairy:	0
Fat:	0.5

Alfredo Sauce

SERVINGS: 8

*Nutritional Info
(per ¹/₂-cup serving):*

Calories:	200
Carbs:	8.7g
Protein:	15.3g
Total Fat:	11.1g

*Food Group
Servings:*

Starch:	0
Fruit:	0
Vegetable:	0
Protein:	1
Dairy:	0.5
Fat:	0.5

INGREDIENTS

2 tablespoons butter

2 tablespoons flour

4 cups nonfat milk, warmed,
   divided

8 ounces Parmesan cheese,
   grated

PREPARATION

Melt the butter in a small saucepan over low heat. Stir in the flour and cook for 2 minutes over medium-low heat, stirring occasionally to keep the mixture from burning. Whisk in half the warmed milk. When smooth, whisk in the rest of the milk. Heat slowly, whisking to prevent lumps from forming and scraping the bottom of the pan to ensure that the sauce doesn't burn. Add the Parmesan cheese to the sauce and stir until smooth. Strain the sauce if necessary to remove any burned particles.

Blackened Seasoning

INGREDIENTS

1 teaspoon white pepper

¾ tablespoon red pepper

1 tablespoon black pepper

4 teaspoons onion powder

2 teaspoons garlic powder

4 teaspoons Mrs. Dash

1 teaspoon dried sage

2 tablespoons dried safflower

4 teaspoons paprika

2 teaspoons gumbo file powder

4 tablespoons dried oregano leaves

8 tablespoons whole-leaf thyme

PREPARATION

Put all the ingredients in a blender and process until fine. Store in an airtight shaker jar.

SERVINGS: 24

Nutritional Info (per 1-teaspoon serving):

Calories:	5
Carbs:	0.4g

Food Group Servings:

Starch:	0
Fruit:	0
Vegetable:	0
Protein:	0
Dairy:	0
Fat:	0

Marinara Sauce

SERVINGS: 32

*Nutritional Info
(per ¼-cup serving):*

Calories:	25
Carbs:	3.9g
Protein:	1.4g
Total Fat:	0.9g

*Food Group
Servings:*

Starch:	0
Fruit:	0
Vegetable:	1
Protein:	0
Dairy:	0
Fat:	0

INGREDIENTS

10 cups (80 ounces)
    canned whole, peeled
    tomatoes, no added salt,
    undrained
2 tablespoons olive oil
2 cups chopped white
    onions
1 tablespoon minced
    garlic

1 tablespoon dried herb
    mix, typically containing
    rosemary, marjoram,
    thyme, and savory
1 teaspoon ground fennel
    seed
¼ cup burgundy wine
2 ounces tomato paste, no
    added salt

PREPARATION

Put the tomatoes in a blender or food processor and pulse until smooth. Heat the oil in a Dutch oven or stockpot over medium-high heat. Add the onions and sauté until soft. Add the garlic, herb mix, and fennel. When the garlic becomes fragrant, add the burgundy wine and stir. Add the tomato paste and cook for 2 minutes. Add the tomato mixture and simmer gently over low heat for 1½ to 2 hours, stirring occasionally. Pour into smaller containers for storage, to allow for adequate cooling in refrigerator or freezer.

Raspberry Vinaigrette

INGREDIENTS

2½ ounces fresh raspberries

1¼ teaspoons clover honey

1 tablespoon water

4¾ teaspoons champagne
    vinegar

5 teaspoons canola oil

PREPARATION

Put the raspberries, honey, water, and vinegar in a blender. With the blender on, slowly add the oil. Blend until fully combined.

SERVINGS: 8–10

*Nutritional Info:
(per 1-tablespoon
serving):*

Calories:	33
Carbs:	2g
Total Fat:	3g

*Food Group
Servings:*

Starch:	0
Fruit:	0
Vegetable:	0
Protein:	0
Dairy:	0
Fat:	0.5

Blue Cheese and Chive Potato Salad

SERVINGS: 4

*Nutritional Info
(per serving):*

Calories:	78
Carbs:	15g
Protein:	2g
Total Fat:	1g
Saturated Fat:	0.5g
Dietary Fiber:	1g
Sodium:	173mg
Cholesterol:	3mg

*Food Group
Servings:*

Starch:	1
Fruit:	0
Vegetable:	0
Protein:	0
Dairy:	0
Fat:	0

INGREDIENTS

$3/4$ pound red potatoes (about 6 small), cubed

8 tablespoons nonfat sour cream

2 tablespoons low-fat (1%) buttermilk

$1/8$ teaspoon ground black pepper

$1/2$ teaspoon cider vinegar

$1/2$ ounce blue cheese, crumbled

2 tablespoons chopped onion

2 tablespoons diced celery

1 tablespoon chopped fresh chives

PREPARATION

Place the potatoes in a Dutch oven or stockpot. Cover them with water, and bring to a boil. Cook 8 minutes, or until tender. Drain and place in a large bowl.

In a medium bowl, combine the sour cream, buttermilk, pepper, and cider vinegar. Stir in the blue cheese. Add the onion, celery, and fresh chives. Pour the mixture over the potatoes; toss gently to coat. Cover and chill.

Coconut Rice

INGREDIENTS

1⅓ cups water

7 tablespoons dry basmati rice

7 tablespoons light coconut milk

½ ounce unsweetened flaked coconut

PREPARATION

Bring the water to a boil in a nonstick saucepan. Stir in the rice and coconut milk. Cover and simmer until the rice is al dente, about 20 minutes. Stir in the flaked coconut before serving.

SERVINGS: 4

Nutritional Info (per serving):

Calories:	151
Carbs:	21g
Protein:	2g
Total Fat:	8g
Saturated Fat:	7g
Dietary Fiber:	1g
Sodium:	6mg
Cholesterol:	0mg

Food Group Servings:

Starch:	1
Fruit:	0
Vegetable:	0
Protein:	0
Dairy:	0
Fat:	1.5

Mediterranean Couscous

SERVINGS: 4

Nutritional Info (per serving):

Calories:	271
Carbs:	48g
Protein:	9g
Total Fat:	4g
Saturated Fat:	0.5g
Dietary Fiber:	4g
Sodium:	30mg
Cholesterol:	0mg

Food Group Servings:

Starch:	2.75
Fruit:	0
Vegetable:	0.25
Protein:	0
Dairy:	0
Fat:	0.75

INGREDIENTS

1¼ cups reduced-sodium chicken broth

1¼ cups dry couscous

½ cup chopped red bell pepper

½ cup chopped yellow pepper

¾ cup chopped white onion

1 tablespoon extra-virgin olive oil

1 tablespoon red wine vinegar

¼ tablespoon ground black pepper

1 tablespoon chopped fresh basil

PREPARATION

Heat the chicken broth and combine it with the couscous in a pan. Let the couscous plump. Crumble it to a uniform consistency, with no lumps.

Heat a nonstick skillet over medium-high heat. Sauté the red and yellow peppers in the skillet until tender-crisp. Remove them from the pan and sauté the onions until browned well.

For the dressing, combine the olive oil, vinegar, black pepper, and basil in a small bowl. Mix well. Combine the fluffed couscous, vegetables, and dressing.

Pesto Pasta

INGREDIENTS

7½ ounces dry whole-wheat
spaghetti

½ cup chopped red bell
pepper

1⅓ cups cannelloni beans,
rinsed and drained

¼ cup Buitoni pesto sauce

PREPARATION

Cook the spaghetti according to the package directions. Toss the drained spaghetti with the chopped peppers and beans. Stir in the pesto.

SERVINGS: 4

*Nutritional Info
(per serving):*

Calories:	332
Carbs:	51g
Protein:	14g
Total Fat:	8g
Saturated Fat:	2g
Dietary Fiber:	10g
Sodium:	304mg
Cholesterol:	5mg

*Food Group
Servings:*

Starch:	3.75
Fruit:	0
Vegetable:	0
Protein:	0
Dairy:	0
Fat:	1

Rice Pilaf with Carrots

SERVINGS: 4

Nutritional Info (per serving):

Calories:	153
Carbs:	25g
Protein:	4g
Total Fat:	4g
Saturated Fat:	1g
Dietary Fiber:	2g
Sodium:	108mg
Cholesterol:	0mg

Food Group Servings:

Starch:	2
Fruit:	0
Vegetable:	0
Protein:	0
Dairy:	0
Fat:	0.5

INGREDIENTS

- 1 teaspoon extra-virgin olive oil
- 1 tablespoon diced white onion
- 1 cup dry brown long-grain rice
- 2 tablespoons minced garlic
- $\frac{1}{4}$ teaspoon white pepper
- $1\frac{1}{4}$ cups reduced-sodium chicken broth
- $\frac{1}{3}$ cup shredded carrots
- $\frac{1}{8}$ tablespoon salt
- 2 tablespoons diced green onion
- 2 teaspoons chopped walnuts

PREPARATION

Heat the oil in a heavy-bottomed saucepan over medium-high heat. Add the onion and sauté until soft. Add the rice and stir until coated with oil. Stir in the garlic and white pepper. Add the broth and bring it to a boil; cover and reduce the heat to low, then simmer for 10 minutes. Stir in the carrots and salt; cover and simmer for 10 minutes more, or until all the liquid is absorbed and the rice is cooked.

Remove from the heat and let stand 5 minutes. Fluff with a fork before serving. Garnish with the diced green onion and chopped walnuts.

Roasted Pepper and Goat Cheese Polenta

INGREDIENTS

1¼ ounces red bell pepper

⅛ jalapeño pepper

1 cup reduced-sodium
  chicken broth

⅓ cup polenta mix

¼ teaspoon white pepper

2 teaspoons chopped parsley

½ ounce soft goat cheese,
  crumbled

1 teaspoon chives

PREPARATION

Preheat the oven to 400° F. Place the red and jalapeño peppers in a small roasting pan and roast until soft.

Bring the broth to a boil in a saucepan over medium-high heat and add the polenta. Stir in the roasted peppers and jalapeños, white pepper, and parsley.

Continue cooking the polenta according to the package directions. When the polenta is cooked, turn it out on a greased baking pan and sprinkle the goat cheese and chives evenly throughout. Allow the polenta to cool.

Cut the polenta into four equal servings, then place it on a greased baking sheet. Bake for 10 minutes, or until golden brown.

SERVINGS: 4

*Nutritional Info
(per serving):*

Calories:	92
Carbs:	13g
Protein:	4g
Total Fat:	2g
Saturated Fat:	1g
Dietary Fiber:	1g
Sodium:	246mg
Cholesterol:	3mg

*Food Group
Servings:*

Starch:	0.75
Fruit:	0
Vegetable:	0
Protein:	0
Dairy:	0
Fat:	0

The Duke Plan is flexible enough for you to indulge in desserts (in moderation). While the following choices represent better, more healthful options than your usual sweet fare, even the healthiest desserts can lack the essential nutrients needed to fuel your weight-loss regimen—and they contain calories not accounted for in your meal plan. If you choose to incorporate a dessert into a day's plan, you may want to compensate for the extra calories by cutting out one snack or eating a smaller portion at a meal.

Items that don't fit into any particular food group, like alcohol and desserts, are counted as miscellaneous calories. Foods with miscellaneous calories should be enjoyed sparingly, as an occasional treat.

Berry Sorbet

SERVINGS: 6

Nutritional Info (per serving):

Calories:	107
Carbs:	29g
Protein:	0.5g
Total Fat:	0.5g
Saturated Fat:	0.5g
Dietary Fiber:	5g
Sodium:	3mg
Cholesterol:	0mg

Food Group Servings:

Starch:	0
Fruit:	0.5
Vegetable:	0
Protein:	0
Dairy:	0
Fat:	0
75 Miscellaneous calories	

INGREDIENTS

½ cup lime juice
⅓ cup sugar
2 tablespoons grenadine syrup
⅓ cup water
12 ounces raspberries
12 ounces strawberries, halved

PREPARATION

Bring the lime juice, sugar, grenadine, and water to a boil in a saucepan over medium heat, and cook until the sugar is dissolved. In a blender or the work bowl of a food processor, purée the berries, then press through a fine sieve to eliminate the seeds. Combine the berry purée and sugar syrup in a bowl. Cover and freeze for 2 hours, or until the center is almost frozen. Remove from the freezer and beat with a hand mixer until smooth. Return to the freezer for 1 hour, or until the center is again almost firm. Remove from the freezer and stir until smooth before serving.

Chocolate Cherry Chews

INGREDIENTS

¼ cup dried cherries

¾ cup cranberry juice

¼ cup unsweetened cocoa
   powder

2 tablespoons sweetened
   condensed milk

2 tablespoons apple butter

1 teaspoon vanilla extract

½ cup shredded coconut,
   divided

PREPARATION

Preheat the oven to 350° F. Lightly oil the baking sheets or coat them with cooking spray; set aside. In a small saucepan, combine the cherries and cranberry juice. Bring to a simmer over low heat and cook, stirring frequently, for 2 minutes, or until all the juice has been absorbed into the cherries. Set aside and cool.

In a mixing bowl, combine the cocoa, condensed milk, apple butter, and vanilla. With an electric mixer, beat until smooth and blended. Add the plumped cherries and half the coconut; stir just until combined. Using 2 small spoons, form and drop 1-inch mounds onto the prepared baking sheet. Sprinkle the remaining coconut over the cookies. Bake for 8 to 10 minutes, until the cookies are no longer sticky and the coconut has begun to brown. Do not overbake; the cookies firm up slightly as they cool. Transfer to a wire rack to cool completely.

SERVINGS: 10

*Nutritional Info
(per serving):*

Calories:	73
Carbs:	13g
Protein:	1g
Total Fat:	2g
Saturated Fat:	2g
Dietary Fiber:	1g
Sodium:	18mg
Cholesterol:	0.5mg

*Food Group
Servings:*

Starch:	0
Fruit:	0
Vegetable:	0
Protein:	0
Dairy:	0
Fat:	0

73 Miscellaneous
   calories

Guilt-Free Chocolate Cheesecake

SERVINGS: 14

Nutritional Info (per serving):

Calories:	202
Carbs:	23g
Protein:	4g
Total Fat:	11g
Saturated Fat:	5g
Dietary Fiber:	0.5g
Sodium:	167mg
Cholesterol:	9mg

Food Group Servings:

Starch:	1
Fruit:	0
Vegetable:	0
Protein:	0.5
Dairy:	0
Fat:	1
30 Miscellaneous calories	

INGREDIENTS

6 ounces semisweet chocolate pieces

12 ounces firm tofu, divided

1 tablespoon honey, divided

1 graham cracker crust

8 ounces reduced-fat cream cheese

$\frac{1}{2}$ teaspoon heat-stable sugar substitute (such as Splenda)

$\frac{3}{4}$ teaspoon vanilla extract

PREPARATION

In a double boiler set over barely simmering water, or in the microwave, melt the chocolate pieces. Place the melted chocolate, 4 ounces tofu, and half the honey in a blender or the work bowl of a food processor. Blend well, then spread the mixture in the graham cracker crust.

Clean the blender or work bowl and add the cream cheese, remaining tofu, remaining honey, sugar substitute, and vanilla. Blend well, then spread over the chocolate layer in the graham cracker crust. Garnish with fresh berries if desired.

Silken Chocolate Pie

INGREDIENTS

12 ounces semisweet
    chocolate pieces

$\frac{1}{3}$ cup coffee liqueur (may
    substitute regular or decaf
    coffee)

8 ounces firm tofu

1 tablespoon honey

1 graham cracker crust

PREPARATION

Melt the chocolate in a double boiler set over barely simmering water, or in the microwave. In a blender or the work bowl of a food processor, process the coffee, tofu, and honey. When smooth, slowly add the melted chocolate. Pulse until smooth and fully incorporated. Using a spatula, spread the chocolate mixture into the graham cracker crust. Refrigerate for 3 hours, or until firm.

SERVINGS: 12

Nutritional Info (per serving):

Calories:	281
Carbs:	38g
Protein:	2g
Total Fat:	12g
Saturated Fat:	7g
Dietary Fiber:	0.5g
Sodium:	151mg
Cholesterol:	0mg

Food Group Servings:

Starch:	1
Fruit:	0
Vegetable:	0
Protein:	0
Dairy:	0
Fat:	0

200 Miscellaneous
    calories

Peach-Cherry Crisp

SERVINGS: 4

*Nutritional Info
(per serving):*

Calories:	189
Carbs:	33g
Protein:	2g
Total Fat:	6g
Saturated Fat:	0.5g
Dietary Fiber:	2g
Sodium:	28mg
Cholesterol:	0mg

*Food Group
Servings:*

Starch:	0
Fruit:	0.5
Vegetable:	0
Protein:	0
Dairy:	0
Fat:	1

70 Miscellaneous
   calories

INGREDIENTS

1 tablespoon cornstarch

¾ cup unsweetened, pitted
   dark cherries, drained,
   juice reserved

2 tablespoons sugar

⅓ cup cherry juice

¾ cup sliced canned peaches

⅓ cup dry rolled oats

3 tablespoons chopped
   walnuts

⅛ teaspoon ground mace

2 teaspoons soft trans-fat-free
   margarine

PREPARATION

Preheat the oven to 350° F. Combine the cornstarch with the reserved cherry juice and stir until dissolved. Heat the mixture gently in a medium saucepan over medium-low heat, stirring
frequently until thickened. Remove from the heat. Stir in the
sugar and cherry juice. Add the peaches and cherries, and combine.

   Combine the oats, walnuts, and mace in a medium bowl. Using
a fork or pastry blender, cut the margarine into the dry ingredients to create a crumbly topping. Spread the fruit mixture evenly
into an 8-inch-square baking pan and cover with topping. Bake 20
to 30 minutes, or until bubbly. Serve hot.

Sweet Potato Pie with Almond Crust

INGREDIENTS

Crust:

2½ cups almond flour

¼ cup liquid egg whites

2 packets heat-stable sugar
  substitute (such as
  Splenda)

1 tablespoon soft margarine

Pie filling:

2 cups cooked mashed sweet
  potatoes

2 large eggs, beaten

¼ cup nonfat milk

1 tablespoon packed brown
  sugar

1½ teaspoons heat-stable
  sugar substitute

½ teaspoon salt

½ teaspoon ground nutmeg

4 tablespoons soft margarine

PREPARATION

Preheat the oven to 325° F. Coat a 9-inch deep-dish pie pan with cooking spray. In a medium bowl, combine the flour, egg whites, and sugar substitute. Slowly add the margarine, pressing the mixture against the sides of the bowl with a large spatula or spoon until the dough forms a smooth ball. Roll out the dough on a lightly floured surface to form a ⅛-inch-thick 12-inch round and place it in the pie pan.

Mix the mashed sweet potatoes, eggs, and milk in a medium bowl. In a separate bowl, combine the sugars and all seasonings. Stir the sugars and seasonings into the potato mixture until thoroughly combined. Pour into the pie shell, spreading evenly. Bake 20 to 25 minutes, until light golden and set. Let cool slightly, cut into wedges, and serve.

SERVINGS: 8

*Nutritional Info
(per serving):*

Calories:	256
Carbs:	22g
Protein:	8g
Total Fat:	16g
Saturated Fat:	2g
Dietary Fiber:	2g
Sodium:	273mg
Cholesterol:	53mg

*Food Group
Servings:*

Starch:	0.75
Fruit:	0
Vegetable:	0
Protein:	1.5
Dairy:	0
Fat:	0
60 Miscellaneous calories	

DUKE DIET SNACK LIST
FOR ALL CALORIE LEVELS, ALL WEEKS

CARROTS WITH LIGHT RANCH DIP
2 large carrots (or 1 cup baby carrots)
with 2 tablespoons light ranch dressing

CHEESE AND CRACKERS WITH TOMATO JUICE
4 small whole-grain crackers, 1 low-fat string
cheese, 1 cup tomato/vegetable juice

OPEN-FACED PEANUT BUTTER SANDWICH
1 slice whole-wheat bread with 2 teaspoons
natural peanut butter

OPEN-FACED TURKEY SANDWICH ON WHEAT
3 ounces lower-sodium deli-style turkey,
2 slices tomato, and 1 tablespoon mustard on
1 slice whole-wheat bread

APPLE AND ALMONDS
1 small apple (2$\frac{1}{2}$-inch diameter) with $\frac{1}{2}$ ounce
almonds (about 11 nuts)

HUMMUS WITH VEGGIES AND CRACKERS
6 small whole-grain crackers and $\frac{1}{2}$ medium
red bell pepper, sliced, with 3 tablespoons
hummus

PEANUT BUTTER AND GRAHAM CRACKERS
2 teaspoons natural peanut butter on two
2$\frac{1}{2}$-inch graham cracker squares

LOW-FAT PUDDING
$\frac{1}{2}$ cup low-fat pudding

APPLE WITH PEANUT BUTTER
2 teaspoons natural peanut butter on 1 small
apple (2$\frac{1}{2}$-inch diameter)

GINGERSNAPS AND MILK
1 cup nonfat milk with 2 gingersnaps

BLUEBERRIES WITH WALNUTS
$\frac{1}{2}$ cup blueberries with $\frac{1}{2}$ ounce walnuts
(about 7 halves)

CHEESE AND CRACKERS
8 small whole-grain crackers with 2 low-fat
cheddar cheese cubes

HARD-BOILED EGG AND ORANGE
1 large hard-boiled egg, plus 1 small (2$\frac{3}{8}$-inch
diameter) orange

COTTAGE CHEESE AND PEAR
$\frac{1}{4}$ cup low-fat cottage cheese and 1 small pear

BAGEL AND CREAM CHEESE
$\frac{1}{2}$ whole-grain bagel with 1 tablespoon low-fat
cream cheese

HUMMUS AND CARROTS
3 tablespoons hummus with 2 large carrots
(or 1 cup baby carrots)

MILK AND CEREAL
1 cup whole-grain cereal and $\frac{1}{2}$ cup nonfat
milk

YOGURT
6 ounces low-fat vanilla yogurt

APPLESAUCE AND MILK
1 cup unsweetened applesauce and 1 cup
nonfat milk

**TOASTER WAFFLE WITH CREAM CHEESE AND
FRUIT SPREAD**
One 4-inch round toaster waffle with $\frac{1}{4}$ cup
low-fat cottage cheese and 1 teaspoon all-
natural fruit spread

CHAPTER TEN

The Duke Diet Exercises

By now, we hope you're sold on the immeasurable value of exercise—and not just for weight loss. Exercise is the ultimate "whole person" treatment, improving cardiovascular health; helping to address high blood pressure and diabetes; increasing flexibility, grace, and agility; easing stress and anxiety; commonly relieving joint pain; and even lifting spirits. Few things that you can do for yourself are better than finding an exercise routine that you really enjoy and sticking to it. You'll be amazed at how quickly you'll feel its effects, and it won't be long before they're visible, too. As one woman who took up our strength training program told us, "Nothing feels as good as looking in the mirror and loving what you see."

At the Duke Diet & Fitness Center, we introduce clients to strength and flexibility work, tailored to their level of fitness, in the very first week of the program, just as we did in chapter 5 of this book. You will find the same strength and flexibility exercises in this chapter and also on www.dukediet.com. On the website, you'll also find additional exercises for each fitness level, plus instructional videos for all of the workout routines, so you can see the moves and hear instructions on exactly how to perform these workouts correctly.

THE FITT PRINCIPLE

We've shown you how we help our clients progress in their fitness routines. We encourage people to move forward and challenge themselves. Our strategy holds to the principle described by the acronym FITT, which stands for *frequency,* the number of times you exercise each week; *intensity,* how hard you work while exercising; *time,* the number of minutes you devote to each session; and *type,* the kind of exercise you are doing. You can apply the FITT principle both to your aerobic activity and to your strength and flexibility training. To use the FITT principle to raise your fitness level, simply change up to any of these four elements one at a time to make your workout more challenging. For example, when it comes to frequency, you might add another session of exercise to your weekly schedule; for intensity, you could increase your walking speed, the number of pounds you lift, or the strength of your resistance tubes; for time, you could add five or ten minutes to each workout session; and for type, you might change your routine from walking to bicycling, or add a Pilates or yoga class. Changing one of these will make a difference, and the new challenge will help keep you motivated. We have built this principle into each of the workouts in each of the levels in this book to keep you challenged. To help you progress, more workouts are available on the website.

WHAT YOU NEED

You don't need to join a gym or invest in expensive or fancy equipment to participate in the Duke Diet Exercise Plan. All you need are five pieces of basic gear that won't take up much space in your closet: a stability ball, a medicine ball, resistance tubes, dumbbells, and a mat. Many department stores have fitness/sports departments where you'll be able to find everything you need.

Stability Ball

Usually made of vinyl, stability or fitness balls are used to strengthen core muscles, improve your balance and coordination, and increase your flexibility. When you sit on one, you have to use your abdominal and back muscles to keep your balance, so you get an almost automatic workout. If you suffer from back pain, you'll find that working with a stability ball can help relieve it because your stomach muscles support your spine and the ball cushions your back evenly and gently.

Stability balls come in different sizes, and it's important both to choose a ball that fits you and to keep it properly inflated. You want a ball that keeps your knees level with your hips when you sit on it. The firmer the ball, the more challenging exercise on it will be.

Here are some general guidelines for choosing the right stability ball for your height:

- Under 4 feet, 6 inches: 30-centimeter (12-inch) ball
- 4 feet, 6 inches to 5 feet, 0 inches: 45-centimeter (18-inch) ball
- 5 feet, 1 inch to 5 feet, 7 inches: 55-centimeter (22-inch) ball
- 5 feet, 8 inches to 6 feet, 2 inches: 65-centimeter (26-inch) ball
- Over 6 feet, 2 inches: 75-centimeter (30-inch) ball

Look for a high-quality stability ball that promises to be burst-resistant and comes packaged with an inflation pump and an instructional video.

Medicine Ball

A medicine ball is simply a ball with weight in it. Depending on how you use it, this exercise tool can build strength, quickness, and flexibility. Medicine balls come in a variety of sizes, designs, and weights and can be used as a substitute for dumbbells. As a rule of thumb, start out with a lighter medicine ball and increase the weight as your fitness improves.

Select a ball that's heavy enough to challenge you but does not limit your control or your range of motion. Try out different medicine balls in the store and choose the weights that feel best to you. Our clients typically start out with one 2-pound and one 4-pound medicine ball.

Some medicine balls bounce; others do not. The bouncing kind lets you perform throwing and catching exercises against a wall and also lets you do certain abdominal strengthening moves. To help you find the right medicine ball, here are the basic types:

- **Gel-filled:** With soft vinyl on the outside, these balls don't bounce. Often used in physical therapy, they are available in a wide range of sizes.
- **Air-filled:** These balls bounce and get bouncier the more air you put in them. This is the type of ball we use for our general resistance exercises.
- **With handles:** These balls are designed to be used in place of dumbbells. Gyms and personal trainers commonly stock them.
- **With a rope attached:** The rope may be permanently attached or removable. These balls are perfect for swinging exercises and core-strengthening rotational exercises.

For the routines in this book, you'll need two basic air-filled medicine balls, a lighter one and a heavier one.

Resistance Tubes

Long used by physical therapists, resistance tubes are pieces of rubber or elastic that can be used for a wide range of exercises. You pull against the resistance of the tubes, using smooth, controlled movements and not letting the elastic snap back on its own; this builds, tones, and strengthens the muscles in your upper and lower body. Working with tubes is nice and easy on the joints. The kind to use for the Duke exercises has a handle on each end and an anchor that allows you to secure it to a door (check the packaging for instructions for using the anchor).

Lightweight and portable, resistance tubes are great for busy travelers. Since they're inexpensive, you can keep an extra set in your car or office and work out as the spirit moves you. Check the packaging to determine which ones are higher or lower in resistance, since there is a lot of variation and colors are not standard across brands.

Start with a tube that's comfortable but challenging to stretch. As you use that tube in your workouts, your muscle strength and endurance will improve and the exercises will grow easier. When you no longer feel as challenged, switch to a tube with higher resistance to increase the intensity of the exercise. As you can see, resistance tubes make it easy to set your own fitness pace. Be sure to examine them regularly for nicks, tears, or punctures that might cause them to snap.

Dumbbells

Dumbbells are small, handheld weights that generally come in pairs—one for each hand—ranging from two pounds to one hundred pounds. Some dumbbells are adjustable, meaning you can easily up their poundage as you need greater challenges. Dumbbells are available in different materials: iron, foam covered, vinyl covered, or rubber encased. There are even water dumbbells, designed for pool exercising, for people with joint problems such as arthritis.

Dumbbells offer some special workout advantages. Just picking them up requires you to engage your abdominal, back, and hip muscles, all of which figure prominently in your overall strength, balance, and posture. They're also very easy to use because, in typical workouts, you move them according to your body's natural range of motion. You can target specific areas of your body very effectively with dumbbells, and since there are hundreds of exercises you can do with them, you'll never be bored.

We suggest that you get a set ranging in weight from two to twenty pounds (or higher if you are a little stronger). You will need enough weight so that you can progressively increase your workout intensity by using heavier weights as your strength builds. It may be wise to go to a local fitness store and try out a few pairs to get a better idea of the weight range that suits your needs before you buy.

Exercise Mat

Working out on a solid surface can be hard on your body, so even if your floors are carpeted, you'll need a good mat for stretching and toning exercises such as yoga and Pilates. Available in many shapes and sizes, mats are made from plastic or rubberized materials. Some fold up, and others roll up. The mats that roll up are the most portable and easiest to store.

A good mat should be at least a half-inch thick, and it should be firm because a too-soft one will not support you well enough. Be sure to choose a mat long and wide enough for your body and activities. It's very important that you choose one that feels good to you, so don't be embarrassed to try out different mats in the store. The salesclerks will have seen people do this before. Be sure to ask which mats are best for the surfaces on which you plan to use them.

If this sounds like a lot of equipment, don't worry. None of it is it very expensive and most of it will last for years. The total cost will likely be less than the price of a couple months' worth of membership in a gym.

THE DUKE DIET EXERCISE PLAN

These easy-to-follow strength and flexibility workouts are designed to be performed at home by Level 1 and Level 2 exercisers. Fitness Prep Level exercisers should wait to begin them until they can comfortably walk 8,000 to 10,000 steps a day, nearly every day for a week. These workouts will train all your major muscle groups. We'll be the first to admit that adding exercise to your daily routine can initially seem daunting, but once you get started and see how much better you feel every time you work out, you'll want to continue. We promise.

During Weeks 1 and 2, perform Workout 1 for your fitness level, and during Weeks 3 and 4, perform Workout 2. Our website (www.dukediet.com) has additional workouts you can try after you complete the ones in this book.

When performing these exercises, be sure to follow the instructions closely and pay attention to the photos and/or website videos to ensure that you use proper exercise form.

STRENGTH TRAINING GUIDELINES

1. Warm up with at least five minutes of light aerobic activity, such as marching or jogging in place, climbing stairs, riding a stationary bicycle, or walking on a treadmill.

2. For Level 1, do one set of twelve to fifteen repetitions of each exercise; for Level 2, do two sets. After four weeks, if you're ready, you can progress to two sets if you're in Level 1 or to three sets if you're in Level 2.

3. Choose an appropriate weight or resistance. It is best to start with a lower weight and see how that feels. If you can easily get to 15 repetitions, it is probably too light. If you cannot get to 12, it is too heavy. There is no real formula for selecting an appropriate weight, but with some careful trial and error, you will find the right level for each exercise. Your muscles should always feel challenged by the last few repetitions of an exercise; as you progress, switch to a heavier resistance or add more repetitions. Rest for about a minute between sets.

4. To increase resistance when using tubing, increase your distance from the anchor point, use two tubes, or shorten the tube by forming a loop to pick up the slack.

5. Perform each exercise slowly and in a controlled fashion; avoid jerky, fast movements.

6. Cool down by performing the designated stretches that follow your routine. Hold each stretch for ten to thirty seconds, without bouncing.

7. For Level 1, perform your strength training workout twice a week; for Level 2, three times a week. Be sure to do the workouts on nonconsecutive days.

8. Employ the FITT principle to progress in your fitness program once you have completed four weeks at Level 2, or log on to www.dukediet.com for additional weeks of workouts. If you are doing a routine twice a week, increase your *frequency* to three times a week. To increase your *intensity,* try using heavier resistances as you get stronger. Increase the *time* of your workout by adding additional sets. To add another *type* of strength building exercise to the mix, you might add Pilates or yoga to your weekly routine, too.

9. Keep track of your progress on the monitoring card in chapter 5 or in your Lifestyle Journal on our website. Record the times you worked out (note the duration for cardio) as well as the number of sets and repetitions you performed.

Chair Squat

Squats build strength in your lower body.
The specific muscles worked are the quadriceps (thighs)
and the gluteals (hips and buttocks).

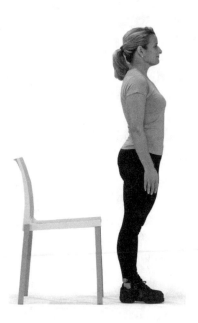

STEP 1: Place a chair just behind you and stand
in front of it with your feet hip- or shoulder-width
apart and your weight on your heels.

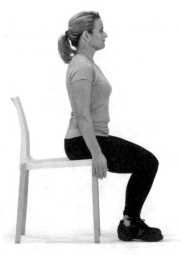

STEP 2: Contract your abs and keep your knees
behind your toes as you bend from the hips and
slowly sit down on the chair. Exhale as you
straighten your legs and return to standing.

TIP: Lift your chest and keep your back straight as you perform the squat.

Regular Push-up

Though many exercisers grimace at the thought of push-ups,
they are very effective at strengthening your arm and chest
muscles, so give them a try. The specific muscles worked
are the triceps (back of the arms), the pectorals (chest),
and the deltoids (shoulders).

**STEP 1: Lie on your stomach
with your hands under your
shoulders. Place your toes or
knees on the floor, depending on
your ability.**

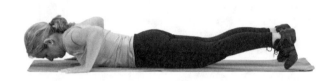

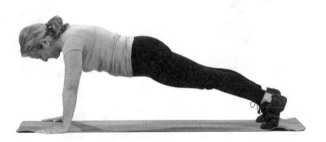

**STEP 2: Push yourself
up, then lower your
upper body until your
elbows form an
approximately 90-
degree angle.**

**STEP 3: Pause, then straighten
your arms to raise your body
without locking your elbows.
Repeat.**

TIP: Keep your forehead down, in line with your spine, as you perform this exercise. Breathe out on the push-up and relax your neck.

Wall Push-up

This is an alternative to the Regular Push-up. Wall Push-ups are great if you don't like to get down on the floor. The specific muscles worked are the triceps (back of the arms) and the pectorals (chest).

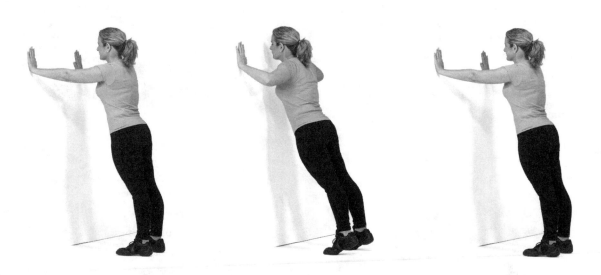

STEP 1: Lean with your hands against a wall, at shoulder height, about shoulder-width apart.

STEP 2: Bend your elbows until they form an approximately 90-degree angle as you push your body toward the wall. Pause.

STEP 3: Straighten your arms without locking your elbows. Repeat.

TIP: Lead with your chest. Your heels can come up off the floor, but be careful not to strain when pushing up.

Seated Leg Extension

This is a good exercise to strengthen the quadriceps
(thigh muscles).

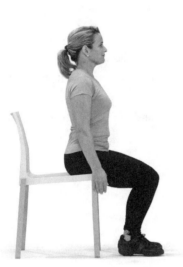

STEP 1: Sit on a chair with
both feet on the floor.

STEP 2: Squeeze the muscles in the front of your
right leg and straighten your knee in front of you,
without locking your knee. Pause, then slowly
return to the starting position. Complete all
repetitions on your right leg before switching to
your left leg.

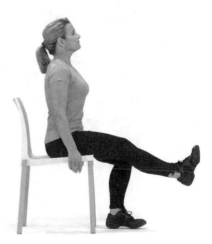

TIP: Go slowly when you straighten your leg; hold 2 to 3 seconds.

Straight-Leg Raise on Mat

This exercise strengthens the hip flexors, the muscles that help you flex your hip—important when you're climbing stairs.

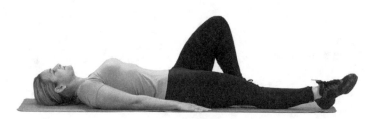

STEP 1: Lie on your back with your left knee bent and your left foot flat on the floor. Extend your right leg and point your toes forward.

STEP 2: Lift your right leg up as far as you can, until your foot points to the ceiling. Pause, then slowly return to the starting position. Repeat with the other leg.

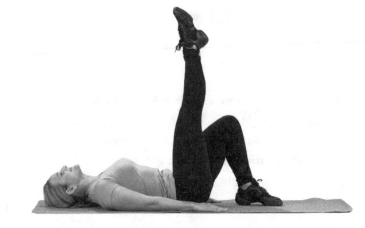

TIP: To make this exercise easier, raise your leg only to the height of the opposite knee.

Hip Bridge on Mat

This exercise helps you strengthen your back.
The specific muscles worked are the gluteals
(hips and buttocks) and the lower back.

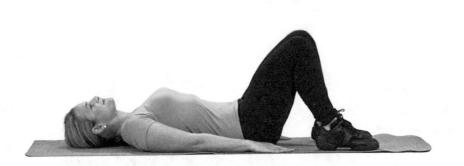

STEP 1: Lie on your back with your knees bent, your feet flat on the floor, and your arms at your sides. Keep your chin pointing toward the ceiling and your abs tight.

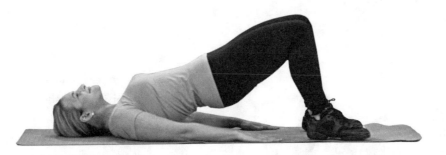

STEP 2: Press your weight down through your heels and exhale as you squeeze your buttocks and lift your hips off the floor. Your body should form a straight line from your knees down to your shoulders. Slowly return to the starting position. Repeat.

TIP: Relax your head and shoulders and breathe out as you raise your hips.

Abs Curl on Mat

You may have heard this before: If your abdominal muscles
are weak, your back will feel it. This is a good exercise
to start working your abs. The specific muscles
worked are the abdominals.

**STEP 1: Lie on
your back with
both knees bent.
Cross your arms
over your chest
or place them
behind your head,
with your elbows out
to the sides. Keep
your spine neutral.**

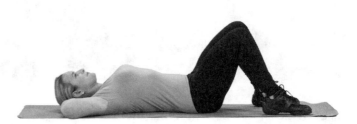

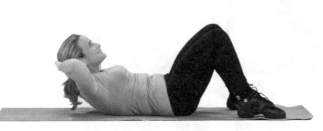

**STEP 2: Engage your abs by
curling up, raising your shoulders
and upper back off the floor
toward your pelvis. Contract at
the top of the movement, pause,
then slowly return to the starting
position. Repeat.**

TIP: Be careful not to pull on your neck as you curl up. To progress, lift your
toes off the floor, while keeping your heels down. This will make you work your
abs a bit harder.

Wall Squat with Stability Ball

This is a key exercise at the Duke Diet & Fitness Center.
It's great for strengthening weak knees and hips. The ball helps
to cushion your back and maintain your form throughout
the squat. The specific muscles worked are the quadriceps
(thighs) and the gluteals (hips and buttocks).

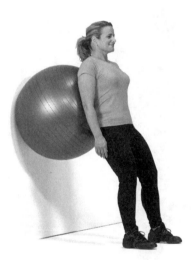

STEP 1: Stand with your lower back against the ball, and the ball between you and the wall. Your feet should be shoulder-width apart.

STEP 2: Push your back into the ball and bend your knees until your thighs are parallel with the floor. Be sure to keep your knees over your ankles. Return to the starting position and repeat.

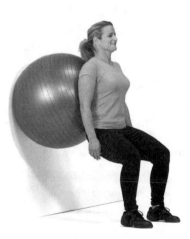

TIP: Don't let your bottom roll back toward the wall.

Standing Chest Press with Resistance Tube

We love any exercise with tubes. Tubes can be as effective as dumbbells or machines for strengthening your muscles. The handles make it easy to hold the tubes, and you'll feel a satisfying burn in your arms as you exercise. The specific muscles worked are the triceps (backs of the arms) and the pectorals (chest muscles).

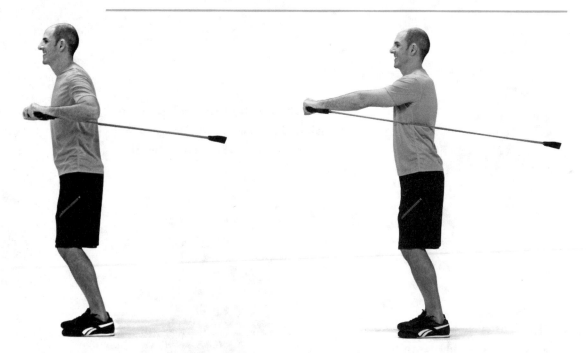

STEP 1: Anchor the tube just above waist height. Facing away from the anchor point, position the tube under your arms at chest height with your palms facing down and your elbows bent at a 90-degree angle.

STEP 2: Press your hands forward and together. Slowly return to the starting position and repeat.

TIP: As you press out, breathe out. Don't let your back arch; keep it straight.

Back Row with Resistance Tube

This is a great exercise for improving the poor upper back posture
many of us fall into when we slump forward
to work on our computers. The specific muscles
worked are the upper back muscles.

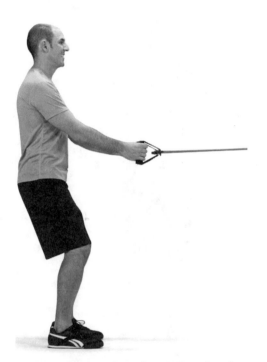 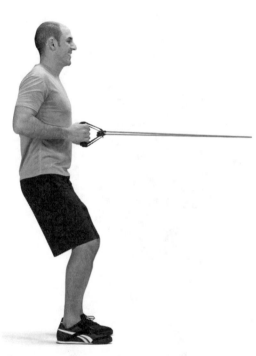

STEP 1: Anchor the tube at waist height. Stand facing the anchor point, with knees slightly bent. Extend your arms in front of your body and hold the tube with a neutral grip.

STEP 2: Squeeze your shoulder blades together; lead with your elbows, and pull the tube back toward the sides of your torso in line with your sternum (breastbone). Return to the starting position and repeat.

TIP: Really focus on squeezing the shoulder blades together.

Biceps Curl
with Resistance Tube

This simple exercise is great for increasing the strength in your arms.
The specific muscles worked are the biceps (front of the arms).

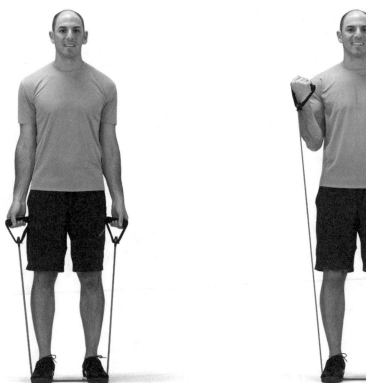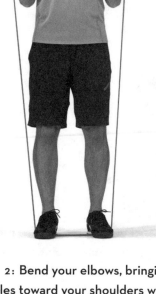

STEP 1: Stand on the tube with both feet. Grasp the handles with your palms forward and your arms fully extended.

STEP 2: Bend your elbows, bringing your knuckles toward your shoulders while keeping your elbows tucked in by your sides. Slowly return to the starting position and repeat.

TIP: Breathe out as you curl up. Keep your wrists in line with your forearms; don't curl them at the top of the movement.

Double Leg Heel Raise with Stability Ball Press-up

This simple exercise is effective for improving balance.
We also like the gentle upper body stretch it provides.
The specific muscles worked are the calves.

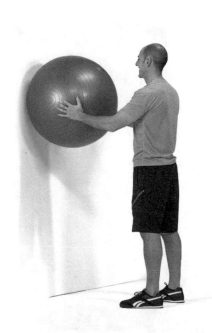 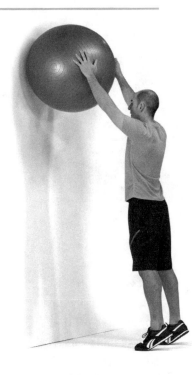

STEP 1: Place the ball at chest height on the wall.

STEP 2: Lift your heels, rising up on your toes while rolling the ball overhead.

STEP 3: Pause, then slowly lower your feet and roll the ball back. Repeat.

TIP: Get a nice upper back stretch by stretching your arms out as you push the ball up the wall.

Abs Curl on Stability Ball

This is one of our favorite starter exercises. The ball makes a comfortable support for your back. The specific muscles worked are the abdominal muscles.

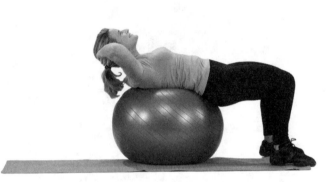

STEP 1: Lie with your lower back on a ball, feet on the floor. Hold your hands behind your ears, with your elbows out.

STEP 2: Contract your abs to lift your upper torso off the ball, keeping your lower back pressed into the ball. Return to the starting position and repeat.

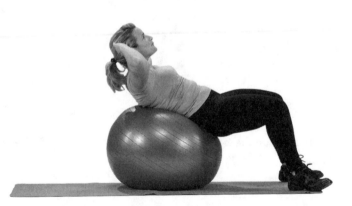

TIP: Pull your belly button toward your spine, lifting your chest toward the ceiling. Inhale on the way down and exhale on the way up.

Total Body Stretch

This is a nice exercise to focus and relax your mind and body.

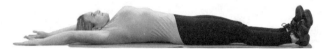

STEP 1: Lie on your back with both arms over your head and extended behind you with your toes pointed to the ceiling. At the same time, extend your arms and legs and pull your toes toward your shins. Take three to five deep breaths and rest.

TIP: Make your body long, as if you're being pulled from both ends in opposite directions. Be sure to breathe.

Lower Back and Gluteals Stretch

This position will help you stretch and relax your lower back.
It focuses on the gluteal muscles as well.

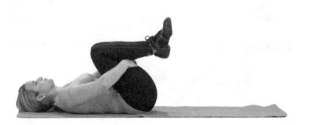

STEP 1: Lie on your back with your knees bent and your ankles together. With your hands behind your knees, pull your legs toward your chest. Take three to five deep breaths and rest.

Hamstrings Stretch

Tight hamstrings can lead to lower back pain.
Give them a nice, deep stretch with the towel.

STEP 1: Lie on your
back with a towel
wrapped behind
one leg.

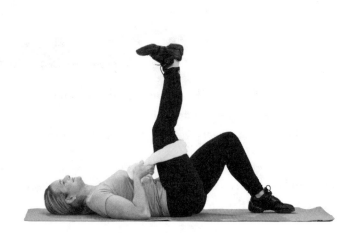

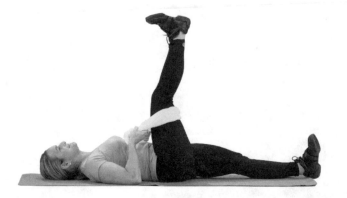

STEP 2: Gently straighten the
opposite leg. Grab both ends of the
towel and lift your extended leg
toward your chest. Repeat the
stretch with the other leg.

Lower Back Stretch with Knees Tilted to One Side

We love the way this stretch targets the muscles around the abs and in the lower back. It focuses on the oblique (side) abdominals, too.

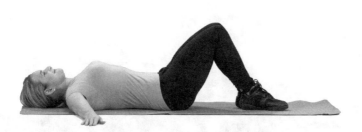

STEP 1: Lie on your back with both knees bent. Extend both arms perpendicular to your body.

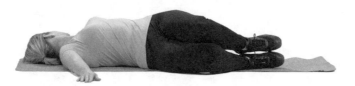

STEP 2: Slowly let your knees fall to one side and turn your head so you're looking over your opposite shoulder and feeling a stretch in your lower back. Repeat the stretch, letting your knees fall to the other side and looking over the opposite shoulder.

Quadriceps Stretch

Another Duke Diet & Fitness Center staple.
This important stretch can help improve knee problems.

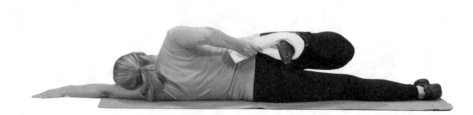

STEP 1: Lie on your side and extend your bottom arm overhead. Bend your top knee and wrap a towel around your ankle. Gently pull your ankle toward your body, feeling a stretch in the front of your thigh. Repeat on the other side.

Modified Hamstrings Stretch

The seated version of the hamstrings stretch also stretches
the muscles around your hips. The towel helps
you keep your back straight.

STEP 1: Sit with your legs
extended in a vee.

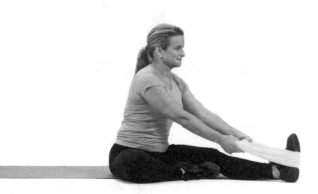

STEP 2: Bend
one leg in toward
your opposite
thigh. Wrap a
towel around the
foot of your
extended leg.

STEP 3: Holding both ends of
the towel, gently pull your body
toward your leg, feeling a stretch
in your lower back, hamstring,
and calf. Repeat on the other leg.

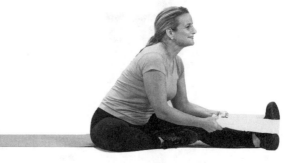

Triceps Stretch

The focus of this stretch is the back of your arms,
but it also helps to flex your shoulder muscles. It is
a great stretch if you play racquet sports.

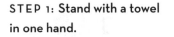

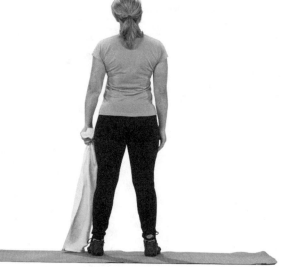

**STEP 1: Stand with a towel
in one hand.**

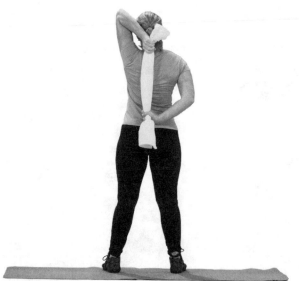

**STEP 2: Extend your arm overhead and
bend at the elbow. With the opposite
arm behind your back, reach for the
towel and gently pull, feeling a stretch in
the back of the extended arm. Switch
arms and repeat the stretch.**

Biceps Curl and Overhead Press with Dumbbells

The "curl and press" movement strengthens muscles in your upper body that you use in your everyday chores. The specific muscles worked are the biceps (front of the arms), the triceps (back of the arms), and the deltoids (shoulders).

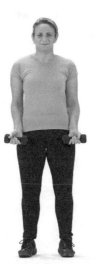

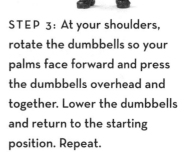

STEP 1: Start out standing with your feet in a comfortable position, holding the dumbbells with your arms fully extended at your sides, palms facing away from your body.

STEP 2: Bend your elbows to curl your fists toward your shoulders.

STEP 3: At your shoulders, rotate the dumbbells so your palms face forward and press the dumbbells overhead and together. Lower the dumbbells and return to the starting position. Repeat.

TIP: Keep your abs tight. Breathe out on the press-up.

Chest Press with Dumbbell Twist on Stability Ball

The chest press is subtle, but it effectively engages your chest muscles. The specific muscles worked are the pectorals (chest), the triceps (back of the arms), and the biceps (front of the arms).

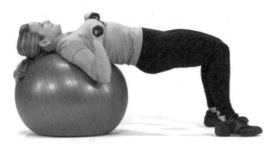

STEP 1: Lie on your back on the ball with your head and shoulders supported and your feet on the floor. Hold the dumbbells at your sides at midchest level, with your elbows flexed. Your palms should face toward your feet.

STEP 2: Press the dumbbells straight up over your chest, turning your hands to touch the ends of the dumbbells together. Return to the starting position and repeat.

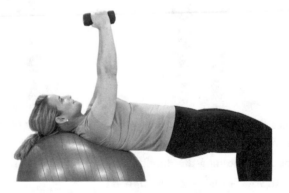

TIP: Hold your hips up and keep your knees over your ankles.

Back Fly with Dumbbells on Stability Ball

This is a great exercise to keep your upper back straight and strong. Use a lighter weight on this one. The specific muscles worked are the upper back muscles.

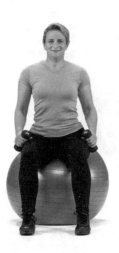 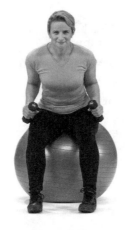 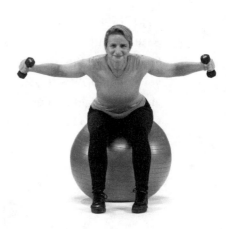

STEP 1: Sit on the stability ball with your arms at your sides, holding one dumbbell in each hand, with your palms facing in.

STEP 2: Bend your torso forward, keeping your back straight, until your chest faces your thighs.

STEP 3: Raise your arms to your sides, with your elbows slightly bent but in line with your shoulders and your palms facing the floor. Hold the weights steady for 2 seconds and keep your head in line with your spine. Release and repeat.

TIP: Don't strain your back as you lean forward; try to keep the natural curve in your lower (lumbar) spine.

Triceps Kickback with Dumbbell

Your triceps help you perform most of your ordinary chores,
such as lifting heavy bags.

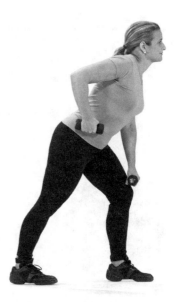

STEP 1: Begin with your feet in a staggered
position, with one foot in front of the other.
Support your torso by placing one hand on
your front thigh, with your elbow slightly bent.
Hold the weight in your other hand at hip level,
with your palm facing your waist.

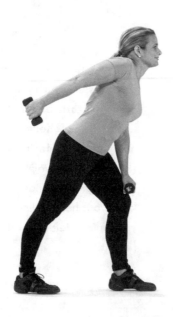

STEP 2: Extend your arm behind you,
contracting your triceps. Pause, then slowly
return to the starting position and repeat for
a full set. Then repeat the exercise on the
other side.

TIP: Go slowly, and don't snap your elbow. Keep your abs tight.

Superman

This is one of our favorite exercises because it focuses
on the muscles of the back and can help improve your posture.
The specific muscles worked are the upper and
lower back and the gluteals (hips and buttocks).

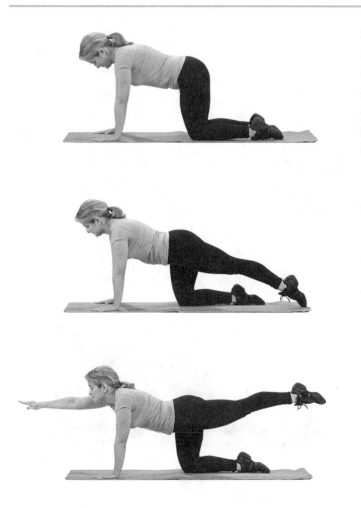

STEP 1: Start by kneeling on the mat with your palms on the floor, under your shoulders, fingers pointing forward.

STEP 2: Extend your left leg backward, resting your toes on the mat. Lift your right arm and extend it in front of you while simultaneously extending your left leg behind you. Return to the starting position and repeat with your left arm and right leg.

TIP: Keep your forehead low and your neck in line with your spine. Breathe out on the lift, stretching long but not high.

Hip Bridge with Stability Ball

Hip bridges work the gluteals (hips and buttocks) and
the lower back muscles. We like to call these areas
the backside of the core muscles.

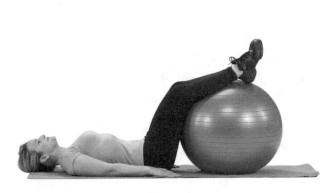

STEP 1: Lie on the mat with your
lower legs and feet resting on the
ball and your arms at your sides.

STEP 2: Lift your
hips off the mat,
squeezing your
buttocks. Hold 2 to
3 seconds. Return to
the starting position
and repeat.

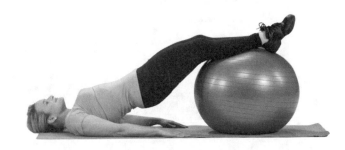

TIP: Breathe as you lift up your hips.

Wall Squat and Overhead Press with Medicine and Stability Balls

Adding the medicine ball press makes this squat a little more challenging. The specific muscles worked are the quadriceps (thigh muscles) and the gluteals (hips and buttocks).

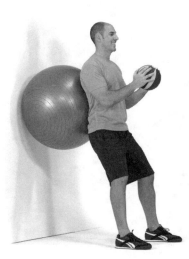

STEP 1: Stand with the stability ball between you and the wall, your lower back against the ball. Your feet should be shoulder-width apart. Hold the medicine ball in front of your face just above shoulder height, your elbows slightly bent.

STEP 2: Push your back into the ball and bend your knees until your thighs are parallel with the floor. Be sure to keep your knees in line with your ankles. At the same time, press the medicine ball over your head until your elbows are extended but not locked. Slowly return to the starting position and repeat.

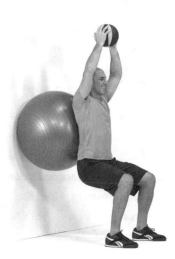

TIP: Keep your chest lifted so your back stays straight. Breathe out as you press up.

Torso Twist with Resistance Tube

We love how this exercise works the waistline. It is fun,
yet challenging. The specific muscles worked are
the oblique (side) abdominal muscles.

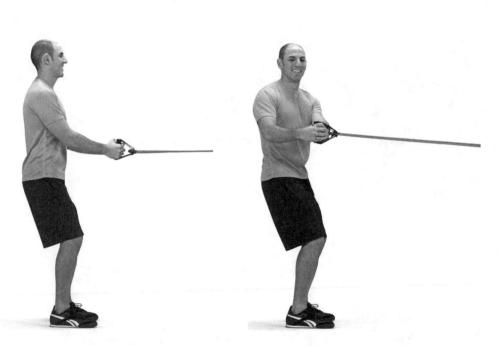

STEP 1: Anchor the tube at waist
height. Facing the anchor point,
stand with your feet slightly wider
than hip-width apart and your
knees slightly bent. Hold the
handles together with both hands.

STEP 2: Rotate your torso (from the
waist up) toward one side while keeping
your arms straight. Return to the starting
position, and then repeat the twist to the
other side.

TIP: If you feel any strain in your back, stop.

Triceps Press
with Resistance Tube

Many of us don't like the "wings" (extra skin and fat) on the backs
of our arms. This exercise will help tighten the triceps muscles
in that area (but it does not burn the fat away).

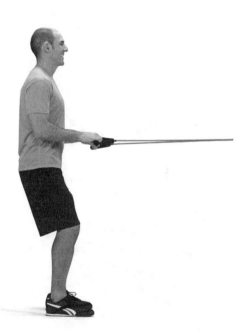 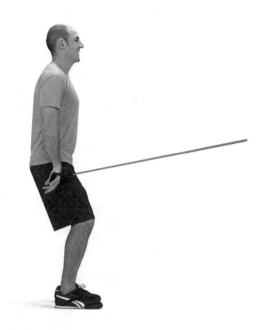

STEP 1: Anchor the tube at waist height.
Grasp the handles with your palms facing
down and your elbows tucked in by your
sides at a 90-degree angle.

STEP 2: Keeping your
elbows fixed at your sides,
press down until your arms
are fully extended. Slowly
return to the starting
position and repeat.

TIP: Keep your elbows next to your sides; only your forearms should move.

Stiff-Arm Pull-down with Resistance Tube on Stability Ball

This one challenges your balance on the ball. It specifically works the muscles of the upper back and the abdominals.

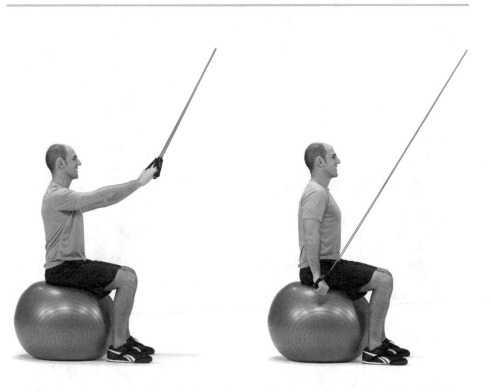

STEP 1: Anchor the tube on the top of a door. Sit on the stability ball or a chair facing the anchor. Grasp the handles with your palms facing down and your arms extended at about a 45-degree angle from your shoulders.

STEP 2: Pull down and back. Focus on squeezing your shoulder blades together. Keep your arms straight. Slowly return to the starting position and repeat.

Leg Extension with Stability Ball

This is a great exercise that works your core muscles while also focusing on your thighs. This exercise specifically works the quadriceps (thigh) muscles.

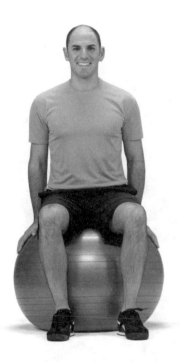 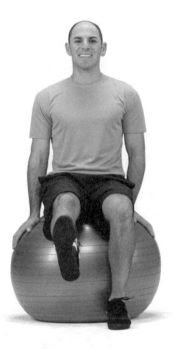

STEP 1: Sit on the ball with both feet on the floor.

STEP 2: Squeeze the muscles in the front of your right leg and straighten your knee in front of you, without locking your knee. Pause, then slowly return to the starting position. Repeat with the other leg.

TIP: Breathe out as you straighten your leg.

Hamstrings Curl
with Stability Ball

This one hits the muscles on the backs of your legs.
You can also really feel the burn in your calves. The specific
muscles worked are the hamstrings and the calves.

STEP 1: Lie with
your back on the
floor and your lower
legs and feet on top
of the stability ball.
Place your arms
along your sides,
with your palms
facing down.

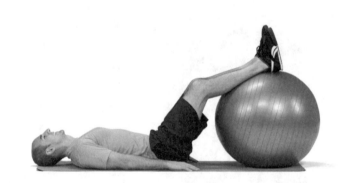

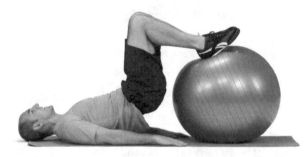

STEP 2: Lift your hips to form a
bridge. Flex your knees while pulling
the ball toward your buttocks. Return
to the starting position and repeat.

TIP: To make this exercise easier, keep your hips on the mat.

Crisscross Crunch with Stability Ball

This is a very challenging abs crunch, which is good not only for your oblique (side) abdominal muscles but also for your balance.

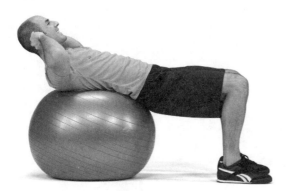

STEP 1: Lie with your lower back on the ball and your feet on the floor. Place both hands behind your ears, supporting your head lightly.

STEP 2: Rotate your torso toward one side while simultaneously lifting the opposite knee, bringing the opposite knee and elbow together.

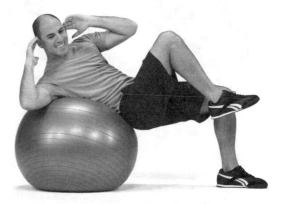

STEP 3: Slowly return to the starting position and repeat, alternating sides.

TIP: If this exercise is too difficult, don't lift your leg. Keep both feet on the floor.

Upper Back and Chest Stretch

Most of us hold stress in our necks and upper backs.
This simple but important stretch relaxes the upper back
and opens up the chest area.

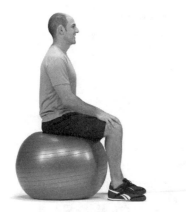 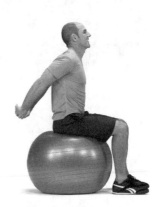

STEP 1: Sitting on the ball, place your feet flat on the floor, shoulder-width apart.

STEP 2: Extend your arms in front of you and interlace your fingers, with your palms facing your body. Press your hands away from your body, rounding your upper back.

STEP 3: Clasp your hands behind your back and lift your arms up behind your body until you feel a stretch in your chest and the front of your shoulders.

TIP: Breathe in as deeply as possible and open your rib cage.

Rotary Torso Stretch

This is a gentle way to stretch the abdominal muscles on your sides (the oblique muscles), while also targeting your lower back.

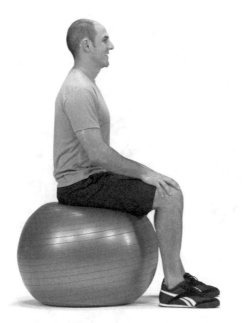 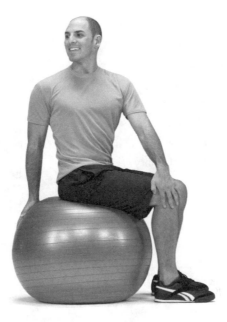

STEP 1: Sitting on the ball, place your feet flat on the floor, shoulder-width apart.

STEP 2: For support, rest your right hand on the ball, behind your body. Place your left hand on your right knee. Rotate your torso to the right, looking over your right shoulder. Reverse hand positions and repeat to the left.

TIP: Be gentle. Lift your chest to straighten your back and twist slowly. If you feel any pain in your back, stop.

Lat-Shoulder Stretch

This is a gentle stretch for your upper back and all along your spine.

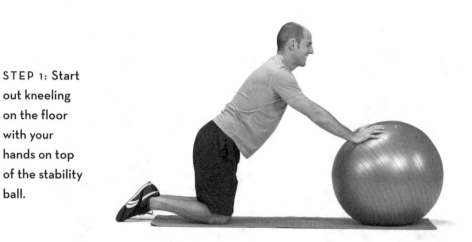

STEP 1: Start
out kneeling
on the floor
with your
hands on top
of the stability
ball.

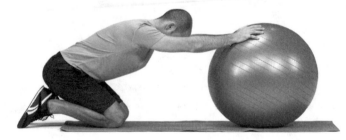

STEP 2: Keeping your hands on
the ball, roll your body back
while lowering your bottom
toward your feet. Drop your
head between your arms. Hold
10 to 30 seconds. Relax.

TIP: Breathe in deeply, then breathe out as you arch your back. Try not to let
the ball roll.

Supported Lower Back Stretch

We love this exercise because it's easy to do in the office,
as well as at home. It focuses on the lower back
and the gluteals (hips and buttocks).

STEP 1: Sit on the stability ball with your legs
wide apart.

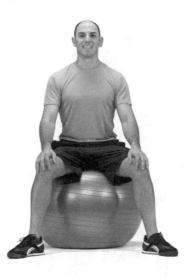

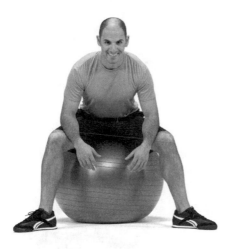

STEP 2: Bend forward, placing your
elbows on your knees.

STEP 3: Move your hands down to your
ankles or to the floor. Breathe and
stretch deeply into your lower back and
gluteals. Hold 10 to 30 seconds.

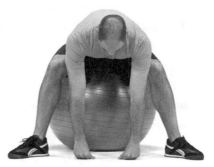

Seated Hamstrings Stretch

This stretch is easy to do anywhere. If your lower back is tight,
your hamstrings need to be stretched as well as your back.
This stretch focuses on the hamstrings and the calves.

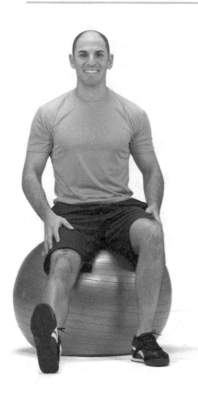

STEP 1: Sitting on the stability ball, place your left foot flat on the floor while straightening your right leg.

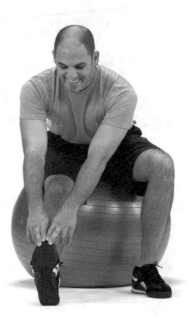

STEP 2: Bending at your hips, extend both hands toward your shins or, if you can reach, pull back on your toes. Flex your right foot until you feel the stretch in your right hamstring. Hold 10 to 30 seconds. Relax. Reverse leg positions and repeat.

Figure 4 Stretch

This is another favorite of ours, which really stretches
your hip muscles. It focuses on the hip flexors
and gluteals (hips and buttocks).

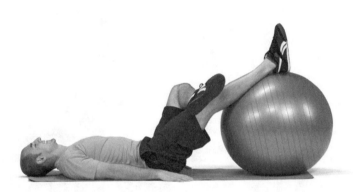

**STEP 1: Start by lying on the floor with your feet on top of the ball. Cross your left
ankle over your right knee.**

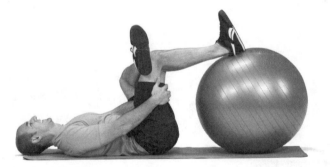

**STEP 2: Pull your right leg gently toward your chest with your hands under your
thigh. Hold 10 to 30 seconds. Relax. Reverse leg positions and repeat.**

TIP: If needed, use a towel to pull your leg closer to your chest.

Hip Flexor Stretch

Tight hip muscles are common when people start to exercise. This is a great exercise to isolate the front of the hip and stretch it gently.

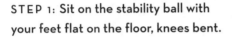

STEP 1: Sit on the stability ball with your feet flat on the floor, knees bent.

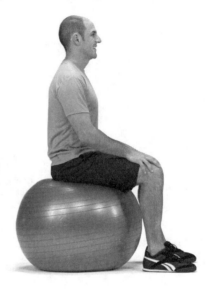

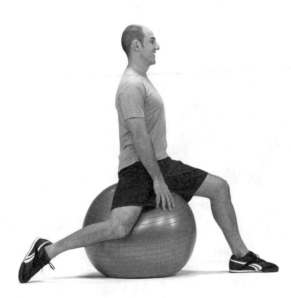

STEP 2: Turn sideways, extending your right leg out behind you. Keep your left knee bent. Press your right hip forward. Hold 10 to 30 seconds, then reverse leg positions and repeat with your right knee bent and your left leg straight.

TIP: Keep your chest up and your back straight.

PART FOUR

The Real World

CHAPTER ELEVEN

Change for a Lifetime

In this chapter, we encourage you to commit to your healthy lifestyle—for life—as so many of our clients at the Duke Diet & Fitness Center have done with great success. For inspiration, you may want to check out the success stories on www.dukediet.com and share in the experiences of some of our patients. Another excellent source of inspiration is the National Weight Control Registry's website, www.nwcr.ws. Established in 1995, the registry tracks some 5,000 people who have shed considerable numbers of pounds and managed to maintain a substantial amount of that weight loss. We want you to see that while it may seem difficult and overwhelming at times—especially in the face of the sometimes considerable obstacles to health we face in our modern world—a great many people do, in fact, achieve lasting weight loss. We truly believe that you can be among them!

As you'll see from the stories on the National Weight Control Registry website, the paths these folks took were varied, and many had struggled over a long period of time to manage their weight. But the message is clear. They found what worked for them just as you will find what works for you. They also found that maintaining a healthier weight got easier with practice. Our patients often tell us the same story: Things that once seemed strange or foreign—or even impossible—became second nature. All it takes is persistent effort and a commitment to try your best each day.

As you move forward with your healthier Duke-inspired lifestyle, we hope that you've gained a new self-confidence. Look at the changes you've already made: You've brought your diet into portion- and calorie-controlled nutritional balance; you've embarked on a sustainable, enjoyable fitness plan; and you've received a whole new toolbox full of behavioral health strategies. You've learned techniques for assessing the core areas of a healthy lifestyle through the Pillars of Lifestyle Change. You've developed strategies for communicating and managing your emotions more effectively, setting achievable goals, and creating action plans—and more. You're probably noticing changes already! Many folks at this point will have settled into a comfortable level of progress with their weight loss, and the goal will be to maintain the new habits they are cultivating and continue losing weight. Those who had less weight to lose may already be close to their target weight. Whatever the case, all you have to do for lasting lifestyle change is keep up the good work.

Part of negotiating the real world will mean eventually shifting from weight loss to weight maintenance. Remember, this is not a new skill for you to learn. It is simply a matter of making minor adjustments in your daily caloric intake until your weight levels off. To do this, you will make calorie adjustments using the same strategies you learned in chapter 2 and in the core four-week program. To slow your weight loss, simply add 50 to 100 calories a day to your meal plan, then see what happens with your weight that week. If your weight loss levels off, then nothing more is needed. If you're continuing to lose weight the following week, add another 50 to 100 calories until you reach the point where your weight is holding steady.

Conversely, if you find your weight loss stalling despite continued efforts to lose, we first encourage you to reinforce the structure in your plan. We generally tell our patients that while plateaus are part of weight loss, the first step is to ensure you are doing all you can. Make sure your portion judgments have not slipped—that you are monitoring your food and activity and are exercising at the level you need to be. If you've done this and your weight loss is still stalled, don't panic. Recognize that this is a natural part of the process. Sometimes your body seems to need to adjust to its new, lower weight. Just stay the course, knowing that if you are doing all you are supposed to be doing, you are getting healthier and more fit, even if the numbers on the scale move a little more slowly for a while. Now the challenge becomes reinforcing your new, healthier habits so that you practice them consistently, accept-

Should I Consider Medication or Surgery?

The strategies in this book are commonly referred to as *therapeutic lifestyle change*, or TLC. Like most weight loss experts, we believe TLC to be the necessary foundation for weight control. But sometimes, despite repeated efforts, people find themselves unable to maintain healthful habits or accomplish lasting weight loss. It may be appropriate for those who meet that description and are suffering from obesity (body mass index of 30 or greater) to *supplement* (not replace) their lifestyle change efforts with anti-obesity medications.

Medications can be helpful when used *in conjunction with* efforts to maintain healthier habits of eating and physical activity. In clinical trials of medication plus lifestyle change, these products have been shown to help people lose approximately 7 to 10 percent of their starting weight over the course of six months (a few percentage points more than those not taking medication but trying to follow a good diet and exercise plan). Studies also show that those continuing on certain medications in the long term (for one to two years) tend to regain less weight than those following a diet and exercise plan alone.

Two medications are currently approved in the United States for long-term use. These medications are not for everyone. Check with your doctor to see whether they might be appropriate for you. But remember—there are no miracle drugs (and we doubt there will be anytime soon). People who achieve the best results use the medications *along with* serious efforts to improve their eating and activity—not *instead of* them! You can visit www.dukediet.com to find out more details.

Surgical approaches to obesity management have been continually refined over the years, and as techniques have improved and surgeons have become more experienced, surgery has generally become safer and more effective. And the results are usually very favorable. We, and our surgical colleagues at Duke, feel that weight loss surgery, like medication, works best when combined with a vigorous lifestyle change effort, and we describe these two approaches as *complementary*. When patients ask me whether they should consider surgery, I usually tell them that it might be an appropriate option to consider if they feel that their "back is against the wall." In other words, if you are severely obese (body mass index 40 or greater), have associated medical problems and an impaired quality of life, and no other options have worked well, it might be a good idea at least to explore surgery. A full discussion about obesity surgery is beyond the scope of this book, but we refer you to www.dukediet.com, to the Duke Weight Loss Surgery Center website, and to the website for the American Society for Bariatric Surgery for more information (see the resources section at the end of this book).

—*Howard Eisenson, M.D.*

The Giver's Challenge

Asking for help was a real challenge for Barry, age fifty-five, one of my clients at Duke. He was in a helping profession himself and worked as a live-in counselor. He was so dedicated to other people's needs that he had lost sight of his own. He found it very difficult to learn to put himself first once in a while, especially when it came to his weight and his health. I challenged Barry to examine the thoughts that came to mind when he was faced with the choice of meeting his own needs versus meeting the needs of others. After considerable reflection, he realized that deep down inside he felt guilty when he put himself first. That small voice inside said words like "That's selfish" or "You're not worth it" if he chose to do what he needed for himself. In time, by using the techniques we teach to help redirect these long-standing thought patterns, Barry was able to develop a new, more accepting dialogue with himself.

He was able to set aside solid blocks of time during which he was focused on his own needs. Eventually, he came to accept that he was just as important and worthy of support as the people he helped, and that he was able to do a better job for others when he made the effort to care for himself as well. Gradually he became comfortable turning to those close to him for help with his concerns.

—*Peter Perlman, M.S.W., Behavioral Health Clinician*
at the Duke Diet & Fitness Center

ing a temporary plateau and understanding that, after a short period, you will probably start to come down from the apparent plateau.

When it comes to your fitness routine, whether your goal is further weight loss or weight maintenance, you should continue to build on the activities you have established. Staying challenged and keeping an interesting routine is important for lasting success. We hope you are continuing to vary your fitness plan—that you keep adding new activities and are finding ways to put more physical effort into your activities of daily living. With the fitness routines, you can continue to progress through the levels. Visit www.dukediet.com for ideas on finding more variety and intensity to keep yourself challenged.

Of course, as we have discussed throughout the book, another element of real-world living is hitting some inevitable snags. But as you've already seen, by having a clear and realistic range of goals (optimal, minimal, and desirable), action plans for getting back on track when you slip, and a strong grasp of the problem-solving skills we have taught, you can deal with *any* challenges that come your way. You have also learned strategies for communicating more effectively, for managing stress and emotions, and for building a strong support system.

THE POWER OF POSITIVE THINKING

In the spirit of moving forward, we want to share a final behavioral health skill that focuses on using your mind to its best advantage. Our thoughts influence not only the way we approach adopting new, healthier habits, but also the way we perceive ourselves and our emotional states. We all experience an internal dialogue that can either support us by pushing us to achieve our goals and rewarding us when we do or work against us with harsh criticism and false, negative assertions. These negative thoughts can take on many forms. They can be about our abilities (for example, *I'm no good at anything*), our sense of self-worth (*I don't deserve to be happy*), or our appearance (*my hips are too big*). Ultimately, this negative dialogue can wear us down and influence how successful we can be at making lasting changes. After all, if our own internal voice is persistently putting us down or predicting failure, how can we possibly expect to succeed? We will show you how to reform that inner critic. Destructive thoughts might be a culmination of the criticism you've received and internalized from family members, teachers, and others you've known or from a society that constantly dictates how a person should look, feel, act, or simply be.

While destructive thinking is not always within your direct consciousness, as you become aware of the internal dialogue you have with yourself throughout the day, you can alter it and redirect your thinking in a more positive direction. Four simple steps can help you alter the path of this negative dialogue. With practice, you will become skilled at challenging negative thoughts and be able to replace that old internal conversation with a new and more positive one.

1. Identify the thought. Think of a destructive thought that you'd like to change. Let's choose *I hate exercise!* Consider how this thought affects your behavior, other thoughts, and emotions. Does it keep you from working out, or at least make you procrastinate so you have to cut short your workday-morning sessions? Does it lead to other negative thoughts about activities you hate? Does it make you feel "lazy" or angry when you start thinking about how much you hate exercise?

2. Stop the thought. Stopping a thought can be as simple as saying "Stop," either aloud or in your mind. Thought stopping allows you to interrupt the negative dialogue and prevent the thought from progressing to *Since I hate exercise, I'll never be any good at it . . . I may as well not bother to work out . . . I'm not working out today.*

3. Challenge the thought. Chances are, your negative thought is not 100 percent true. So take a stand and challenge it. Is it really *all* exercise that you hate or just aerobics class at your health club, where you have trouble following the routines and think the "gym bunnies" are judging you? Maybe you've been overdoing it lately and actually just hate feeling so sore the next day. Maybe you've forgotten how much you like walking or biking outdoors and have been forcing yourself to take an aerobics class because you signed up for a gym membership. Explore the facts so you can use them in the next step.

4. Replace the thought with a more adaptive one. Think like the captain of the debate team. Come up with a rational argument against the negative thought. If your thought is *I hate exercise!,* but that really applies only to aerobics class, replace the thought with *I don't hate all exercise; I only hate aerobics class, where I feel judged.* Maybe there are other activities at the gym that you'd enjoy more, like taking Pilates or using the elliptical trainer or the stationary bicycle.

Negative thoughts come in all shapes and sizes. Rather than go through a long list, let's highlight a couple of tendencies that we frequently see in our patients.

All-or-Nothing Thinking

All-or-nothing thinking means exactly what it says—that you tend to see everything as right or wrong, black or white, with no shades of gray. If you don't work out a full hour at the gym, the session is a waste of time. If you eat an extra dessert, you tell yourself, *I ate off plan—I've blown it. I may as well wait until next week to start over.* Or if you skip one exercise session, you think, *Since I didn't go to aerobics class today, I'm a total failure.* Yes, we know, some of those sure sound familiar, don't they?

There is a solution to all-or-nothing thinking: Look for the middle ground. We have shown you how to set three levels of goals, including minimal ones, so forgiveness is built into our program. Now work on building forgiveness into your thinking, too. Tell yourself: *Any activity is better than none. I met my minimal goal, so I was successful. I can adjust my meal plan later in the day, or over the next few days, to offset my little slip, instead of doing even more calorie damage by giving up on the plan for the rest of the day or week. I know I am not perfect—but who is?*

We like to refer to this as simply thinking (and doing) "the next right thing."

Discounting the Positive

Another common pattern we see is not giving credit where credit is due—ignoring or minimizing your accomplishments. Maybe you lost less weight than you hoped this week, so you dismiss the success you did achieve—that you lost some weight, made healthy choices, were more active, and so on. Or perhaps friends compliment you on looking thinner, but all you can think or, worse yet, say out loud is "I have a long to way to go."

You can counter this type of negative thinking by being sure to take a moment *every* day to recognize your accomplishments. Perhaps list them on a piece of paper, star them on your monitoring card, or record them in your

Lifestyle Journal on our website. Use this record of successes to redirect negative thoughts.

Perfectionism

Another common destructive thought pattern is perfectionism. While it's a form of all-or-nothing thinking, it's so common among our clients and it undermines so many of our core strategies—like setting reasonable, achievable goals for weight loss, eating, exercise, and stress management—that it warrants its own discussion.

Perfectionism is believing that you must be (or appear to be) perfect and that the only acceptable outcome for anything you undertake is excellence. People are driven to perfectionism for lots of reasons; we find that one of the more common ones is underlying fear of failure, judgment, or rejection.

Let's face it, in small doses, perfectionism is useful, pushing us to aim higher for success. However, when it's more pronounced, perfectionism has many negative repercussions. Perfectionists tend to set impossible goals. They're afraid to experiment with creative problem solving. In fact, they can become so paralyzed by fear of failure that they may avoid getting started at all. They're reluctant to try new activities or recipes, afraid to try to reach out to a support network, unwilling to go after that new job or promotion they've secretly dreamed about. They feel that nothing they accomplish is ever good enough.

In its milder forms perfectionism can be expressed as procrastination, but at its worst it can send some people's self-esteem spiraling downward, and the intensity of this feeling may lead to hopelessness or depression.

When it comes to weight loss, perfectionists quickly grow discouraged if they don't see immediate results. They may resort to extreme dieting or just give up, believing that they'll never lose weight or be healthy and enjoy being active. As with other kinds of destructive thinking, a logical approach can counter perfectionism. Try taking these steps:

- Create a list of pros and cons: How does perfectionism help and/or hinder you?
- List your fears about imperfection and its potential consequences. Counter them with rational responses.
- Brainstorm—and even write down—the good that sometimes comes from making mistakes. What have slipups taught you?

- Think of people you know and respect, then list the ways in which they're imperfect. Aren't we all? Even the most successful and admired people make mistakes.
- Try to recall times when you were successful, despite making mistakes.
- List the people in your life on whom you can rely for "reality checks," alerting you when you're too hard on yourself or pointing out what you're doing well.
- Above all, love and accept yourself, and believe that success doesn't mean that you have to be perfect at everything.

If you struggle with destructive thinking, try practicing the simple steps outlined here and applying them every day, in various situations in your life. You will find that you can shift your thinking from destructive to productive and turn your thoughts into your strongest ally in your healthy lifestyle.

SUPPORT FOR LIFE

As you move toward lasting weight loss and health, it will be more important than ever to keep your support troops rallied around you. Use these tips, along with the other support and communication strategies provided earlier, to continue to benefit from the valuable assistance of others.

1. Take responsibility. You need to take the lead in creating an environment that is conducive to weight management. Even if your family, friends, and coworkers want to support you, it may be hard for them to do so if you don't explain your needs. Take some time to think about what support means to you and how you would like others to assist, comfort, and encourage you over the long term.

2. Get specific. Once you determine the kind of support you need, create a list of clear-cut requests for your prospective supporters. Vague requests like "I wish you'd be more supportive" will not be explanatory enough. Here are a few examples of areas in which clear communication with supporters might be helpful:

- Eating more slowly than usual. Though perhaps an important part of your plan for mindful, less automatic eating, eating slowly could irritate dining companions who don't realize why you are doing it.

- Waking up early to exercise. Exercising in the morning can be a great way to adhere to your fitness program, but it could prove stressful to a partner who doesn't understand why bed and wake times are changing, or who finds it difficult to adapt.
- Being asked how many pounds you have lost. Perhaps your supporters are trying to be helpful, but their comments come across as prying or criticism.
- Avoiding old snacking habits. Yes, you are responsible for making your own choices about food, but sometimes those wishing to support you need help understanding that making changes can be so much easier in an environment where you are not constantly tempted.

List your clear-cut requests on a separate sheet of paper or record them in your Lifestyle Journal on our website.

3. Identify supporters and request their help in a positive way. Set aside some time to talk privately with each prospective supporter about your needs in a systematic way. It will be hard for people to remember what you want if you pepper them with random requests. Needless to say, indirect or critical comments such as "So-and-so is lucky that she has a husband who really understands her situation" will unfairly put the other person on the defensive without providing any constructive information about your needs.

4. If necessary, seek outside assistance. Some people find it helpful to join an established weight loss support group. Others turn to professionals for help. You can sign up to work with one of our Duke Diet & Fitness Online coaches or find a registered dietitian, personal trainer, or local weight management program. Professionals who are knowledgeable about and sensitive to weight-related issues can add the support and guidance you need to achieve long-term success.

5. Be patient. Just as you may experience setbacks in trying to maintain your new lifestyle, others may occasionally lapse into unsupportive behavior. Remember that your supporters are also learning, and their habits may be just as hard to change as your own. Any long-term adjustments require time, patience, and effort on everyone's part. At the same time, consider how you might model behaviors that help others to be more supportive. Everyone has needs, and by giving effective support ourselves (listening, empathizing, encouraging, and so on) we might just find that it comes back to us more often.

6. Take a leap of faith. Recognize that you need and deserve the help of others on your continuing journey. If you are uncomfortable asking for help, simply take it slow. Start by making small requests for support at first As these more modest needs are met, you will grow comfortable asking for more. As with all the changes you're making on the Duke Plan, think in terms of setting small, achievable *support goals* and create action plans to achieve them.

7. Show Your Appreciation. Finally, don't forget to show appreciation to the supporters who have helped you. Your thanks will not only strengthen your relationship with them but also reinforce their supportive behavior and increase the likelihood that they will support you in the future.

KEEP HOPE ALIVE THROUGH CHALLENGES

On the road of your new life, you're bound to stumble once in a while. Remember that feeling challenged doesn't mean that you're losing the battle. You wouldn't abandon your car if you got a flat, sell your house because of a wasp's nest in the rain gutter, or walk out on your job or marriage after a few rocky days. You'd cope: fix the tire, evict the wasps, talk to your boss, or take a revitalizing weekend getaway with your spouse or partner. Your own physical and emotional well-being deserve the same conservation efforts.

Challenge is an inevitable fact of life. You have the strength and the skills to confront it and overcome it. If you need extra support now and then, revisit the techniques in this book or check www.dukediet.com for additional strategies, online Q&As with Duke experts, and conversations with your fellow dieters—or, if you like, even some virtual sessions with a Duke-trained life coach. Believe in yourself. You're worth it!

Life Change That Lasts

At age twenty-six, I was seriously overweight. By the time I was twenty-nine, I'd shed a lot, but I had trouble keeping it off. I kept yo-yoing for years. I'd pack on major pounds, lose them, and then start the cycle all over again. It was my wife who first did the Duke program, and her success inspired me to give it a shot.

Since 1986—that's twenty-one years!—I've managed to hold my weight at 190 pounds, without the ups and downs I've experienced in the past. Now I feel that I can participate more fully in every aspect of my life. I can even keep up with my now-supercharged wife!

The way I look at food has definitely changed. Now I see it as something to plan for and enjoy. Before, I never exercised, but now I get in at least three hours a week, and I aim for more. I also wear a pedometer and try to get my steps in every day. Since I live in Manhattan, it is easy to walk, and I walk a lot. This helps when I am very busy and have to miss the occasional exercise session—since I know I am still very active in my daily life.

You name the diet, and I've tried it. Nothing worked for me until Duke, so stick with it—it will work for you! What you need, as I did, is a new way of life that promotes activity, balance, and health. What I found helped me most was tracking my calories and exercise. That kept me focused—the simple equation of calories in, calories out!

Wait, maybe that's too simple. The behavioral health part helped me *a lot,* too. I realized early on that practical problem-solving and goal-setting strategies were a key. It took a while, but I got pretty good at reducing my stress load, too.

Of course, food was an important part of my life and still is. It made a big difference that I loved the recipes in the Duke Plan and didn't have to suffer the boredom of all those diets that tell you to eat nothing but skinless broiled chicken breasts, fish, and vegetables. You'll actually enjoy what you eat on the Duke Diet!

Good luck—but you won't need it! If you put your faith in the plan, you'll succeed.

—*John, age 63*

CHAPTER TWELVE

A Final Word

Writing this book has been as much of a journey for us as reading and learning from it have probably been for you. We sincerely hope that we have helped you in your quest for better health and that the wide range of strategies we have shown you will lead you to lasting success. We feel honored that you have chosen our plan and proud to know we have given you something real—something that doesn't offer the false promises so many popular diets do, but instead forges a path to lasting lifestyle change. We trust you're feeling better, have lost weight, and are taking more pride in how you look. Wonderful! Perhaps you need a little more time to get into the rhythm—that's okay, too. We know you can do it!

When we were first approached with the suggestion that we write a book, we were both excited and a little hesitant—excited because we saw it as an incredible opportunity to reach the many individuals who are unable to attend our residential program, and hesitant because we were well aware of the challenges involved in conveying the thirty-eight years' worth of knowledge and experience that is the Duke Diet & Fitness Center residential program. Patients spend from a week or two up to several months in our facility. They eat all their meals here, they exercise daily, they meet regularly with our treatment staff, and they enjoy membership in a diverse community, which includes people of all ages and weights, from all over the world and from all walks of life. They share many life experiences, as well as the goals of gaining better health and a more active, more satisfying life, by learning to control their weight, eat well, exercise regularly, and practice better self-care. We are continually impressed by how powerful the residential aspect of our pro-

A Message *from* Dr. Binks

The process of writing this book has often been an occasion for self-reflection on the path my career has taken. I am reminded of the reason I decided to become a psychologist in the first place. I occasionally tell patients this story, and they are always surprised to learn that my goal in becoming a psychologist was actually to treat obesity. I was helping out at the time in a personal training center and remember the exact moment I made the decision. I was working with a middle-aged woman named Jan, who was extremely out of shape. She was also feeling bad about herself. Her self-esteem and her physical health were at an all-time low. In fact, she had difficulty exercising for more than fifteen minutes at a time and was feeling defeated by her body.

Over the course of a month or two, I was witness to what can only be described as a remarkable triumph. We adjusted Jan's eating habits to a healthy, balanced structure. We added five minutes at a time to her aerobic exercise routine, we started her with stretching, and we worked toward strength training with weights. In a short time, I saw Jan's mood begin to shift and the sparkle return to her eyes. It was amazing! A little while later, Jan and the rest of our team competed together in a powerlifting competition! For several years thereafter, Jan continued to inspire every newcomer to the gym. It was then that for the first time I saw as clear as a bell the link between healthy body and mind. There have been many Jans in my years of working in the field. While not all triumphed in athletics, each shared a similarly inspiring story. I genuinely hope you find your triumph as you begin to take the Duke Plan journey to better health!

—*Martin Binks, Ph.D.*

gram can be and how well our participants take care of each other by providing mutual support and encouragement and sharing inspirational stories, humor, wisdom, and practical ideas with each other—not only while they are on the program, but long after they leave. One of our challenges was to create such an experience for you in this book. Another was to express our belief in your ability to succeed while remaining honest in acknowledging the challenging task ahead.

We hope we have succeeded. We have shared the *actual* curriculum we use with our patients, including recipes for the meals we *really serve* and the exercises we *really teach*. We also hope we have inspired you by sharing the experiences of *our clients*—sometimes in their own voices and sometimes in the vignettes shared by *our staff*. We know that different people learn in different ways and that it can be helpful to have multiple resources available, so we have invited you to supplement your experience with the Duke Diet & Fitness Online Weight Loss Program. There, you will encounter others dedicated to changing their lives once and for all, and find expanded meal and exercise plans, additional information, and more frequently asked questions answered by us and our colleagues.

Like our clients at the Diet & Fitness Center, you may very well find that, as your approach to a healthy lifestyle evolves, you get something new out of the program each time you revisit it. You might see something fresh in these pages every time you read through them or find new inspiration from your friends online. We encourage you to go back and look for these new "pearls." It's a great way to stay motivated. Many of our patients choose to come back to Duke for regular visits, not because they feel they have to, but because they find the renewed contact motivating and invigorating. In fact, as Dr. Binks was leaving the center one night recently, a longtime attendee at the program was telling him how much he enjoys returning to reconnect with the Duke community. He expressed that each time he attends a class—even if he's been in it before—or talks with someone else going through the program about things he already knows, he always hears something he had not heard before, something to keep him inspired and moving forward.

Rather than suggesting to you that we have some secret to share, we have tried to show you that almost everything we teach is drawn from a vast body of scientific knowledge about obesity and associated health problems, nutrition, physical fitness, and behavioral health—a body of knowledge accumulated thanks to the efforts of countless researchers and practitioners world-wide, to whom we owe a great debt. We have no essential dietary formula to reveal, no nutritional supplements to sell, no one-size-fits-all, perfect plan. In short, we did not want to give you the idea that there is some sort of magic bullet, as so many weight loss programs would have you believe. You cannot simply wave a wand and be thin. Nevertheless, what we see and hear from those who follow the program is that our approach does contain a certain magic—that it has opened their eyes to a whole new way of viewing weight control. We have the expertise to translate the seemingly massive amounts of often confusing health information and present this to you in a coherent, consistent, and, above all, practical way. We have what we feel is a time-tested ability to help you learn to tailor and adapt the plan to fit *your* needs, so that you can accomplish your goals of losing weight, becoming healthier, and getting more fit!

For that reason, we have gone beyond meal plans and exercise routines by giving you tools to evaluate a wide range of factors unique to you that influence your health. Frankly, we sometimes wonder if *lifestyle change* seems too superficial a term. What we are really referring to is a *life* change. We have challenged you to make an honest appraisal of your life, your priorities, and your relationships. We have looked at improving communication and coping more effectively with emotions and stress, and, most important, we have taught you the skills to adapt to changing circumstances. We have encouraged you to expand your horizons, give priority to your health, and enlist the support you need in attaining special goals—improved health and weight control!

Life is full of twists and turns. These are a part of what makes the human experience exciting and rewarding. The same intelligence, creativity, resourcefulness, courage, and determination that have served you well so many times before in so many areas of your life will work to your advantage now. We know that weight and health are important to you and we hope you take the guidance provided here and apply it successfully—but don't make it your *entire* life! Life is about so much more than calories in and calories out. It's about friends, family, joy, and celebration. It's about experiencing things to their fullest and seeking new adventures. It's about expanding your horizons and getting the most out of every day while living in balance and health. We can't stress this enough. So as you move forward with this blueprint for

The Last Word from Dr. Eisenson

Over the years, my father, Sam, has taught me many valuable lessons, both by his words and by his example. Among my dad's great pleasures were puttering in our yard or taking long walks in the woods near our home, simply enjoying the natural surroundings.

I recall one of his favorite teachings during these activities was that "plants love to grow, and if we don't get in the way, they will." He enjoyed spotting tiny tree seedlings in the lawn, in a flower bed, or on a woodland path and transplanting them to a spot where he thought they might flourish undisturbed. Some of these tiny seedlings (he called them "potchkes," which I suspect is a term drawn from mangled Yiddish) did indeed like to grow, and they demonstrated that by developing into large and sturdy trees, which now grace the yard of every home he ever inhabited.

I have adopted my dad's expression, but modified it slightly for use with my own clients. I often observe to them that the body likes to be healthy—and that it usually will, if we "don't get in the way." I believe this, because I have seen, over and over, remarkable transformations among the people we serve at the Duke Diet & Fitness Center. I can't recall how many times I have heard patients say, "I feel like I've gotten my life back." Frankly, I never tire of hearing it—and I think what a great privilege it is to be able to do this kind of work.

—*Howard Eisenson, M.D.*

healthy living, don't lose sight of the fact that losing weight and practicing healthy habits should help you live your life more fully—it shouldn't take away from it.

We sincerely hope that, together, we have accomplished some good work here, that we have helped provide you with valuable knowledge, useful skills, and, most important, the realistic optimism and confidence that will serve you well as you proceed on your own journey toward making your life as healthy and fulfilling as possible. We are grateful for the opportunity to have worked with you, and we wish you good health and happiness.

Acknowledgments

DR. EISENSON AND DR. BINKS WOULD LIKE TO ACKNOWLEDGE THE FOLLOWING PEOPLE:

It has been our honor and our privilege, by authoring this book, to bring the Duke Diet & Fitness Center (DFC) Plan to a much wider audience than we could ever hope to reach in our residential program. The book would not have been possible without the hard work and diligent contributions of nutrition manager Elisabetta Politi and fitness manager Gerald Endress, who helped with the challenging task of translating into book form the extensive nutritional and fitness information, the practical guidance, and the encouragement that transform lives at the DFC every day. To the extent that we have succeeded in that effort, they deserve great credit.

With a deep sense of gratitude, we also wish to recognize our many other colleagues at the center whose daily work exemplifies the caring, the commitment, the teamwork, and the expertise for which the DFC has become widely recognized. While we regret that we cannot recognize by name all of our superb team, there are many who must be mentioned, including medical director Dr. Ron Sha, Barbara Dean, Donna Yates, Launa ("CheChe") Casto, Bobby Cale, Tina Leiter, Kaye Gardner, Keith Moore, Dina Lumia, John McCall, Peter Perlman, Roger Vandergrift, Brian Housle, Tara House, Kathy Murray, Cindy Hayden, Kim Turk, Neva Avery, Lucie Knapp, Lamont Adams, Susanne Jackson, Deb Reardon, Joel Newton, Linda Pickett, Marit Derrer, Leslie Gaillard, Beth Tierney, Michelle Mosberger, Dr. Amy Wachholtz, Dana Alston, Linda Rocafort, Christine Tenekjian, Lil Williams, Rob Emory, Sandy Gribbin, Sadye Paez, Susan Peterson, and Karen Ziegler.

We also acknowledge the efforts of many professionals who are not based at the DFC but who serve our clients with dedication and skill, helping to make our program a place of hope and of healing. These include massage therapists, physical therapists, and other consultants in many health care specialties at Duke and in the local community. Among this group we honor the late cardiologist Dr. Fred Cobb, who is greatly missed by so many friends, colleagues, and patients.

A special thanks also to the entire Bon Appetit team, who manage, under the leadership of their gifted and dedicated general manager and executive chef, Andrew Craven, to serve healthy, delicious meals, three times a day, seven days a week, 365 days a year, to a rather discriminating clientele who know a thing or two about food. In addition to talented sous-chefs Tyrone Hall and Connor Tucker, we must recognize Amanda Fox, known to "generations" of DFC participants, who has served up a generous measure of warmth and kindness with every platter during her twenty years at the DFC.

We wish particularly to thank our editor, Caroline Sutton at Ballantine Books, and we owe an enormous debt of thanks to Elisa Petrini for helping us write the book. Their combined senses of humor coupled with their impeccable expertise were essential to the success of this project. We will always remember the many marathon conference calls and e-mails with too much work to do in too little time! But as Dr. E. said early in the process, and as we both believe, there is little that people of ability and goodwill, working together, cannot accomplish. We thank our Duke colleagues Molly O'Neill, Dorothea Bonds, Dr. Robert Taber, Doug Stokke, and Dr. Richard Liebowitz for their various critically important roles in launching this collaboration and in helping to ensure its success.

Many people at the Random House Publishing Group contributed to publishing this book on a very tight schedule. We would especially like to thank Gina Centrello, Libby McGuire, Kim Hovey, Brian McClendon, Kate Blum, Mark Maguire, Nancy Delia, Gene Mydlowski, and Christina Duffy. We could not have done this without you.

Similarly, we want to acknowledge the many contributions from the entire team at Waterfront Media, who managed to produce a book and launch a website simultaneously and at full throttle. Specifically, we thank our editorial team, Katharine Davis, Liz Humphreys, Margaret O'Malley, Roseann Foley Henry, Shira Isenberg, Jen Laskey, and Rebecca Rudy, as well as the rest of the Waterfront team, Genevieve Futrelle, Eleanor Berwick Meyer, Nerissa Wels, Francis Banbury Namuk, Robby Thompson, Karim Farag, and Greg Jackson.

We also thank our agent, Richard S. Pine, Inkwell Management, for his support and guidance.

Much of what we do at the Duke Center, and have tried to accomplish in this book, is to select and organize, in a helpful, practical way, information drawn from the efforts of so many researchers and practitioners who have worked and are working today, to advance knowledge in the treatment of obesity and related health concerns. Many of these individuals have devoted entire careers to these challenging pursuits.

There are far too many of them to be acknowledged by name, but we are mindful of our extraordinary debt to them all.

And finally, but most important, we wish to acknowledge, and deeply thank, the many clients from our time at the DFC and from elsewhere, with whom we and our colleagues have been privileged to work. So many of them have challenged, taught, encouraged, and motivated us by including us in critical moments of their life journeys, and by inspiring us with their courage.

DR. EISENSON WOULD LIKE TO THANK THE FOLLOWING PEOPLE:

The Duke Diet & Fitness Center would not have existed, and this book would not have been written, without the vision and wisdom of Dr. E. Harvey Estes, who established the DFC in 1969, early in his tenure as chairman of Duke University's Department of Community and Family Medicine. Subsequent chairs, Dr. George R. Parkerson, Jr., and Dr. J. Lloyd Michener, continued to nurture the program. All of these gentlemen have provided me with valuable guidance and support throughout my career. Perhaps most instrumental in my transition from a community-based family practice to the DFC in 1999 was the encouragement of my longtime friend and valued colleague Dr. Kathryn Andolsek, professor in the Department of Community and Family Medicine and associate director for graduate medical education at Duke. Her example, her caring, and her amazing passion and energy continue to inspire me. I am grateful to Dr. Michael Hamilton, my predecessor as DFC director and my mentor during my early association with the program. Under his leadership the DFC flourished. Michael was motivated by a fascination with the challenges of treating obesity and by a deep desire to be of help to those who suffer with this condition. His very genuine warmth and kindness toward all created an atmosphere of caring at the DFC that we strive to honor today. I appreciate others no longer at the center, and too numerous to mention, whose hard work has contributed greatly to the success of our program. Here I recognize and thank a few with whom I have had the pleasure of working most closely, including Franca Alphin, Michele Hudgins, Dr. Siegfried Heyden, and Dr. Rob Sullivan.

And finally, I am grateful for my wonderful, extended family, whose generosity, support, wisdom, humor, courage, patience, and love enrich my life and my work.

DR. BINKS WOULD LIKE TO THANK THE FOLLOWING PEOPLE:

I would like to acknowledge the opportunity to do obesity research that was afforded me through my work with Dr. Christopher A. Capuano at Fairleigh Dickinson University early in my career. I would also particularly like to acknowledge the substantial influence of Dr. Patrick M. O'Neil, of the Weight Management Center at the Medical

University of South Carolina. Pat introduced me to the vast community of obesity researchers I have come to know and admire, taught me how to combine meaningful clinical care and evidence-based treatments, and clearly shaped my career. For that, I will always be grateful. I would also like to thank Dr. Michael Hamilton, whom I met several years before coming to the DFC. His belief in me as a fresh postdoctoral fellow and his support of me since that time have been so influential in the way my career has unfolded. I thank him for helping me find my place at Duke. I want to echo the sentiments of Dr. Eisenson in acknowledging all who have contributed to the thirty-eight-year history of the DFC. I would also like to thank Dr. Richard Surwit, chief of the Division of Medical Psychology, and Dr. Ranga Krishnan, chair of the Department of Psychiatry and Behavioral Sciences, at Duke, for their ongoing support. I wish to express my sincere gratitude to my staff at the DFC—the Behavioral Health and Lifestyle Coaching teams—for their contribution to the behavioral program, for their dedication to excellence in client care, and for rising to the occasion in support of the success of this project. I truly feel honored to work with such a wonderful group of professionals.

Finally, I want to thank my family for their unwavering support and love. My mother, Kathleen, and father, John, have inspired me with their faith, wisdom, strength of character, and generosity. My brother, Paul, is a true friend whose support and encouragement I value so very much. To Kaye I owe an enormous debt of gratitude. She is a constant and steady support who accepted all that had to be done and sacrificed to accomplish this project. I am so lucky to have her by my side; it means the world to me. Nothing can ever be achieved that is as meaningful as the love of those close to you. I love you all very much.

Bibliography

Blumenthal, J. A., M. A. Babyak, K. A. Moore, W. E. Craighead, S. Herman, P. Khatri, R. Waugh, M. A. Napolitano, L. M. Forman, M. Appelbaum, P. M. Doraiswamy, and K. R. Krishnan. "Effects of Exercise Training on Older Patients with Major Depression." *Archives of Internal Medicine* (1999), 159(19): 2349–56.

Borg, G., "Perceived Exertion as an Indicator of Somatic Stress." *Scandinavian Journal of Rehabilitation Medicine* (1970), 2(2): 92–98.

Canadian Society for Exercise Physiology. Physical Activity Readiness Questionnaire (PAR-Q), 2002, www.csep.ca.

Centers for Disease Control and Prevention. Physical Activity for Everyone: Making Physical Activity Part of Your Life: Overcoming Barriers to Physical Activity. www.cdc.gov/nccdphp/dnpa/physical/life/barriers_quiz.pdf.

Dunn, A. L., B. H. Marcus, J. B. Kampert, M. E. Garcia, H. W. Kohl III, and S. N. Blair. "Comparison of Lifestyle and Structured Interventions to Increase Physical Activity and Cardiorespiratory Fitness: A Randomized Trial. *Journal of the American Medical Association* (1999), 281: 327–334.

Jakicic, J. M., R. R. Wing, B. A. Butler, and R. J. Robertson. "Prescribing Exercise in Multiple Short Bouts versus One Continuous Bout." *International Journal of Obesity and Related Metabolic Disorders* (1995), 19: 893–901.

Rolls, B. J., L. S. Roe, A. M. Beach, and P. M. Kris-Etherton. "Provision of Foods Differing in Energy Density Affects Long-Term Weight Loss." *Obesity Research* (2005), 13: 1052–1060.

Suggested Reading

Allen, D. *Getting Things Done: The Art of Stress-Free Productivity.* New York: Penguin Books, 2001. This book offers helpful strategies for successfully managing what often feel like unmanageable demands on your time and your energy.

Beck, A. T., A. J. Rush, B. F. Shaw, and G. Emery. *Cognitive Therapy of Depression.* New York: Guilford Press, 1979. We include this book to acknowledge the vast contribution that Dr. Beck's cognitive therapy techniques have made to the field of psychology and to lifestyle change interventions in general.

Borushek, A. *The Calorie King: Calorie, Fat and Carbohydrate Counter.* Costa Mesa, California: Family Health Publications, 2007. Also check out their website at www.calorieking.com. We find this to be a helpful resource to assist in determining the nutritional contents of foods.

Burns, D. *Feeling Good: The New Mood Therapy.* New York: HarperCollins, 1980. We recommend this book not only to those who are dealing with depression, but also as a general resource to expand upon what we teach about changing thoughts that interfere with health and wellness goals.

Cash, T. F. *The Body Image Workbook: An 8-Step Program for Learning to Like Your Looks.* Oakland, California: New Harbinger Publications, 1997. This is an excellent resource from one of the foremost authorities on body image. It provides excellent workbook exercises that help people move toward accepting their bodies.

Covey, S. R. *The 7 Habits of Highly Effective People.* New York: Free Press, 1989, 2004. This is a popular guide that has helped many people to clarify their goals and accomplish personal change.

Craighead, L. W. *The Appetite Awareness Workbook: How to Listen to Your Body and Overcome Bingeing, Overeating, and Obsession with Food*. Oakland, California: New Harbinger Publications, 2006. Our patients benefit from learning to reconnect with hunger cues (as we teach at the DFC). This is a good additional resource to expand upon those skills.

Craske, M. G., and D. H. Barlow. *Mastery of Your Anxiety and Worry: Workbook*. 2nd and 4th eds., New York: Oxford University Press, 2006. This is among the more common recommendations we make to clients who experience anxiety. Although it is not a replacement for professional intervention, the skills taught in these books are valuable in learning to effectively manage emotions.

Jansen, J. *I Don't Know What I Want, But I Know It's Not This: A Step-by-Step Guide to Finding Gratifying Work*. New York: Penguin Books, 1993. This book helps people explore their values, goals, and job expectations, which may direct them to a more satisfying career.

Kabat-Zinn, J. *Wherever You Go, There You Are: Mindfulness Meditation in Everyday Life*. New York: Hyperion, 2005. A user-friendly introduction to mindfulness that teaches how to bring this practice into everyday life. The book offers a variety of meditation practices and exercises.

Kimiecik, J. *The Intrinsic Exerciser: Discovering the Joy of Exercise*. New York: Houghton Mifflin, 2002. This is a favorite recommended reading for clients. It teaches ways to begin to associate pleasure with exercise through the help of an inspirational four-step plan for becoming a successful lifelong exerciser.

Netzer, C. T. *The Complete Book of Food Counts*. 5th ed., New York: Dell Publishing, 2000. This is an excellent guide to finding the nutrition content of commonly purchased foods, including brand-name and restaurant foods.

Patterson, K., J. Grenny, R. McMillan, and A. Switzler. *Crucial Conversations: Tools for Talking When Stakes Are High*. New York: McGraw-Hill, 2002. This book presents a plan for powerful and effective communication around difficult issues. It teaches how to communicate in a way that not only strengthens relationships but gets the best results. These techniques are applicable to business as well as personal relationships.

Rolls, B., and R. A. Barnett. *The Volumetrics Weight-Control Plan*. New York: HarperTorch, 2000. This book provides information on a key concept from a renowned expert and is highly recommended to enhance your understanding of healthy eating in a way that helps you to feel satisfied on fewer calories.

Siler, B. *The Pilates Body: The Ultimate At-Home Guide to Strengthening, Lengthening, and Toning Your Body—Without Machines*. New York: Broadway Books, 2000. This is a helpful guide to Pilates.

Surwit, R., A. Bauman, and J. Skyler. *The Mind-Body Diabetes Revolution: A Proven New Program for Better Blood Sugar Control.* New York: Marlow & Company, 2004, 2005. Dr. Surwit explains why mind-body techniques are important in the control of diabetes, with examples from over twenty-five years of research. He then presents an easy-to-follow six-week program designed to teach the average client how to use the power of the mind to help control this chronic disease.

Willett, W., and M. Katzen. *Eat, Drink, and Weigh Less: A Flexible and Delicious Way to Shrink Your Waist Without Going Hungry.* New York: Hyperion, 2006. This is a succinct restatement of Willett's nutritional guidance, paired with easy and interesting recipes from Katzen's extensive experience.

Willett, W., and P. J. Skerrett. *Eat, Drink, and Be Healthy: The Harvard Medical School Guide to Healthy Eating.* New York: Free Press, 2005. This book provides clear, readable, and evidence-supported guidance on good nutrition.

Resources

COOKBOOKS

We recommend that you buy cookbooks that provide nutritional analyses of the recipes. Here are some other criteria to look for when purchasing a cookbook:

- Is the serving size listed? Is it reasonable?
- Do the recipes call for *a lot* of fat, such as cream, margarine, and butter?
- Can you find the ingredients in your local store?
- Can the recipes be made in a reasonable amount of time?
- Are the recipes easy to read and categorized so that you can find the type of dish you want to cook?

The nutrition staff at the Duke Diet & Fitness Center recommends the following cookbooks to our clients:

American Diabetes Association Month of Meals, Quick and Easy Menus for People with Diabetes, third edition, American Diabetes Association (2002).

American Heart Association Low-Fat, Low-Cholesterol Cookbook: Heart Healthy, Easy-to-Make Recipes That Taste Great, second edition, American Heart Association, Ballantine Books (2002).

Diabetic Meals in 30 Minutes—Or Less!, Robyn Wess, MS, American Diabetes Association, (1996, paperback edition 2006).

Healthy Cooking for Two (or Just You): Low-Fat Recipes with Half the Fuss and Double the Taste, Frances Price, RD, Rodale Press (1995, paperback edition 1997).

Lean and Luscious, Bobbie Hinman and Millie Snyder, Prima Lifestyles (1995).

Lean and Luscious Favorites, Bobbie Hinman and Millie Snyder, Prima Lifestyles (1997).

Lean and Luscious and Meatless, Bobbie Hinman and Millie Snyder, Prima Lifestyles (1998).

Moosewood Restaurant Low-Fat Favorites: Flavorful Recipes for Healthful Meals, Pam Krauss, Clarkson Potter (1997).

New Vegetarian Cuisine: 250 Low-Fat Recipes for Superior Health, Linda Rosensweig and the Food Editors of *Prevention* magazine, Rodale Press (1994, paperback edition, 1996).

Not Just Cheesecake: A Yogurt Cheese Cookbook, second edition, Shelley Melvin, Triad Publishing Company (1997).

Quick and Healthy Low-fat, Carb Conscious Cooking, Brenda Ponichtera, RD, Scaledown Press (1994).

Quick and Healthy Volume II: More Help for People Who Say They Don't Have Time to Cook Healthy Meals, Brenda Ponichtera, RD, Scaledown Press (1995).

Skinny Spices: 50 Nifty Homemade Spice Blends and 100 Low-Cal Recipes That Make Any Meal Delicious, E. L. Klein, Surrey Books (1993).

COOKING WEBSITES

Cooking Light

www.cookinglight.com

This site provides daily food and fitness updates, healthy recipes, and nutrition advice from the editors of *Cooking Light* magazine.

Eating Well

www.eatingwell.com

This site covers food, recipes, nutrition, and wellness advice, cooking how-tos, and healthy diets for weight loss, high cholesterol, and diabetes management.

NEWSLETTERS

Berkeley Wellness Letter

www.wellnessletter.com

University Health Publication Services, Berkeley School of Public Health, University of California

Nutrition Action Health Letter
www.cspinet.org/nah/index.htm
Center for Science in the Public Interest

Tufts University Health and Nutrition Letter, Tufts Media
http://healthletter.tufts.edu/

HEALTH WEBSITES

The Web is a wonderful place to find reputable and accurate information, but it's also a place where misinformation abounds. While this list is not exhaustive by any means and we apologize to any reputable sources we have missed, these are sites we regularly recommend to clients and colleagues, as they are good sources of health information.

American College of Sports Medicine (ACSM)
www.acsm.org
This site is sponsored by a primary sports medicine and exercise science organization and is a good source of evidence-based information and fitness resources.

American Diabetes Association (ADA)
www.diabetes.org
This is a nonprofit health organization providing diabetes research, information, and advocacy.

American Dietetic Association (ADA)
www.eatright.org
This organization is made up of food and nutrition professionals; its site provides comprehensive nutrition information and resources.

American Heart Association (AHA)
www.americanheart.org
This is a national voluntary health agency whose mission is to reduce disability and death from cardiovascular diseases and stroke. It is an excellent source of information on heart-healthy living.

American Obesity Association (AOA)
www.obesity.org
This organization is focused on changing public policy and perceptions about obesity. It has recently joined with NAASO, The Obesity Society. AOA is an authoritative source for policy makers, media, professionals, and clients on the obesity epidemic.

American Society for Bariatric Surgery (ASBS)

www.asbs.org

This is a good source of information about weight loss surgery.

Centers for Disease Control and Prevention (CDC)

www.cdc.gov

The CDC is one of the thirteen major operating components of the Department of Health and Human Services (HHS). Since it was founded in 1946 to help control malaria, the CDC has remained at the forefront of public health efforts to prevent and control infectious and chronic diseases, injuries, workplace hazards, disabilities, and environmental health threats. There you can search for all sorts of valuable health information including that relating to weight control.

NAASO, The Obesity Society

www.naaso.org

This is the leading scientific society dedicated to the study of obesity. Since 1982, it has been committed to encouraging research on the causes and treatment of obesity, and to keeping the medical community and public informed of new advances.

National Institutes of Health (NIH)

www.nih.gov

NIH is the nation's medical research agency, a part of the U.S. Department of Health and Human Services; it is the primary federal agency for conducting and supporting medical research. It provides an excellent resource for those wishing to find out more about ongoing clinical trials and general information about government health programs.

National Library of Medicine, Medline Plus: Obesity

www.nlm.nih.gov/medlineplus/obesity.html

National Institutes of Diabetes and Digestive and Kidney Diseases (NIDDK)

www.niddk.nih.gov

The NIDDK conducts and supports research on many of the most serious diseases affecting public health, including much of the clinical research on the diseases of internal medicine and related subspecialty fields, as well as many basic science disciplines.

U.S. Environmental Protection Agency (EPA)

www.epa.gov

This site is an excellent place to find accurate information on food contamination (for example, mercury levels in fish) and other environmental health concerns.

U.S. Food and Drug Administration (FDA), Center for Food Safety and Applied Nutrition
www.cfsan.fda.gov
The FDA site provides information on food and drug regulatory policies and concerns (for example, nutrition and safety labeling).

Index

National Dairy Council, 152
National Weight Control Registry, 393
nerve damage, 191
nutritional power foods, 150–153
Nutrition Lookup, 26, 107
nuts
    fats in, 40–41, 152, 228
    roasting, 229

oats, 152–153
obesity
    definition of, 13–14
    exercise and, 50, 52
    medication for, 395
    surgery for, 395–396
omega-3 fatty acids, 37, 41, 42, 151–152
Onion Ragout, 270
Open-Faced Egg and Cheese Sandwich, 242
Open-Faced Egg and Ham Sandwich, 243
Open-Faced Egg, Ham, and Cheese
    Sandwich, 244
Open-Faced Ham and Turkey Reuben, 288
osteoporosis, 50
overeating
    continuum of, 149
    high-risk situations for, 192
    lifetime habit of, 81
    reasons for, 144
    stress-related, 206
    trigger foods and, 158, 179
overweight, definition of, 13–14

pain
    back, 205, 347
    chest, 73
    with exercise, 77, 156
    in joints, 60, 71, 73, 156, 345
Peach-Cherry Crisp, 342
pedometers, 61, 74, 123
Pepper-Crusted Beef Tenderloin with
    Horseradish Sauce, 317
peppers, 222, 229
perfectionism, 10, 400–401
Perlman, Peter, 396
Pesto Pasta, 335
phytochemicals
    in chocolate, 151
    in cooked vegetables, 34
    in vegetables, 32, 33
Pilates
    for flexibility, 62, 79
    function of, 63

mat for, 349
    as mind-body activity, 55
    for relaxation, 210
    for strength training, 128, 351
    as warm-up, 124
Pillars of Lifestyle Change
    basis of, 82–83
    body image and self-image, 86–87
    emotional well-being, 88–92
    environment, 83–84
    professional life and social life, 87–88
    reexamining, 96
    stress management, 84–86
    support system, 92–95
    in Week 2, 136
Pizza Hut, 190
Politi, Elisabetta, 20, 180
Pomegranate, Steak, and Spinach Salad, 271
Pork Chops with Bourbon Mustard Glaze,
    318
Pork Medallions with Orange-Rosemary
    Sauce, 319
Pork Tenderloin with Apple Chutney, 320
portion control
    calories and, 116
    in Duke Diet, 221
    by repackaging foods, 120
    in restaurants, 182, 183
    serving size and, 26–29
    weighing food for, 222
Potato-Crusted Salmon, 321
poultry
    in fast food, 187–188
    portions of, 183
    protein from, 42, 224
power foods, 150–153
prediabetes, 6, 7, 190, 191
pregnancy, 43, 173
prehypertension, 206
problem solving, 100–101, 205, 207
professional life and social life, 87–88
protein
    calories in, 25, 26
    cooking techniques for, 224–226
    in dairy foods, 230
    digesting, 23
    in Duke Diet, 41–43
    in eggs, 151
    in fast food, 187–190
    in fish, 151
    hunger management and, 31
    in soy, 153

Duke Diet & Fitness
Online Weight Loss Program

www.dukediet.com

Lose Weight Online

The Online Difference

Interactive Weight Loss . . .
Your online program includes a daily Meal Planner, a personalized Fitness Plan, a Weight Tracker, and more!

Enhanced Support . . .
People who participate in online programs benefit from daily motivation and community support.

Daily Expert Advice . . .
The world-renowned experts at the Duke Diet & Fitness Center answer member questions online and give up-to-date diet info to help guide you to weight loss.

Special Offer:
As a thank-you for purchasing *The Duke Diet,* we're giving you a **FREE TRIAL** of the online program. Customize your weight loss plan now by visiting us at

www.dukediet.com/book

This is a limited-time promotion. Offer expires April 30, 2009.

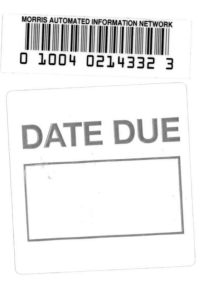